Integrative Men's Health

Integrative Medicine Library

Published and Forthcoming Volumes

SERIES EDITOR

Andrew Weil, MD

Donald I. Abrams and Andrew Weil: Integrative Oncology
Timothy Culbert and Karen Olness: Integrative Pediatrics
Daniel A. Monti and Bernard D. Beitman: Integrative Psychiatry
Victoria Maizes and Tieraona Low Dog: Integrative Women's Health
Gerard Mullin: Integrative Gastroenterology
Randy Horwitz and Daniel Muller: Integrative Rheumatology, Allergy, and Immunology
Stephen DeVries and James Dalen: Integrative Cardiology
Robert Norman, Philip Shenefelt, and Reena Rupani: Integrative Dermatology
Myles Spar and George Munoz: Integrative Men's Health
Robert A. Bonakdar and Andrew W. Sukiennik: Integrative Pain Management

Integrative Men's Health

EDITED BY

Myles D. Spar, MD, MPH
Director of Integrative Medicine
Simms-Mann Health and Wellness Center
Venice Family Clinic Clinical Instructor
UCLA School of Medicine
Integrative Medicine and Men's Health Specialist
West Hollywood, California

George E. Muñoz, MD
Chief Medical Officer
The Oasis Institute
an Integrative, Preventative and Precision Medicine Clinic
Founder and Chief Medical Officer
Arthritis: Osteoporosis Research and Treatment Center, Inc.
Miami, Florida

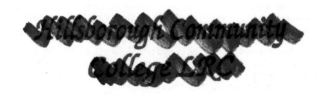

Hillsborough Community
College LRC

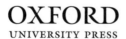

OXFORD
UNIVERSITY PRESS

OXFORD
UNIVERSITY PRESS

Oxford University Press is a department of the University of Oxford.
It furthers the University's objective of excellence in research, scholarship,
and education by publishing worldwide.

Oxford   New York
Auckland   Cape Town   Dar es Salaam   Hong Kong   Karachi
Kuala Lumpur   Madrid   Melbourne   Mexico City   Nairobi
New Delhi   Shanghai   Taipei   Toronto

With offices in
Argentina   Austria   Brazil   Chile   Czech Republic   France   Greece
Guatemala   Hungary   Italy   Japan   Poland   Portugal   Singapore
South Korea   Switzerland   Thailand   Turkey   Ukraine   Vietnam

Oxford is a registered trademark of Oxford University Press
in the UK and certain other countries.

Published in the United States of America by
Oxford University Press
198 Madison Avenue, New York, NY 10016

© Oxford University Press 2014

All rights reserved. No part of this publication may be reproduced, stored in a
retrieval system, or transmitted, in any form or by any means, without the prior
permission in writing of Oxford University Press, or as expressly permitted by law,
by license, or under terms agreed with the appropriate reproduction rights organization.
Inquiries concerning reproduction outside the scope of the above should be sent to the Rights
Department, Oxford University Press, at the address above.

You must not circulate this work in any other form
and you must impose this same condition on any acquirer.

Library of Congress Cataloging-in-Publication Data
Integrative men's health/edited by Myles D. Spar, George E. Muñoz.
p. ; cm.—(Integrative medicine library)
Includes bibliographical references and index.
ISBN 978–0–19–984379–4 (alk. paper)
I. Spar, Myles D., editor of compilation.   II. Muñoz, George E., editor of compilation.
III. Series: Weil integrative medicine library.
[DNLM: 1. Integrative Medicine.   2. Men's Health.   3. Complementary Therapies. WA 306]
RA777.8
613'04234—dc23   2013027789

This material is not intended to be, and should not be considered, a substitute for medical or other
professional advice. Treatment for the conditions described in this material is highly dependent on the
individual circumstances. And, while this material is designed to offer accurate information with respect
to the subject matter covered and to be current as of the time it was written, research and knowledge
about medical and health issues is constantly evolving and dose schedules for medications are being
revised continually, with new side effects recognized and accounted for regularly. Readers must therefore
always check the product information and clinical procedures with the most up-to-date published product
information and data sheets provided by the manufacturers and the most recent codes of conduct and safety
regulation. The publisher and the authors make no representations or warranties to readers, express or
implied, as to the accuracy or completeness of this material. Without limiting the foregoing, the publisher
and the authors make no representations or warranties as to the accuracy or efficacy of the drug dosages
mentioned in the material. The authors and the publisher do not accept, and expressly disclaim, any
responsibility for any liability, loss or risk that may be claimed or incurred as a consequence of the use and/
or application of any of the contents of this material.

1 3 5 7 9 8 6 4 2
Printed in the United States of America
on acid-free paper

This book is dedicated to our teachers at the University of Arizona Center for Integrative Medicine, to trailblazers in the field of men's health, and to our families, who have supported our work on this project over many years.

A special thank you goes to the editors at Oxford University Press and to the chapter authors.

Lastly, we dedicate this book to our families: Dr. Spar's children Clio and Canaan and husband, Danny, and Dr. Muñoz's children George, Sindi, Jake, Samantha, and Alexandra and partner Michele for their loving support and spiritual teaching, and who have all contributed to the joy, and therefore the health, of these two men in boundless ways.

FOREWORD

ANDREW WEIL, MD

Series Editor

Until recently, "men's health" was solely the concern of urologists. From that narrow perspective, many of the most serious health risks that men face as they go through life are not apparent. Men are much less likely than women to seek medical attention for symptoms they develop. They are more likely to engage in risky behaviors and to be in abusive relationships with drugs and alcohol. And they do not live as long as women, for reasons we do not yet understand.

In my experience men are also less accepting of natural remedies and alternative and complementary therapies and less knowledgeable about nutritional influences on health. In the United States, women are the main buyers of books on health and the consumers most demanding of integrative medical services. I have seen many couples over my years in practice; typically, it is wives who try to get husbands to eat more fruits and vegetables, to practice relaxation methods, or to seek counseling for emotional problems.

Because of its emphasis on the whole person and attention to all aspects of lifestyle, integrative medicine is ideally suited to address the health concerns of men. The publication of *Integrative Men's Health* is a milestone in the development of this specialty of clinical practice. I believe it will give practitioners useful information and resources to provide better care for male patients. I congratulate the editors on assembling a strong team of contributors and covering many topics relevant to men's health that are still not adequately taught in conventional medical training.

Tucson, Arizona
August, 2013

PREFACE

M en die younger than women. Average life expectancy is over 5 years more for women than for men in the United States, and of the top 10 causes of death in the United States, men are winning in nine of them (WHO Statistics, 2007; CDC Vital Statistics Report, 2011). An integrative approach provides a holistic model that can effectively address prevention and treatment for many of the conditions that disproportionately affect and kill men.

Integrative medicine takes into account all influences on health including physical, emotional, social, and spiritual factors. The physical influences are viewed holistically and are taken to include influences on overall health and disease from stress, poor diet, inflammation, lack of proper nutrients, and overall imbalance. Such an approach, which focuses on health and prevention as well as optimization of performance in all realms, has been developed for women over the past 20 years, but has not been as fully developed for the benefit of the health of men.

Men have unique health concerns, from high rates of cardiovascular disease, to sexual dysfunction and prostate disorders, to repercussions of low testosterone. Historically, men's health has been relegated to be all that is not women's health. Gradually, the recognition that men have gender-specific health issues has emerged and can be seen in the growing body of research in the field. Departments of andrology have cropped up first in Europe, Asia, and Australia and now in North America, which involve urologists working along with primary care physicians and endocrinologists to treat men, teach students, and engage in research.

This text on integrative men's health brings together some of the top clinicians, educators, and researchers in the most important realms of this new field. It starts by looking at whole-systems approaches impacting the health of men, including nutrition, botanicals and vitamin supplements, the mind–body connection, spirituality, and the impact of physical activity on morbidity and mortality of men. The next chapters look at the approach to men's health taken by traditional Chinese medicine, Ayurvedic medicine, and homeopathy, as these fields have an inherent understanding of the impact of gender on health and illness. Following these chapters, an integrative approach to the divisions of medicine most relevant to the health concerns of men is explored including integrative cardiology, rheumatology, gastroenterology, oncology, dermatology, and urology, as well as an integrative approach to male sexual function and low testosterone. The chapter on healthy aging incorporates many of the aspects of integrative medicine with a specific focus on reducing the impact of aging on the body and mind, and the chapter on toxins explores the influence of the environment on the health of men and the ways any negative influences may be attenuated using integrative approaches.

It is our hope that readers of *Integrative Men's Health* will understand the unique health needs of men, especially as such needs contribute to morbidity and mortality in a significant way. On a deeper level, the reader can expect to obtain an understanding of a comprehensive, holistic, and truly integrated approach to diagnosis, prevention, and treatment of many of the conditions most important to men.

CONTENTS

CONTRIBUTORS

Christina Adams, MD
Integrative Cardiologist
Scripps Center for Integrative
    Medicine
Scripps Clinic/Green Hospital
La Jolla, California

Ronald Boyer, MD
President
Center for Education and
    Development of Clinical
    Homeopathy
Edgemont, Pennsylvania

Bruce B. Campbell, MD
Chair, Department of Executive Health
Associate Clinical Professor of Medicine
Tufts University School of Medicine
Lahey Clinic
Burlington, MA

Frederic C. Craigie, Jr., PhD
Family Medicine Institute
Augusta, Maine

Joel S. Edman, DSc, FACN, CNS
Clinical Nutritionist
Edman Nutritional Services
The Resiliency Center, LLC
Ambler, Pennsylvania

Rachel Freidman, MD
Fellow, Integrative Medicine for the
    Underserved
Santa Rosa Family Medicine Residency
    Program
Santa Rosa, California

Mary L. Hardy, MD
Wellness Works
Stiles Integrative Oncology Program
    at UCLA
Los Angeles, California

Joel J. Heidelbaugh, MD, FAAFP, FACG
Clinical Associate Professor
Departments of Family Medicine and
    Urology
University of Michigan Medical
    School
Ann Arbor, Michigan

David Kiefer, MD
Assistant Clinical Professor of
    Medicine
The Arizona Center for Integrative
    Medicine University of Arizona
    College of Medicine
Tucson, Arizona

Janet Konefal, PhD, MPH
Associate Professor of Clinical Psychiatry
Department of Psychiatry &
  Behavioral Sciences and Assistant
  Dean for Complementary and
  Integrative Medicine Chief Division
  of Complementary Medicine
University of Miami Miller School of
  Medicine
Miami, Florida

John E. Lewis, PhD
Associate Professor Department of
  Psychiatry and Behavioral Sciences
University of Miami Miller School of
  Medicine
Miami, Florida

Brad S. Lichtenstein, ND, BCB
Chair of Homeopathy Department
School of Naturopathic Medicine
Bastyr University
Kenmore, Washington

Tieraona Low Dog, MD
Director of the Fellowship in
  Integrative Medicine The Arizona
  Center for Integrative Medicine
  University of Arizona College of
  Medicine
Tucson, Arizona

Walter W. Mills, MD, MMM, ABHIM
Associate Clinical Professor
Department of Family and
  Community Medicine
UCSF School of Medicine Program
  Director Santa Rosa Kaiser Family
  Medicine Residency Program
Vice Chair Kaiser Regional Integrative
  Medicine Program
Santa Rosa, California

Martin M. Miner, MD
Co-Director of the Men's Health
  Center
The Miriam Hospital
Department of Family Medicine and
  Urology
Warren Albert School of Medicine
Brown University
Providence, Rhode Island

Jose Luis Mosquera, MD, DABIM
Associate Professor of Clinical
  Medicine
Program in Integrative Medicine
University of Arizona School of
  Medicine
Clinical Director of Integrative
  Medicine
St. Michael's Medical Center
Newark, New Jersey

Alexandra Muñoz, MS
Pre-Doctoral Fellow
Department of Molecular and Genetic
  Toxicology
Nelson Institute for Environmental
  Medicine
NYU School of Medicine
New York, New York

Ajay Narola, MD
Resident, Internal Medicine Jersey
  Shore University Medical Center
Neptune, New Jersey

Robert A. Norman, DO
Founder, Owner, and CEO
Dermatology Healthcare, LLC
Tampa, Florida

S. Devi Rampertab, MD
Assistant Professor of Medicine
Rutgers–Robert Wood Johnson
    Medical School
New Brunswick, New Jersey

Neal Rouzier, MD
Director
Preventive Medicine Clinics of the Desert
Palm Springs, California

Philip D. Shenefelt, MD
Professor, Dermatology and
    Cutaneous Surgery
University of South Florida
Tampa, Florida

Christopher J. Suhar, MD
Medical Director
Scripps Center for Integrative
    Medicine
Scripps Integrative Medicine and
    Cardiovascular diseases
Scripps Clinic/Green Hospital
La Jolla, California

Eduard Tiozzo, PhD
Postdoctoral Research Associate
Department of Psychiatry and
    Behavioral Sciences
Division of Complementary and
    Integrative Medicine
University of Miami Miller School of
    Medicine
Miami, Florida

Eric Yarnell, ND
Professor
Department of Botanical Medicine
    Bastyr University
Kenmore, Washington

Integrative Men's Health

1

Introduction to Integrative Health and Medicine for Men

JOSE LUIS MOSQUERA

Men's health today is facing unmet needs and emerging global challenges. Men in this 21st century are dealing with complex and multidimensional health concerns well beyond our recognized biological differences and significantly shorter life spans. Today, men have higher rates than women in virtually all the leading causes of death and are less likely to visit a doctor, get regular preventative checkups, or lead health-promoting lifestyles. Premature mortality in younger men and boys from communicable diseases, violence, and lack of health care access is occurring in this country and worldwide at alarming rates. Changing socioeconomic and political environments in postindustrialized societies are creating troubling physical and mental health disparities in men of all ages. A new health care model with a spotlight on these and many other men's health issues is desperately needed. This timely book shows how integrative medicine can partner in healing these male health care disparities and improve outcomes for all men, which in turn will better the health of the women children, and communities in their lives.

Integrative medicine, a new medicine for the 21st century focusing on therapeutic relationships, health, and healing, is transforming the future of health care and is the ideal approach to collectively address and formulate therapeutic strategies on the many issues specific to men's health. In response to the deeply troublesome and uncompassionate chaos in our fractured health care system, integrative medicine is emerging as a sustainable model of relationship-centered health care focusing on prevention and health-promoting lifestyle choices, which foster healing and wellness. Using evidence-based scientific methods and research, integrative medicine is a health care model driven by inquiry and open to new paradigms, combining conventional therapies with complementary and alternative therapies while seeking natural and safer health solutions for each patient. It is a "high touch," less-high-tech-dependent, individualized patient-centered care model that empowers patients to actively participate in their health and healing. This is accomplished by developing an understanding of all factors that influence health, wellness, and disease, including mind, body, spirit, and community.

Bringing you these concepts and principles of integrative medicine is the core purpose of this book's expert group of authors on men's health. Many are experienced clinicians as well as esteemed colleagues, researchers, and educators in their respective specialties. Conventional and alternative therapeutic modalities in men's health are presented in relationship to the whole person and comprehensively examined for their risks, benefits, and science. Some integrative therapies such as acupuncture and hypnotherapy are very skill specific, which makes them difficult to replicate in the usual Western science models mostly used for drug trials (i.e., randomized, blinded, and placebo controlled). In these as well as other effective alternative therapies presented in this text, such as Ayurvedic medicine, a "sliding scale of evidence" is an additional and more appropriate method to consider the benefits and risks of therapies. In this evaluation standard, the greater the potential of a treatment to cause harm, the stricter the standards of evidence it should be held to. Examples of a greater potential for harm would be the banned pain medication Vioxx, a nonsteroidal osteoarthritis medication and painkiller that was removed from the market only after years of being implicated in multiple deaths and heart attacks and discovery of major flaws in the approval process by the U.S. Food and Drug Administration (FDA). The use of stem cell transplants for breast cancer patients in the early 1990s was another scientifically scrutinized therapy that turned out to provide disastrous and deadly results after FDA approval.

Although integrative medicine as described previously is more than the use of complementary modalities, it does include such use when clinically warranted. There are clearly opportunities for the use of nutritional supplementation, mind–body approaches, and acupuncture or herbal therapy, for example, in clinical situations where Western medicine is not able to provide optimal solutions or where side effects from Western treatment can be mitigated. For example, multiple studies have supported the vast overuse of medications like antibiotics, where millions of prescriptions are written annually to treat self-limiting viral illnesses and end up creating serious drug reactions and resistant bacteria instead of cures. More than 2 million patients experience adverse drug reactions (ADRs) in U.S. hospitals annually, and the overprescribing and abuse of painkillers, antidepressants, and antibiotics are leading causes of both morbidity and mortality throughout the United States. Prescription drug abuse has become a leading cause of mortality throughout the United States in young men (ages 15 to 40). Abuse of tranquilizers, antidepressants, and especially opioid painkillers has reached epidemic proportions, being reported in staggering numbers by state health officials and emergency rooms. Clearly, a new strategy is desperately needed to change the direction of these and other men's health outcomes. The integrative men's health approach in this book is designed to maximize safe and effective care while also promoting the body's natural ability for self-healing and reducing risk. Empowering men with the knowledge and wisdom of this book's expert authors is an ideal step in achieving better health outcomes.

In the traditional Western medicine model, men's health as a specific field of recognition and importance has until recently received anemic recognition and marginal attention by most health professionals. This lack of response by the medical community has occurred despite the huge impact of male health disparities on public health outcomes here in the United States and globally. Much of this generalized apathy toward men's health results from the reductionist model that shaped our modern study of health sciences, in which we break down our body and study its parts, focusing on its systems and pieces while ignoring the whole person in body, mind, and spirit. When it comes to certain medical emergencies and pathophysiologic diagnoses of specific illnesses, reductionism serves us well, but when therapeutic strategies are required for treatment of chronic illness or achieving balanced health and wellness via prevention and health promotion, it fails in its very design to address the care of the individual and whole person. With male health, much of the current health orthodoxy has been to focus on the male genitourinary system, sexual function (i.e., prostatic disease and sexual health), heart (cardiac and circulatory disease), and cancer risk (lung, colon, prostate). Still today many hospitals and medical centers are designed with separate wards or sections devoted to a specific body system. There is the orthopedic floor, the urology floor, the cardiac care floor, the diabetic floor, and so on. Although this specialty care may be necessary, it usually lacks communication with other essential areas of the whole-person lifestyle, which can be vital to facilitate healing. Oftentimes that 60-year-old man lying in his hospital bed waiting for his prostatectomy or cardiac surgery does not receive the benefit of the patient-centered whole-person care that integrative medicine has proven to deliver in a desired, safe, and effective model with better outcomes. Well beyond that prostate gland removal or postbypass painful thoracotomy scar, statins, and other heart medications are the nutritional, spiritual, and mental health needs so essential to promote healing during his hospital stay and well after he leaves the hospital setting and resumes his daily life. Still today, many doctors receive little or no training in nutrition and self-healing strategies, an integral part of nearly all healing foundations. Teaching and giving patients simple tools like breathing exercises, meditation practices, and nutritional strategies can markedly improve their overall health scores. Providing these patients with programs in healthy aging, physical activity, proven supplements, and mind–body therapies such as mindfulness-based stress reduction (MBSR) addresses the lifestyle management factors so essential to continued healing and prevention of chronic and disabling disease. Many of the integrative therapies presented in this book have become very useful tools for me during my 25 years of clinical practice in providing male patients with optimal care and outcomes.

The other possible explanation for the lack of focused attention on men's health issues is that because men have made up the majority of research subjects in most modern scientific studies of diseases that are present in both men and women, men's health was seen as anything that was not specifically women's health. However, this limited view misses the importance of developing a greater understanding of conditions that are especially important to men given their unique presence in men (erectile dysfunction, low testosterone, prostate disease, etc.) or their disproportionate impact on men (cardiovascular disease and death due to lifestyle factors). Furthermore, a unique field of male health is needed to better understand how to address the needs of men, who present differently than women even when suffering from the same conditions as women. Men with depression often act withdrawn or aggressive as opposed to sad, for example. Men do not seek out preventive care as readily as women. These types of gender differences in disease presentation and attitude make it crucial that the field of men's health mature from the "all that is not women's health" model.

Our expertise as integrative physicians is rooted in working with Dr. Andrew Weil, the founder and director of the Center for Integrative Medicine at the University of Arizona College of Medicine. As the leading medical pioneer of integrative health and an iconoclastic figure in medicine, his vision in recognizing and transforming the failures of Western health care models places him as one of the most important medical figures of modern times. In recent years Dr. Weil has continued to spearhead the educational advancement of integrative medicine, and the program has expanded to national and international prominence and practice of what Dr. Weil would like to someday be called just "good medicine" that is practiced by all health professionals. His center at the University of Arizona is widely recognized as the global educational leader in the field by creating fellowships, residencies, medical school consortiums, and online courses available to all health professionals. In addition, evidence-based research studies and integrative book series such as this one are only a few of the areas that have evolved from the wisdom and vision of Dr. Weil's life work to improve the health care of all people. From the simplicity and benefit of his breathing exercises to practicing behavioral change through the contemplative sciences or understanding how food can be your best medicine, his vision of integrative health is here and succeeding.

Obesity is one of the strongest risk factors for many of the diseases of most concern to men, including cardiovascular disease, diabetes, hypertension, and even prostate cancer. Men have higher rates of obesity than women (Flegal, Carroll, Ogden, & Curtin, 2010; Ogden, Carroll, Curtin, Lamb, & Flegal, 2010; U.S. Department of Health and Human Services, 2010) with concomitantly higher rates of many diseases associated with obesity. "Food as medicine" or nutritional therapy is a cornerstone of integrative men's health and a powerful therapeutic tool. Changes in dietary habits can be very challenging for men, both young and old, but once that motivational trigger is found to change unhealthy habits, food can often become the best medicine. In boys with allergies and asthma, diets eliminating dairy products can bring dramatic improvement to their condition; in young men with irritable bowel syndrome, nutritional strategies may include mindful eating, proper chewing of food, taking probiotics, and eating whole food quantities of fiber and protein at shorter intervals during the day. Foods using soy and other plant-based proteins are often suggested to replace animal fat and red meat in the diets of men with prostate disease, whereas a Mediterranean-style diet is often useful to curb the chronic inflammation associated with so many diseases of aging. These include chronic arthritis, neurodegenerative conditions like Alzheimer's disease, heart disease, and cancer. For males who live in poverty, the focus shifts to getting the healthiest calories from affordable sources and treating their nutrition or lack thereof from a psychosocial and practical perspective. Much reform is needed as misdirected government farm subsidies in this country place the worst-quality food calories in the bodies of poorer people who cannot afford to buy from local organic farmers and suffer with greater rates of diseases like diabetes and obesity. Nutritional management is a fundamental therapeutic plan included in all areas of men's health described in this book. Let's briefly examine and summarize a few of these important areas by the authors in the following chapters.

Cardiovascular disease in men has been and remains the leading cause of death in this country over the last century. Some estimates place cardiovascular disease as the leading cause of male death worldwide by the year 2030. This is mostly the result of a "Westernization" of our U.S. dietary habits and lifestyle, which creates and increases the known risk factors of obesity, diabetes, high blood pressure, and high cholesterol levels. Integrative cardiology for men focuses on these lifestyle changes, which, as seen with the research and studies of Dean Ornish, MD, can actually reverse coronary artery disease (CAD) within months. The ability to reverse CAD with lifestyle changes cannot be overstated, especially when stenting coronary arteries and prescribing statins has never been scientifically proven to prolong the lives of these patients. If risk factors such as tobacco use are not addressed with preventative and health-promoting behavior, medications alone are less likely to sustain a man's healthy heart. Environmental, cultural, and behavioral factors must be addressed, especially in regions of the world adopting Western diets and habits of processed and refined foods filled with damaging amounts of fructose, salt, and excessive caloric intake. Such is the case among Southeast Asian and Russian men, where CAD is rising at alarming rates with these harmful dietary habits, tobacco use, and sedentary lifestyles. In the United States, rates of heart disease have been in decline, with regional disparities. West Coast men have lower rates of CAD than East Coast men, and minorities such as Latinos increase their CAD rates when they move to the United States, with increasing rates of obesity, diabetes, and metabolic syndrome. The integrative health model is an ideal approach to address the psychosocial, behavioral, and dietary habits that strongly contribute to cardiovascular disease in these men.

The field of men's oncology can also receive great benefit from integrative medicine. Many recent surveys cite that the majority of cancer patients seek and use complementary and alternative medicine (CAM). Remember that CAM is only one part of the integrative approach to oncology. Lifestyle and nutritional changes can help prevent the majority of men's cancers. Cessation of tobacco use and eliminating red meat and animal fats from the diet are basic examples of how to reduce lung, colon, and prostate cancer risks. The range of integrative approaches can include acupuncture/traditional Chinese medicine (TCM), botanicals, mind–body, and the transcendent realm of spirituality. Acupuncture has proven scientific benefits for helping chemotherapy-induced nausea and vomiting and overall well-being. Mind–body techniques such as hypnotherapy, visual imagery, and MBSR help patients feel an improved sense of well-being, which is emerging as an important scientific indicator in many CAM studies, especially in the practice of contemplative sciences. Essential to the field of integrative oncology is the following principle: Although there may not be absolute cures, healing can always occur, at all stages of disease, for patients with cancer. These integrative approaches offer men the ability to overcome the fears of disease and take control of their lives and spirit.

When it comes to men's health, many will automatically focus on two issues: prostate disease and sexual health. Prostate disease includes benign prostatic hypertrophy (BPH), prostatitis, and cancer, whereas sexual health involves erectile dysfunction, low testosterone, and male andropause. All can greatly benefit from the integrative health approaches discussed in this book. Prostate cancer is a condition with a wide spectrum of effects on men's health, from a very manageable non-life-threatening condition to a very aggressive and deadly form. This range of disease depends on several factors, including family history, age, harmful eating habits and lifestyle choices, environmental toxins, and the stage and cellular pathology (Gleason's score) of each case. African Americans, especially those who are obese and who smoke, suffer in greater numbers than Latinos or White Caucasian men. Absolute prostate-specific antigen (PSA) values remain controversial in their significance unless they are coupled with digital prostate exams and show significant change in repeated exams. Advanced surgical robotics and radiation therapies have high success rates in treating most prostate cancers, but developing the integrative strategies in this book to prevent disease can dramatically reduce the chances of developing prostate cancer and also help in recovery from disease.

Are we prescribing too much Viagra, Levitra, and Cialis? Absolutely! If we spend more time with these men and peel away at the layers of lifestyle and behavioral risk factors, many can learn to have satisfying sexual health without these erectile dysfunction medications. Furthermore, sexual dysfunction can be a warning sign of systemic cardiovascular disease. Sexual health in men is often multifactorial, with risk factors like tobacco use, substance abuse, diabetes, vascular disease, depression, and andropause being some of the most frequent contributors. I find that failure to cope with stress and the resulting chronic anxiety and depression are seen often in these settings. Marital or relationship conflicts, which can often underlie sexual health disorders, should be openly presented and discussed with each patient. An integrative-based physical exam and hormonal blood tests will likely provide the diagnostic keys and basis for therapeutic strategies.

Neurodegenerative diseases and the field of integrative neurosciences are finally merging. Common diseases in men like Alzheimer's disease, stroke, Parkinson's disease, and demyelinating illnesses like multiple sclerosis and amyotrophic lateral sclerosis all seemed to fit perfectly into the reductionist model of Western medicine of diagnostic testing, yet in the last 20 years we have been experiencing a revolution of newly researched findings in mind–body medicine with the emerging and transformative concept of neuroplasticity. Neuroplasticity is the ability of the brain and nervous system to change structurally and functionally as a result of environmental change and input without pharmacologic intervention. Research now demonstrates how contemplative practices like meditation and mindfulness-based training can actually change our central nervous system and subsequently affect our stress response and immunity. The importance of these mind–body relationships cannot be overstated in developing therapies for these chronic inflammatory and immune-mediated conditions. The work of researchers like Dr. Richard Davidson at the University of Wisconsin Medical School and Dr. Esther Sternberg at the National Institutes of Health (NIH) in the area of contemplative practices and integrative neural immune function are bringing new insight into the neural, immune, and hormonal factors of neurodegenerative diseases, from their causation to the use of mind–body therapies in treating them.

Mind–body therapies in men's health can provide supportive treatment options with excellent results. The mind–body connection has been clearly established through scientific research, and understanding of it continues to evolve. Hypnotherapy and visual imagery are proven resources in helping a range of behavioral conditions and in healing from illness, and contemplative practices are emerging as excellent ways to help our stress responses and balance our minds. MBSR is a powerful tool of contemplative practice being taught to patients with chronic illness, health professionals, and even those in the military. It focuses on the Buddhist idea of compassionate and nonjudgmental living in the moment and is a method scientifically validated by the work of Dr. Jon Kabat-Zinn at the University of Massachusetts School of Medicine. Creating a mindful society could be transformative in addressing men's health issues.

Motivational interviewing techniques, journaling, and meditation are also very useful tools in the integrative arsenal of mind–body medicine. Listening to patients and providing open-ended advice and support has become a lost art in medicine. When it comes to introductions and interviews with health professionals, male patients will often project a strong defensive posture often mired in denial and fear. As a result, men can sometimes be more difficult patients, but when provided with some of these mind–body tools and techniques, they become willing participants in their healing.

With the alarming rates of obesity and diabetes in men, particularly in minorities such as Latinos and African Americans and in lower socioeconomic groups, exercise programs are an essential part of an integrative plan to promote health and wellness. Poor nutritional habits and sedentary lifestyles underlie obesity of epidemic proportions here in the United States and in other countries adopting a Western "fast food" lifestyle. Exercise should begin in infancy, with parents and/or caregivers promoting physical exploration of the environment while facilitating movement skills and promoting musculoskeletal development. Men of all ages who exercise 30 minutes or more daily benefit from improved cardiovascular health and suffer from less depression and anxiety.

Older men suffer from the normal aging process of muscle mass loss or sarcopenia, usually after age 50, but this process can begin as early as age 30. Morbidity and mortality rates rise higher in men who do not exercise as they age. An unsound body clearly makes healing and disease cures more challenging. Learning and practicing a physical activity can be an enjoyable lifelong commitment to promote health and wellness; whether it's taking a brisk walk daily or rigorously training for a triathlon, either physical activity will bring healthy rewards.

For men, healthy aging and longevity varies greatly with their environment, culture, and socioeconomic status both in this country and globally. Disparities between the longevity of men and women exist both here in the United States and globally. Men continually lag in longevity. Communicable diseases, injuries, suicide rates, and violent deaths all occur at significantly higher rates in men. The male response to stress, negative emotions, and sadness is complex and not entirely understood, but the increased mortality rates and disparities are alarming. When the former Soviet Union broke apart, the socioeconomic instability caused men's life spans there to plummet at much greater rates than women's. Men are more likely than women to engage in risky behaviors like smoking, drinking excessive amounts of alcohol, and using illicit drugs. Mental health conditions such as depression are underdetected and undertreated in men, resulting in worse outcomes than in women. Health education and sociocultural programs to help men embrace rather than deny aging are essential ways to reduce the longevity gaps between men and women. In places like Sardinia and Iceland, the life span gaps between genders averages less than 3 years, whereas in places like Latvia, the gap is over 11 years, with men in that region living an average of 66 years and women living 77 years.

Violence, unemployment, and illicit drug use all are factors in the deaths of working-class men (ages 15 to 64). The premature deaths of working-class men around the world have reached epidemic proportions. According to European Union statistics from a 2011 report of 27 European countries, there were 630,000 deaths annually for men in this group, compared to 30,000 for women of the same age. In the United States, similar statistical disparities exist. Disenchanted and disenfranchised groups of young men globally are protesting to be heard and integrated as educated and contributing human beings to their societies. These protests, however, are often met with violence and lead to unattended mental stress and illness. Drug abuse, especially prescription drug abuse of painkillers, sedatives, anxiolytics, and antidepressants, has become a leading cause of mortality in young men ages 20 to 45 in many U.S. states. All of these factors are destroying a vital part of the male population: the young, healthy, working man. The impact and consequences on societies and families are profound.

African American men's health statistics are especially grim when compared to both Black women and Caucasian men of similar ages. African American women outlive African American men by 7 years in this country, whereas the average difference is 5 years in all ethnic groups. The largest gap in mortality is in the high school– and college-age population (15 to 24 years), where a disproportionate majority of deaths in this age group are African American males. Sadly, the majority of these deaths are preventable and usually the result of violent homicide, accidents, or suicide. Homicide is the leading cause of death for this age group in African American males, who are nine times more likely than their Caucasian peers to be homicide victims. Drowning is also a leading cause of death for young Black males (10%), with twice as many drowning deaths reported annually compared to White men. Later in life high blood pressure, smoking, lung cancer, and prostate cancer are all disproportionately higher in Black men.

Although African American men use tobacco more often, suffer disproportionately with higher rates of prostate cancer, and have lower life expectancies than White men, Hispanic or Latino men surprisingly outlive both non-Hispanic Black and non-Hispanic White men. Hispanic males' life expectancy at birth is 77.9 years (overall life expectancy for all Americans is 77.7), but once they reach the age of 65, their average life expectancy in the United States jumps to 84 years. For Hispanic women reaching age 65, their life expectancy reaches 86 years, also outdistancing White and African American women. These startling differences exist despite Hispanics in America having poor access to our health care system and some of the lowest rates of health insurance in the country for any minority group in all age groups. Reasons for this health outcome paradox in U.S. Hispanics are not entirely clear, but several factors have recently emerged to explain these unexpected statistics. Hispanics smoke less and subsequently have lower rates of tobacco-related cancers. Strong community and family support along with faith-based beliefs and prayer may be additional contributory reasons.

In contrast to the better health older Hispanics in the United States enjoy, younger Latino males are experiencing soaring rates of diabetes, HIV, mental illness, and violent deaths. These rising rates coincide with some of the lowest high school graduation rates among all minorities, limiting employment opportunities and access to higher education. Younger Hispanic and African American males both share increased mortality when compared to Caucasian males of similar age groups.

To address these disparities in male ethnic groups, this book also includes chapters with a variety of complementary and alternative therapies that are safe and effective. Understanding and developing spirituality in male patients can often support and improve healing of disease. A majority of men believe that religion, faith, and prayer help them and family members cope with illness. Spirituality may not involve a formal religion but instead represent a journey of experience and connection to one's life and its meaning. As physicians, we should be prepared to understand and engage male patients in discussions of their spirituality. For men, issues of forgiveness, punishment, and reconciliation become important questions that can bring clarity and meaning to their souls.

TCM has been practiced for over 2,000 years in East Asia and in the 21st century has become a popular therapy here in the United States and other developed countries. When discussing TCM, most health professionals think of acupuncture, the purposeful insertion of needles at cutaneous and subcutaneous sites understood to correspond to established meridians or channels of body energy. This use of needles at points to produce a "Da Qi" sensation is one of the various parts of TCM. These parts include palpation, tongue and pulse diagnosis, Moxa (heated points), herbal remedies, and communication rapport with the practitioner and patient. Traditional Chinese medicine has now become a well-studied model in Western medicine with proven benefits in areas of pain management, nausea from chemotherapy, and a variety of musculoskeletal conditions such as arthritis of the knees or back and musculo-ligamentous strain or spasms. Functional magnetic resonance imaging studies and measurement of neuron modulation in acupuncture patients are beginning to provide the scientific evidence to confirm its effectiveness in a host of conditions. Other holistic traditional-based therapies discussed in this book proven to be safe and effective include Ayurveda and homeopathy. Scientific evidence for these therapies has always been challenged, yet historical outcome studies for them are impressive. Their shared holistic and integrative approach is likely a major supportive reason for their safe and effective results.

All the therapies in this book, both conventional and alternative, are discussed and presented using evidence-based medicine within the broader concept of men's health promotion and prevention of men's illness. This concept, a defining principle of integrative medicine, is vital and key to understanding the core mission of integrative men's health. Until very recent times, men would seldom receive the benefit of specific targeted health prevention and promotion of their well-being. Men's health today is a Global contrast with, with successful models of integrative health emerging in places like Sardinia and Japan while places like South Africa war-torn Afghanistan, or regions in the United States suffer huge disparities reflecting a broken system in dire need of repair.

Disparities of male health in our postmodern, postindustrialized societies actually began less than a century ago. Amazingly, back in 1920 male and female mortality statistics were fairly equal. Many of the disparities in male morbidity and mortality began during the Great Depression and World War II, continuing through the second half of the 20th century to the modern day. Communicable diseases like HIV, malaria, and tuberculosis have been responsible for millions of deaths annually and have ravaged the lives of men in the prime working ages of their lives, particularly in the African continent. Wars, violence, and mental illness have also led to countless fatalities and permanently injured younger men. Many of these issues have viable solutions, which can begin with understanding the preventative strategies and therapies mentioned throughout this book. Several of these chapters will focus on understanding and utilizing specific complementary and alternative therapies alongside conventional medicine. Chapters are also devoted to psychosocial determinants of men's health such as environmental impact and risk-taking behaviors. Throughout this book there is true expert advice to help in the search to regain wellness and balance, activate inner and natural healing responses, age more healthily, and prevent chronic illness. The final chapter addresses the future of men's health.

The spotlight must remain brightly lit on men's health. It is essential to sustain recent advances and to erase the existing disparities with integrative health strategies. Young men in this country and around the world continue dying at disproportionate rates from violence, communicable diseases, and risky behaviors, and men over age 65 are facing escalating rates of chronic disability and morbidity in a failing and unsustainable health care system that is in reality a financially motivated disease management system. There is clearly a profound necessity and a rising demand for a better and deeper communication with men about their health issues. These omnipresent growing disparities clearly indicate the urgent need for an informed self-awareness and compassionate solutions to permeate the field of men's health. This field is now finally undergoing a true "zeitgeist," and with the expert authors and integrative medicine pioneers in this book, you have joined in the emerging consciousness and mindful attention to improve men's health here in the United States and around the entire globe.

REFERENCES

Flegal KM, Carroll MD, Ogden CL, Curtin, LR. Prevalence and trends in obesity among US adults, 1999–2008. JAMA. 2010;303(3):235–241.

Ogden CL, Carroll MD, Curtin LR, Lamb MM, Flegal, KM. Prevalence of high body mass index in US children and adolescents, 2007–2008. JAMA. 2010;303(3):242–249.

U.S. Department of Health and Human Services. Final review, Healthy People 2010: Nutrition and overweight. Available from: http://www.cdc.gov/nchs/data/hpdata2010/hp2010_final_review_focus_area_19.pdf.

2

Nutritional Therapies for Men's Health

JOEL S. EDMAN AND MYLES D. SPAR

ood nutrition is an important foundation for optimal health and well-being for men, as well as for an integrative medicine therapeutic approach to symptoms and disorders that may be common in men. Nutrition in this context includes using specific dietary guidelines, including health-promoting foods, using targeted nutritional supplements, and addressing any other important issues that would be necessary to develop an effective and individualized nutritional program.

As an overall lifestyle component, nutrition may be a more difficult intervention to address with men for a number of reasons. From a public health standpoint, it is well established that men are less aware, proactive, and assertive than women when it comes to their health care. Nutrition, as a lifestyle approach, can also be more complicated and challenging to deal with (than exercise, for example) because there are many approaches and controversies that can be challenging to sort out. Various diets make claims touting benefits for losing weight, building muscle mass, increasing energy, and/or combatting fatigue and include elements that may be contradictory, such as caveman-inspired higher protein diets and juice-based or raw diets. It gets very confusing for the medical practitioner, let alone the layman. Finally, behavioral changes (including timing of meals, determining macronutrient ratios, learning to cook new foods, and finding where to shop for them) associated with dietary recommendations may be difficult for anyone to make given resources, time, and motivational constraints.

Because this chapter describes integrative nutritional therapies, it is important to outline a few key differences between medical nutrition therapy practiced in an integrative or complementary and alternative medicine (CAM) clinical practice in comparison to a dietetics and/or conventional medicine setting. One primary difference is that integrative nutritionists or practitioners are much more likely to recommend therapeutic diets (e.g., vegetarian, rotation/elimination, sugar free, or lower carbohydrate), at least for a specific period of time, because they can be an important part of an integrative program. Another important distinction is that nutritionists and integrative medical practitioners are much more likely to recommend nutritional supplements to go along with therapeutic diets, whereas most dieticians and conventional medical doctors are often not trained in the use of nutritional supplements and have little experience with their therapeutic potential. This chapter will focus on the diet portion of nutritional recommendations, with the following chapter focusing on supplements.

Dietary Guidelines

Healthy dietary guidelines may best be exemplified by the anti-inflammatory diet, inspired by the Mediterranean diet and food choices that are generally associated with Mediterranean dietary patterns. Research supports these guidelines in the prevention and adjuvant treatment of diseases such as obesity, diabetes, heart disease, cancer, and neurocognitive decline associated with aging (Hu & Willet, 2002), because the mechanism of inflammation has been shown to be the common pathway leading to these disease processes. Anti-inflammatory diets generally emphasize fish, vegetables, whole grains, beans or legumes, and fruit while limiting meat and poultry (see the Anti-Inflammatory Food Pyramid in Figure 2.1). In so doing, the diet encourages healthy types and amounts of protein and healthy or low-glycemic-index/glycemic-load complex carbohydrates. In addition, the diet emphasizes healthy fats such as olive oil, nuts and seeds, and avocado, which contain high levels of monounsaturated fat, as well as omega-3 fatty acids from these foods and many types of fish. Finally, all of these natural foods contribute to significant phytonutrient intake, which has increasingly been found to have significant biochemical and physiological benefits.

Most nutritionists, dieticians, and medical practitioners would agree on these basic nutritional approaches and principles. In fact, the Mediterranean-style diet has been shown to decrease inflammatory markers and improve cholesterol levels and has been associated with a decreased recurrence of cardiovascular disease among survivors of heart attacks (de Lorgeril and Salen, 2011; Esposito et al., 2013).

Recent research and commentary suggests that aging is an inflammatory process. This is in addition to the current understanding that obesity and cardiovascular disease (CVD) are inflammatory conditions, and that CVD is the leading cause of mortality and morbidity for men. Most research suggests that omega-3 fatty acids have the most significant anti-inflammatory effects and that carbohydrates can be major contributors to inflammation and obesity. Studies show that replacing carbohydrates even with saturated fats leads to decreased

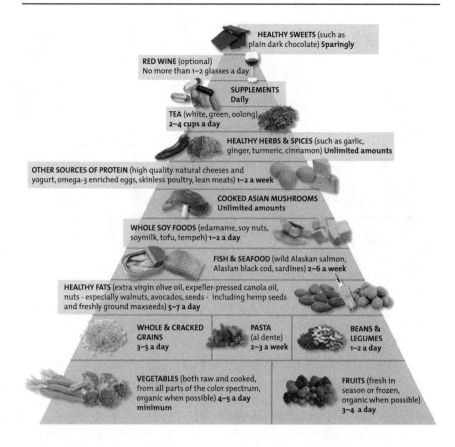

FIGURE 2.1. Dr. Weil's anti-inflammatory diet pyramid.

HEALTHY SWEETS
How much: Sparingly
Healthy choices: Unsweetened dried fruit, dark chocolate, fruit sorbet
Why: Dark chocolate provides polyphenols with antioxidant activity. Choose dark chocolate with at least 70% pure cocoa and have an ounce a few times a week. Fruit sorbet is a better option than other frozen desserts.

RED WINE
How much: Optional, no more than 1–2 glasses per day
Healthy choices: Organic red wine
Why: Red wine has beneficial antioxidant activity. Limit intake to no more than 1–2 servings per day. If you do not drink alcohol, do not start.

SUPPLEMENTS
How much: Daily

Healthy choices: High-quality multivitamin/multimineral that includes key antioxidants (vitamin C, vitamin E, mixed carotenoids, and selenium); coenzyme Q10; 2–3 g of a molecularly distilled fish oil; 2,000 IU of vitamin D3
Why: Supplements help fill any gaps in your diet when you are unable to get your daily requirement of micronutrients.

TEA
How much: 2–4 cups per day
Healthy choices: White, green, oolong teas
Why: Tea is rich in catechins, antioxidant compounds that reduce inflammation. Purchase high-quality tea and learn how to correctly brew it for maximum taste and health benefits.

HEALTHY HERBS & SPICES
How much: Unlimited amounts
Healthy choices: Turmeric, curry powder (which contains turmeric), ginger and garlic (dried and fresh), chili peppers, basil, cinnamon, rosemary, thyme
Why: Use these herbs and spices generously to season foods. Turmeric and ginger are powerful, natural antiinflammatory agents.

OTHER SOURCES OF PROTEIN
How much: 1–2 servings a week (1 portion is equal to 1 ounce of cheese, 1 eight-ounce serving of dairy, 1 egg, 3 oz cooked poultry or skinless meat)
Healthy choices: High-quality natural cheese and yogurt, omega-3-enriched eggs, skinless poultry, grass-fed lean meats
Why: In general, try to reduce consumption of animal foods. If you eat chicken, choose organic, cagefree chicken and remove the skin and associated fat. Use organic, reducedfat dairy products moderately, especially yogurt and natural cheeses such as Emmental (Swiss), Jarlsberg, and true Parmesan. If you eat eggs, choose omega-3-enriched eggs (made by feeding hens a flaxmeal-enriched diet) or organic eggs from free-range chickens.

COOKED ASIAN MUSHROOMS
How much: Unlimited amounts
Healthy choices: Shiitake, enokidake, maitake, oyster mushrooms (and wild mushrooms if available)
Why: These mushrooms contain compounds that enhance immune function. Never eat mushrooms raw, and minimize consumption of common commercial button mushrooms (including crimini and Portobello).

WHOLE SOY FOODS
How much: 1–2 servings per day (1 serving is equal to ½ cup tofu or tempeh, 1 cup soymilk, ½ cup cooked edamame, 1 ounce of soynuts)
Healthy choices: Tofu, tempeh, edamame, soy nuts, soymilk

Why: Soy foods contain isoflavones that have antioxidant activity and are protective against cancer. Choose whole soy foods over fractionated foods like isolated soy protein powders and imitation meats made with soy isolate.

FISH & SEAFOOD
How much: 2–6 servings per week (1 serving is equal to 4 oz of fish or seafood)
Healthy choices: Wild Alaskan salmon (especially sockeye), herring, sardines, and black cod (sablefish)
Why: These fish are rich in omega-3 fats, which are strongly anti-inflammatory. If you choose not to eat fish, take a molecularly distilled fish oil supplement that provides both EPA and DHA in a dose of 2–3 g per day.

HEALTHY FATS
How much: 5–7 servings per day (1 serving is equal to 1 teaspoon of oil, 2 walnuts, 1 tablespoon of flaxseed, 1 ounce of avocado)
Healthy choices: For cooking, use extra virgin olive oil and expellerpressed organic canola oil. Other sources of healthy fats include nuts (especially walnuts), avocados, and seeds—including hemp seeds and freshly ground flaxseed. Omega-3 fats are also found in cold water fish, omega-3-enriched eggs, and whole soy foods. Organic, expeller-pressed, higholeic sunflower or safflower oils may also be used as well as walnut and hazelnut oils in salads and dark-roasted sesame oil as a flavoring for soups and stir-fries.
Why: Healthy fats are those rich in either monounsaturated or omega3 fats. Extravirgin olive oil is rich in polyphenols with antioxidant activity and canola oil contains a small fraction of omega-3 fatty acids.

WHOLE & CRACKED GRAINS
How much: 3–5 servings a day (1 serving is equal to about ½ cup cooked grains)
Healthy choices: Brown rice, basmati rice, wild rice, buckwheat, groats, barley, quinoa, steel-cut oats
Why: Whole grains digest slowly, reducing frequency of spikes in blood sugar that promote inflammation. "Whole grains" means grains that are intact or in a few large pieces, not whole wheat bread or other products made from flour.

PASTA (al dente)
How much: 2–3 servings per week (1 serving is equal to about ½ cup cooked pasta)
Healthy choices: Organic pasta, rice noodles, bean thread noodles, and part whole wheat and buckwheat noodles like Japanese udon and soba
Why: Pasta cooked al dente (when it has "tooth" to it) has a lower glycemic index than fully cooked pasta. Low-glycemic-load carbohydrates should be the bulk of your carbohydrate intake to help minimize spikes in blood glucose levels.

BEANS & LEGUMES
How much: 1–2 servings per day (1 serving is equal to ½ cup cooked beans or legumes)

Healthy choices: Beans like Anasazi, adzuki, and black, as well as chickpeas, black-eyed peas, and lentils
Why: Beans are rich in folic acid, magnesium, potassium, and soluble fiber. They are a lowglycemicload food. Eat them wellcooked either whole or pureed into spreads like hummus.

VEGETABLES
How much: 4–5 servings per day minimum (1 serving is equal to 2 cups salad greens, ½ cup vegetables cooked, raw, or juiced)
Healthy choices: Lightly cooked dark leafy greens (spinach, collard greens, kale, Swiss chard), cruciferous vegetables (broccoli, cabbage, Brussels sprouts, kale, bok choy, and cauliflower), carrots, beets, onions, peas, squashes, sea vegetables, and washed raw salad greens
Why: Vegetables are rich in flavonoids and carotenoids with both antioxidant and antiinflammatory activity. Go for a wide range of colors, eat them both raw and cooked, and choose organic when possible.

FRUITS
How much: 3–4 servings per day (1 serving is equal to 1 medium-size piece of fruit, ½ cup chopped fruit, ¼ cup of dried fruit)
Healthy choices: Raspberries, blueberries, strawberries, peaches, nectarines, oranges, pink grapefruit, red grapes, plums, pomegranates, blackberries, cherries, apples, and pears—all lower in glycemic load than most tropical fruits
Why: Fruits are rich in flavonoids and carotenoids with both antioxidant and anti-inflammatory activity. Go for a wide range of colors, choose fruit that is fresh in season or frozen, and buy organic when possible.
Additional Item:

WATER
How much: Throughout the day
Healthy choices: Drink pure water or drinks that are mostly water (tea, very diluted fruit juice, sparkling water with lemon) throughout the day.
Why: Water is vital for overall functioning of the body.

weight, and replacing carbohydrates with polyunsaturated fatty acids (PUFAs) such as omega-3 leads to a decrease in insulin resistance (Taubes, 2008).

Assessing the propensity of carbohydrates to promote inflammation is best done through use of the glycemic load. This measure takes into account both the glycemic index of particular foods and the amount of that food included in a serving. Thus, a high-glycemic-index food such as grapes actually confers a lower overall glycemic load because the number of grams of grapes generally consumed in one serving is relatively low compared to the number of grams of pasta consumed, which has a lower glycemic index but a higher glycemic load

(Atkinson, Foster-Powell and Brand-Miller, 2008). The glycemic load actually predicts the amount by which blood sugar will rise after a meal. This is important with regard to inflammation, as sugar itself is inflammatory. The higher the average glucose, the more glucose molecules attach to proteins in the body, creating proinflammatory molecules called advanced glycation end-products (AGEs).

DIETARY APPROACHES AND FUNCTIONAL ASPECTS OF DIET

Beyond these food and dietary guidelines, two primary dietary approaches are frequently addressed in integrative medicine: (a) abnormal glucose tolerance, insulin resistance, and hypoglycemia, addressed through a balance of macro-nutrients and other factor-specific guidelines described later, and (b) elimination or rotation diets for food intolerance or food allergy. Depending on the symptom or disorder, various levels of dietary guidelines could be recommended and/or a combination of these approaches may be used.

Insulin resistance is a significant and growing problem that leads to over-weight and obesity, diabetes, hypertension, lipid abnormalities, cardiovascular disease, cancer, and neurocognitive decline. Therefore, dietary guidelines and other approaches that lower insulin resistance would contribute to weight loss and a decreased risk of morbidity associated with these disorders. These include (a) limiting or avoiding sugars and refined carbohydrates; (b) balancing meals for protein, healthy fats, and complex carbohydrates; (c) limiting caffeine; (d) eating smaller, more frequent meals and snacks; (e) stretching and exercising regularly; (f) utilizing effective stress management strategies; and (g) taking specific nutrients or nutritional supplements that influence insulin resistance, such as magnesium and chromium. It is possible that abnormal glucose tolerance in underweight people (hypoglycemia) and insulin resistance in overweight or obese people reflect a continuum that can be addressed in similar ways. Some of the most important recommendations are to eat more regular meals and snacks of smaller sizes and avoid prolonged periods of not eating and to minimize processed foods (refined grains and hydrogenated oils) that lead to overeating and increased blood sugar levels.

Rotation and elimination diets can be useful for stomach and intestinal disorders (irritable bowel syndrome [IBS], inflammatory bowel disease [IBD], and gastroesophageal reflux disease [GERD]), migraine headaches, autoimmune disorders, chronic inflammatory or pain disorders, skin conditions, allergies, and other diseases. These diets can be applied in three primary ways: (a) a rotation diet (making sure not to repeat the same foods more than once in a 4-day cycle); (b) a "level 1" elimination diet (avoiding sugars, dairy, wheat, alcohol, and caffeine); and (c) a "level 2" elimination diet (avoiding foods from level 1 plus other potentially offending foods such as peanuts, soy, other gluten grains [rye, barley, and oats], corn, citrus, eggs, and any other foods that may be suspected to cause symptoms). The patient's or client's ability and willingness to comply even for a short time is important to consider. Generally the patient needs to adhere to an elimination diet for a period of at least 3 weeks to determine if there is any improvement in symptoms. Once improvements are noticed, foods can be added back into the diet one by one to help determine which food, when added back, causes a resurgence of symptoms. This approach may also be helpful for chronic conditions of uncertain origin and/or when there are few therapeutic options, such as for IBS, dermatitis, and arthritis.

EFFECTIVE AND/OR POPULAR DIETARY APPROACHES

There are a range of dietary approaches that are available to men who are trying to lose weight and eat more healthfully. Although there may be some overlap, they can be generally categorized as (a) healthy and low fat—including the Mediterranean diet, the DASH diet, Weight Watchers, and whole foods types of diets; (b) vegetarian or plant-based diets—including the Ornish diet, the macrobiotic diet, strict vegetarianism, or a vegan diet or raw foods diet; (c) lower or low-carbohydrate diets—including the Atkins diet and the South Beach diet; (d) balanced calorie deficit diets—including Weight Watchers; (e) prepared foods diets—including NutriSystem and Jenny Craig; and (f) genetically optimal diets such as Paleo or individualized diets based on a patient's specific blood type or genetic profile.

An in-depth discussion of each of these diets is beyond the capacity of this book, but the Paleo diet (aka caveman diet) is especially popular among men, and the Ornish diet has rigorous research data showing its effectiveness among those with heart disease, so those will be discussed further.

The Paleo diet has been promulgated by Loren Cordain, PhD, and is very popular among participants of CrossFit training programs. The basic premise is that certain foods that humans have been eating for the longest time in the history of our species are optimal because changes in food have happened faster than our bodies' ability to evolve to handle such foods. Optimal foods include the types of foods humans would have eaten 10,000 years ago as hunter-gatherers, before the advent of larger communities and farming. Fruits, vegetables, nuts and seeds, and lean animal protein make up the bulk of the diet. Grains, anything manufactured or artificial, legumes, refined sugars, and dairy products are not included in the diet. Some studies have shown improvement in glucose tolerance, weight, waist circumference, and blood pressure with the Paleo diet (Frassetto et al., 2009). The limitation to these studies is that they are largely based on small samples, sometimes without control groups. Most of the evidence for the Paleo diet comes from studies showing that elements of this diet are beneficial, but that is not proof that the whole diet together is beneficial (Lindberg et al., 2007; Osterdahl et al., 2008).

The very low-fat diet, as made famous by Dean Ornish, MD, includes 15% of calories or less from fat. Dr. Ornish has published several intervention trials showing the benefits of such a diet for heart disease and cholesterol (Ornish et al., 1998). Long-term effects of such a low-fat diet are still not known, and the practicality of people adhering to such a strict limitation on fat intake is a concern. A larger study of such a diet in a real-world population of Medicare beneficiaries is currently being planned.

The challenge to nutritionists is to target the optimal diet and supplement programs that can produce results yet are not so difficult that they cannot be adhered to. Lower carbohydrate approaches can be helpful and healthy for weight loss and CVD risk reduction. Lower carbohydrate diets should, however, be included within an integrative medical program that includes physical fitness and stress management, as well as targeted nutritional supplementation. Another general consideration is that prepared-food weight loss programs must be accompanied by educational and behavioral training so that individuals can maintain results and lifestyles once they are no longer getting the purchased foods.

This comprehensive weight loss and health promotion process requires dialogue and understanding, as well as informational and practical support. Finally, the guidelines should be recommended for a finite period of time such as 3 to 12 weeks to see if results are achieved if it is a fairly restrictive or challenging program. An example recommendation could be to avoid or rotate sugar, wheat, dairy, and alcohol for 4 weeks and see what results are produced.

Nutritional Supplementation

The consideration for the use of nutritional supplements in clinical practice is, to a certain degree, a question of philosophy and practice orientation. For practitioners of integrative or complementary medicine, supplements work well within the framework of natural approaches that include diet, exercise, stress management, and other modalities such as acupuncture or massage. Geriatric practice can be particularly responsive to targeting key supplements in order to avoid adding to the number of other medications already being taken and potential adverse effects or interactions.

The Dietary Supplement Health and Education Act (DSHEA) passed by Congress in 1994 is the primary legislation that regulates all aspects of supplements, including manufacturing, quality control, labeling, and marketing. There is a vast range of supplements that practitioners may recommend or that patients may opt to try on their own. Categories of supplements include vitamins, minerals, fatty acids, amino acids, antioxidants, probiotics and prebiotics, herbs and botanicals, enzymes, hormones, glandulars, functional foods and food concentrates, homeopathic remedies, and others.

Although it is always ideal to get essential nutrients from food, there are many reasons a supplement may benefit a patient, including the patient's poor dietary choices, variations in soil nutritional content, micronutrient losses from food processing and cooking, and genetic polymorphisms or variations in individual nutrient requirements (Oakley, 1998). Several models can be used to understand how supplements can benefit the patient population, including (a) nutritional deficiency, (b) subclinical nutritional deficiency, (c) biological response modifiers, and (d) mass action effects (Ames, 2004). It is the overt nutritional deficiency that is well defined and most often utilized in medical and nutritional practice. Classic examples are iron and vitamin B_{12} deficiencies that produce clinical symptoms, can be identified through laboratory analyses, and can be supplemented and monitored for symptom and assay changes.

More challenging is the evaluation of the other three research models in which there are varying levels of supportive evidence from in vitro, animal, and clinical research. For example, a perceived subclinical magnesium deficiency is the reason many integrative medicine practitioners recommend magnesium despite normal serum or red blood cell magnesium levels (Olerich and Rude, 1994). Magnesium is a cofactor for over 300 enzymes and is a calcium channel blocker. Research supports magnesium's influence in hypertension, diabetes and glucose tolerance, allergies, migraines, muscle cramps, constipation, neurocognitive function, and possibly other disorders (Swain & Kaplan-Machlis, 1999; Ueshima, 2005). Because magnesium is often inadequate in the diet and can be depleted by chronic disease, it may be prescribed by primary health care providers to help address a range of symptoms.

Omega-3 fatty acids or fish oil supplements are a good example of biological response modifiers. Supplements can enhance dietary influences, as described in the previous dietary section, and can effectively alter the synthesis of pro-inflammatory versus anti-inflammatory eicosanoids. Similar to magnesium, omega-3 fatty acids are potentially beneficial in a range of disorders due to their anti-inflammatory effects and impact on cellular membrane fluidity and function because of their effect on membrane fatty acid composition (Yehuda et al., 2005). Like magnesium, there is no established nutritional status measure,

Table 2.1: Framework for Recommending Supplements

Healthy diet as a foundation
Evidence base that includes a sound rationale and mechanism
Positive benefit-to-risk ratio
Defined dose and time frame to assess effects
Targeted populations to treat such as (a) patients with adverse or inadequate responses to medication, (b) patients or families who would like to try nutrition and/or natural therapies before taking pharmaceuticals, or (c) elderly patients who are already taking many medications

although some studies have quantified blood levels of specific omega-3 fatty acids or omega-3–to–omega-6 fatty acid ratios (Tiemeier et al., 2003).

With regard to "mass action" effects, Ames and colleagues have written an excellent review on the biochemical influences of high-dose vitamins on enzyme binding and activity (Ames, 2004). As many as 50 genetic diseases and many genetic polymorphisms have shown improvement through nutritional supplementation, with other polymorphism effects to be determined as their identification and clinical effects are more thoroughly understood.

Despite the challenges presented, supplements can be effectively utilized in patient care once a reliable source of products is identified. Table 2.1 describes an effective framework from which supplements can be recommended.

There are some dietary or nutritional supplements that can be safely recommended and may be beneficial. Table 2.2 presents some of the most important and useful supplements. A more in-depth discussion of particular supplements can be found in Chapter 3.

Common Men's Health Issues

Specific medical conditions and the dietary approaches that can modify them can be found throughout this book in the corresponding chapters. For those clinical issues not covered in their own chapters, we discuss here the recommended nutritional approaches.

OVERWEIGHT, OBESITY, INSULIN RESISTANCE, METABOLIC SYNDROME, AND CARDIOVASCULAR DISEASE

Overweight and obesity pose the most important health risks to men because they contribute to diabetes, hypertension, hyperlipidemia, heart disease, cancer,

Table 2.2: Important and Useful Dietary Supplements

Supplement	Rationale
Multivitamin and mineral	Despite some conflicting results, research has suggested that multivitamin and mineral supplements may reduce the risk for heart attacks and certain types of cancer, as well as reduce C-reactive protein and infection rates in diabetics and the elderly (Barringer et al., 2003; Church et al., 2003; El-Kadiki & Sutton, 2005; Fuchs et al., 2003; Holmquist et al., 2003). Taking a multivitamin and mineral every day can reinforce healthy behaviors that contribute to a healthy lifestyle.
Omega-3 fatty acids or fish oil	Health benefits of fish were described earlier in this chapter. It should also be noted that fish oil is now endorsed by the American Heart Association for the prevention of cardiovascular disease (CVD). There are at least six mechanisms by which omega-3 fatty acids reduce CVD risk: (a) anti-inflammatory, (b) hypolipidemic, (c) antithrombotic, (d) cytokine inhibition, (e) antiarrhythmic; and (f) endothelial-derived nitric oxide stimulation (Holub & Holub, 2004).
Calcium, magnesium, and vitamin D	Important for bone health and the many important aspects of magnesium influence that were listed earlier. Also, there is some recent provocative research suggesting that vitamin D may be involved in immune function and cancer, autoimmune disorders, insulin resistance, and possibly other disorders, especially in the elderly (Holick, 2006).
Probiotics	Have been shown to be helpful for symptoms such as constipation and diarrhea, and they are very safe (Boyle et al., 2006). They may also be helpful for irritable bowel syndrome (IBS), inflammatory bowel disease (IBD), atopic disease, and *Clostridium difficile* infections with a yeast supplement, *Saccharomyces boulardii* (Katz, 2006).
Glucosamine sulfate and chondroitin sulfate	Good research suggests that glucosamine and chondroitin sulfate can help reduce stiffness and pain in osteoarthritis (Richy et al., 2003).
Coenzyme Q10	Coenzyme Q10, or ubiquinone, is an important part of the oxidative phosphorylation chain leading to mitochondrial adenosine triphosphate synthesis. HMG-CoA reductase inhibitors or statins lower circulating levels of CoQ10, but the consequences are not well understood. Perhaps the most common symptom would be muscle cramps. Supplementation may be warranted especially in susceptible populations such as those over 65 years of age or those with congestive heart failure (Witte et al., 2005).

neurocognitive decline, and aging. It is therefore important to focus on two primary nutritional goals, which are to develop a healthy dietary/nutritional regimen and to achieve a healthy weight and/or fitness level. To reach these goals, there are several factors that are important to address, including (a) developing a health care team and/or a support network, (b) finding an approach that is manageable over the long term and successful, and (c) identifying and addressing barriers that come up and prevent someone from achieving a healthy weight and/or fitness level. Research consistently suggests that which dietary approach is followed (although this does need to be carefully considered) may be less important than following it strictly or as required to achieve desired results. In addition, the coaching philosophy, which is based on the "stages of change" behavioral model and is consistent with integrative medicine philosophy, appears to be a helpful adjunct that can lead to success.

It is particularly important to be persistent because research suggests that people may try a weight loss program four to five times before they are successful. Still other research indicates that successful long-term weight loss requires 5 days per week of aerobic exercise and weight training.

Other factors may be involved with insulin resistance that needs to be addressed. Decreasing insulin resistance will help to reverse the range of modifiable CVD risk factors such as hypertension, elevated triglycerides and abnormal lipids, and diabetes, all of which are associated with metabolic syndrome and CVD risk. The same guidelines discussed previously regarding the anti-inflammatory diet and lower glycemic load diets will help to lower insulin resistance. Supplements that further help include therapeutic doses of cinnamon, selective kinase response modifiers (SKRMs) such as acacia bark (Minich et al., 2010), chromium, and α-lipoic acid.

DEPRESSION

There are several dietary factors that can be important in depression and should be understood and addressed. These include dietary composition and intake of omega-3 fatty acids (Lin and Su, 2007) and folate (Tolmunen et al., 2004). Although the dietary contributions of these nutrients are important, it should be appreciated that these should be augmented with supplements to get the maximal benefit, especially when addressing ongoing depressive symptoms or trying to prevent a recurrence. As described more clearly in the supplement section, omega-3 fatty acid intake has been shown to decrease susceptibility to depression and may be helpful as adjuvant therapy.

The supplements with the most significant influence on depression include (a) omega-3 fatty acids; (b) S-adenosyl methionine; (c) St. John's wort—which is most beneficial for mild to moderate depression but potential interactions with medications must be addressed; and (d) vitamin D—which is helpful for seasonal depression but more recent evidence suggests benefits for other forms of depression. Finally, both diet and supplements should be included within a comprehensive and individually designed integrative medicine approach.

Fitness and Optimizing Recovery

There are no specific dietary recommendations for men looking to optimize muscle recovery or growth after resistance training. However, there is good evidence that the timing of meals and mix of macronutrient intake is important.

Carbohydrate plus protein in combination within 2 hours of finishing exercise is important for replenishing glycogen stores and building muscle. Some studies have shown that a ratio of approximately 4 g carbohydrate for every 1 g protein may be the optimal ratio, with a goal of about 1 g carbohydrate per kilogram body mass after vigorous endurance training. The danger of not eating within 2 hours is that the glycogen stores may not be replenished fully in preparation for the next bout of fitness training. Protein is important to help repair torn muscle fibers, especially after resistance training. A combination of faster absorbing and slower absorbing proteins is especially beneficial, such as a mix of casein and whey protein. One particular favorite postworkout food is chocolate milk, because of its particular ratio of carbohydrates and proteins.

Assessment of Nutritional Status

Current guidelines on recommended nutrient intake are based on federal Recommended Daily Allowance (RDA) levels. These levels were developed to provide guidance on the avoidance of frank nutritional deficiency and related diseases such as pellagra or scurvy. The RDA says nothing about optimal nutritional intake. In fact, given the variety of genetic profiles, levels of activity, gender differences, and hormonal and body-type differences, it is nearly impossible to recommend optimal intake at the population-wide level. Therefore, integrative practitioners often aim to assess the individual patient's nutritional status. Some nutrient levels are easily measured in a serum sample, such as 25-(OH) vitamin D, but some nutrients are more difficult to assess because they are largely intracellular, such as magnesium.

Various labs will perform nutritional assessments looking at white blood cell (WBC) intracellular levels of nutrients or the functional status of nutrients (looking at WBC function in a cell with normal levels of each nutrient as compared to a patient's WBC function). Although these tests may be helpful in identifying suboptimal levels, the results may vary depending on daily nutritional variation. It is as important to treat signs and symptoms and the nutritional deficiency that could be causing them as it is to target specific test results.

Summary and Conclusions

Nutritional interventions are a large part of an integrative health approach to men, especially with regard to prevention of heart disease and metabolic syndrome. The most important elements of a healthy nutrition program with these goals include an aim to maintain healthy weight using an anti-inflammatory, Mediterranean-style diet.

Specific diets such as elimination diets, the Ornish low-fat diet, and the Paleo-style diet may be helpful for particular individuals, depending on their goals and health risks.

REFERENCES

Ames B. Supplements and tuning up metabolism. J Nutr. 2004;134(11):3164S–3168S.

Atkinson FS, Foster-Powell, K, Brand-Miller JC. International tables of glycemic index and glycemic load values: 2008. Diabetes Care. 2008:31(12);2281–2283. Summary at website: http://www.health.harvard.edu/newsweek/Glycemic_index_and_glycemic_load_for_100_foods.htm

Barringer TA, Kirk JK, et al. Effect of a multivitamin and mineral supplement on infection and quality of life. A randomized, double-blind, placebo-controlled trial. Ann Intern Med. 2003;138(5):365–371.

Boyle RJ, Robins-Browne RM, et al. Probiotic use in clinical practice: what are the risks? Am J Clin Nutr. 2006;83(6):1256–1264;quiz 1446–1447.

Church TS, Earnest CP, et al. Reduction of C-reactive protein levels through use of a multivitamin. Am J Med. 2003;115(9):702–707.

de Lorgeril M, Salen P. Mediterranean diet in secondary prevention of CHD. Public Health Nutr. 2011 Dec;14(12A):2333–2337.

El-Kadiki A, Sutton AJ. Role of multivitamins and mineral supplements in preventing infections in elderly people: systematic review and meta-analysis of randomized controlled trials. BMJ. 2005;330(7496):871.

Esposito K, Kastorini CM, et al. Mediterranean diet and metabolic syndrome: An updated systematic review. Rev Endocr Metab Disord. 2013;14(3):255–263.

Frassetto LA, Schloetter M, et al. Metabolic and physiologic improvements from consuming a Paleolithic, hunter-gatherer type diet. Eur J Clin Nutr. 2009;63(8):947–955.

Holick M. Vitamin D. Its role in cancer prevention and treatment. Prog Biophys Mol Biol. 2006;92(1):49–59.

Holmquist C, Larsson S, et al. Multivitamin supplements are inversely associated with risk of myocardial infarction in men and women—Stockholm Heart Epidemiology Program (SHEEP). J Nutr. 2003;133(8):2650–2654.

Holub DJ, Holub BJ. Omega-3 fatty acids from fish oils and cardiovascular disease. Mol Cell Biochem. 2004;263(1–2):217–225.

Hu FB, Willett WC. Optimal diets for prevention of coronary heart disease. JAMA. 2002;288:2569–2578.

Katz JA. Probiotics for the prevention of antibiotic-associated diarrhea and Clostridium difficile diarrhea. J Clin Gastroenterol. 2006;40(3):249–255.

Lin Py, Su KP. A meta-analysis review of double-blind, placebo-controlled trials of antidepressant efficacy of omega-3 fatty acids. J Clin Psychiatry. 2007;68(7):1056–1061.

Lindeberg S, Jönsson T, et al. A paleolithic diet improves glucose tolerance more than a Mediterranean-like diet in individuals with ischemic heart disease. Diabetelogica. 2007;50(9):1795–1807.

Minich DM, Lerman RH, et al. Hop and acacia phytochemicals decreased lipotoxicity in 3T3-L1 adipocytes, db/db mice, and individuals with metabolic syndrome. J Nutr Metab. 2010;2010. pii: 467316. Epub 2010 May 18. http://www.ncbi.nlm.nih.gov/pmc/articles/PMC2915809/?tool=pubmed

Oakley GP Jr. Eat right and take a multivitamin. N Engl J Med. 1998;338: 1060–1061.

Olerich MA, Rude RK. Should we supplement magnesium in critically ill patients? New Horizon. 1994;2(2):186–192.

Ornish D, Scherwitz LW, et al. Intensive lifestyle changes for reversal of coronary heart disease. JAMA. 1998;280:2001–2007.

Ornish D. All references for the Ornish Diet can be found at http://www.ornishspectrum.com/proven-program/the-research/

Osterdahl M, Kocturk T, et al. Effects of a short-term intervention with a Paleolithic diet in healthy volunteers. Eur J Clin Nutr. 2008;62(5):682–685.

Richy F, Bruyere O, et al. Structural and symptomatic efficacy of glucosamine and chrondroitin in knee osteoarthritis: a comprehensive meta-analysis. Arch Intern Med. 2003;163(13):1514–1522.

Swain R, Kaplan-Machlis B. Magnesium for the next millennium. South Med J. 1999;92(11):1040–1047.

Taubes G. *Good Calories, Bad Calories: Challenging the Conventional Wisdom on Diet, Weight Control and Disease*. Random House, New York, 2008.

Tiemeir H, van Tuijl HR, et al. Plasma fatty acid composition and depression are associated in the elderly: the Rotterdam Study. Am J Clin Nutr. 2003;78(1):40–46.

Tolmunen T, Hintikka J, et al. Dietary Folate and the risk of depression in Finnish middle-aged men: a prospective follow-up study. Psychother Psychosom. 2004 Nov–Dec;73(6):334–339.

Ueshima K. Magnesium and ischemic heart disease: a review of epidemiological, experimental, and clinical evidences. Magnes Res. 2005;18(4):275–284.

Witte KK, Nikitin NP, et al. The effect of micronutrient supplementation on quality-of-life and left ventricular function in elderly patients with chronic heart failure. Eur Heart J. 2005;26(21):2238–2244.

Yehuda S, Rabinovitz S, et al. Essential fatty acids and the brain: from infancy to aging. Neurobiol Aging. 2005;26(1):98–102.

NUTRITION POSTEXERCISE:

- J Appl Physiol 1994;76:839–845.
- J Appl Physiol 1994;76(2):839–845, Copyright © 1994 by American Physiological Society

3

Dietary Supplements and Men's Health

TIERAONA LOW DOG AND DAVID KIEFER

Introduction

There are many chapters in this book that provide specific guidance with regard to the use of dietary supplements (DSs) for particular health conditions. Thus, to reduce repetition, we will provide background information regarding the safety and quality of DSs, as well as a brief overview of some of the DSs commonly used by men. Resources that can assist clinicians on the appropriate use of DSs for general preventive health or for specific diagnoses are provided at the end of this chapter.

Dietary supplements, according to the Dietary Supplement Health and Education Act of 1994 (DSHEA), are products intended to supplement the diet and may contain one or more of the following ingredients: a vitamin, a mineral, a botanical, an amino acid, or another dietary substance, or a combination of these ingredients or their extracts. By definition, DSs are intended for oral ingestion in pill, capsule, tablet, or liquid form and do not include topical or injectable preparations. Since the passage of the DSHEA, the marketplace has grown from roughly 4,000 products to more than 29,000. Given this dramatic increase and the sheer number of products, it is understandable that consumers and health care professionals alike have difficulty navigating the supplement marketplace.

DSs are used by most Americans, with some surveys indicating use by up to 70% of the population (Timbo et al., 2006). This phenomenon is not unique to the United States. Sales in the global dietary supplement industry reached $187 billion in 2010, buoyed by rising sales in traditional markets like the United States and the European Union (EU) and in emerging markets like China and India. Although women are more likely than men to take DSs, men do make up a considerable part of the marketplace, especially in certain populations.

For example, in one group of men with prostate cancer, 73% reported taking a dietary supplement (Wiygul et al., 2005). Many athletes use DSs to improve performance and endurance. One study of 440 Canadian athletes found that within the previous 6 months, 87% reported having taken three or more DSs, primarily sports drinks, multivitamin and mineral preparations, protein powders, and meal replacement products (Lun et al., 2012). Like women, many men use DSs for general health maintenance. According to a survey conducted by the Council for Responsible Nutrition in 2008, 50% of adult men 18 and older living in the United States were taking a multivitamin. A study of men over the age of 40 living in New Zealand found that 47% reported using at least one daily supplement and 30% took two or more supplements (Bacon et al., 2011). The most common supplements used were vitamins or minerals (49%), followed by nutritional oils (22%; including fish oils, 13%) and glucosamine/chondroitin preparations (13%). Supplements were mainly taken for nonspecific prophylaxis or health maintenance (58%), although 21% of respondents cited treatment of or symptom alleviation for a medical condition.

Consumers generally perceive DSs as safe and most use them without consultation from a health care provider. Clinicians, on the other hand, often cite safety concerns regarding quality (i.e., adulteration, contamination) and the potential for DS–drug interactions. These concerns appear to be somewhat justified. A large national survey reported that 72% of people using herbal remedies were also taking prescription drugs and 84% were taking over-the-counter preparations (Gardiner et al., 2007). Clinicians should be aware that some patients *preferentially* combine DS and prescription medications. A survey of multiethnic herbal medicine users reported that 40% believed that combining herbs with drugs had a synergistic effect (Kuo et al., 2004). Although authoritative information on DS–drug interactions is scarce, the risk is particularly concerning for medications that have a narrow therapeutic index or are critical to the well-being of the patient. Not surprisingly, anticoagulant medications, especially warfarin, are the drugs most often identified as having the highest risk for DS–drug interactions (Qato et al., 2008). Less discussed in the literature is the possibility of a beneficial DS–drug interaction, in other words, a DS that may reduce the adverse effects of a prescription medication or augment its effectiveness. For example, there are a number of studies that demonstrate that milk thistle extract (*Silybum marianum*) reduces drug-induced hepatotoxicity (Post-White et al., 2007).

The issue of adulteration and contamination is also a legitimate concern and complicated by the fact that finished products adulterated with pharmaceuticals can be very hard to detect using traditional laboratory analysis. Men are the primary consumers of two of the three categories of products, bodybuilding and sexual enhancing agents, that are most commonly adulterated in the marketplace. The third category is weight loss supplements, used by both women and men. In one study, 14 of 20 dietary supplements marketed as natural slimming products were adulterated; eight contained sibutramine (4.4 to 30.5 mg/capsule), five contained sibutramine (5.0 to 19.6 mg/capsule or tablet) in combination with phenolphthalein (4.4 to 66.1 mg/capsule), and one was adulterated with synephrine (19.5 mg/capsule; Vaysse et al., 2010). In another study, 35 out of 105 botanical dietary supplements tested were adulterated with drugs including glibenclamide, sibutramine, and sildenafil (Chen et al., 2009). Almost 10% of Chinese herbal medicine products randomly purchased in Chinatown, New York, were adulterated with Western pharmaceuticals including promethazine, chlorpheniramine, diclofenac, chlordiazepoxide, hydrochlorothiazide, triamterene, diphenhydramine, and sildenafil (Miller & Stripp, 2007). Clearly, clinicians should inquire about the use of any DSs but should be particularly diligent about asking male patients if they are taking any supplements for erectile dysfunction, libido, or weight loss or to increase muscle mass.

Heavy metals can be present as a contaminant, such as when herbs are harvested in highly polluted areas, though they are sometimes intentionally added to traditional Chinese medicines or Ayurvedic preparations. In some cases, it is thought that the metals improve the effectiveness of the formula. Some formulae contain lead or mercury ingredients, such as minim or cinnabar. Clinicians must also be alert to potential heavy metal toxicity in patients using traditional herbal medicines. One fifth of both U.S.-manufactured and Indian-manufactured Ayurvedic medicines purchased via the Internet were found to contain detectable lead, mercury, or arsenic (Saper et al., 2008). All metal-containing products exceeded one or more standards for acceptable daily intake of toxic metals. Among the metal-containing products, 95% were sold by U.S. websites and 75% claimed Good Manufacturing Practices.

In June 2008, the Food and Drug Administration's new current good manufacturing practices (cGMPs) went into effect. These new regulations were developed in an effort to strengthen regulations that would ensure the purity, quality, strength, and composition of DSs being sold in the marketplace. All companies, no matter their size, had to come into full compliance with the cGMPs by June 2010. Hopefully, with enhanced inspection of manufacturing facilities and strict enforcement of cGMPs, the quality of DSs will improve, which will also increase the safety of DSs by reducing the risk of adulteration and contamination.

Selected Micronutrients in Men's Health

Many men take a daily multivitamin/mineral (MVI) supplement for general health purposes. There is tremendous variation in MVIs in the marketplace, with some providing 70% to 150% of the daily value (DV) of most vitamins and minerals and others containing up to 3,000% of the DV for some nutrients. It is therefore difficult to determine the long-term risks and benefits from taking MVIs in the general population. Clinicians should always ask patients to bring their supplements with them to appointments for review. There remains considerable debate regarding the safety of some of the nutrients commonly found in MVIs, such as selenium and vitamin E, when it comes to men's health. Initiated in 2001, the Selenium and Vitamin E Cancer Prevention Trial (SELECT) was a phase III, randomized, placebo-controlled human trial to investigate the chemopreventive effects of selenium (200 µg/day from L-selenomethionine), vitamin E (400 IU/day of all-rac-α-tocopheryl acetate), or their combination on prostate cancer (Lippman et al., 2009). Compared with placebo, the absolute increase in risk of prostate cancer per 1,000 person-years was 1.6 for vitamin E, 0.8 for selenium, and 0.4 for the combination (Klein et al., 2011). These results are in sharp contrast to previous research, the positive results of which spurred the SELECT trial. Questions continue to be raised about the type of vitamin E and selenium used in SELECT. For instance, this research protocol used all-rac-α-tocopherol, even though research shows that different stereoisomers of vitamin E have different biologic activities (Ledesma et al., 2011). The Nutritional Prevention of Cancer (NPC) study showed a significant reduction in prostate cancer when taking 0.5 g of high-selenium brewer's yeast (Clark et al., 1996); however, the SELECT trial used L-selenomethionine, which is only one of more than 20 selenium-containing species in brewer's yeast. In addition, the dose of vitamin E in the SELECT trial was eightfold higher than that used in the Alpha-Tocopherol, Beta-carotene Cancer Prevention (ATBC) study, which showed a 32% reduction in prostate cancer and 41% decrease in prostate mortality (Heinonen et al., 1998). Would using a broader range of vitamin E compounds or brewer's yeast have changed the outcome of the trial? That's impossible to know. But until we have more information, clinicians might want to counsel patients to select an MVI that provides 100 IU of vitamin E as a mixture of tocopherols and selenium in the form of brewer's yeast.

Another mineral of controversy in men's health is calcium with regard to prostate cancer. Separating out the potential effects of calcium versus dairy is difficult. A meta-analysis examined the impact of calcium, vitamin D, and dairy products upon prostate cancer risk using pooled data from 45 studies and over 26,000 participants (Huncharek et al., 2008). They examined both cohort studies and case-control studies and concluded that there was no association between calcium (relative risk [RR] = 1.06) or milk intake (RR = 1.06) and risk of prostate cancer. Data from the European Prospective Investigation into Cancer and Nutrition study (EPIC) found that high intake of calcium from dairy products was positively associated with risk of prostate cancer (RR = 1.2) in 142,000 men over nearly a 9-year period; however, there was no association detected between *nondairy* calcium and increased risk of prostate cancer (Allen, 2008). When 672 men were randomly assigned to either 1,200 mg/day of calcium carbonate or placebo for 4 years in a colorectal adenoma chemoprevention trial, after a mean follow-up of 10.3 years, there were 33 prostate cancer cases in the calcium-treated group and 37 in the placebo-treated group (Baron et al., 2005). At this time, if there is a relationship between calcium and prostate cancer, it appears that it is related to dairy consumption. The Institute of Medicine (IOM) has set the recommended daily intake for calcium from all sources for men at 1,000 mg/day from ages 19 to 70 and 1,200 mg/day for those 71 years and older.

While vitally important for bone health, vitamin D is also important for immune, reproductive, cardiovascular, and neurological health. Men are at risk for osteoporosis, especially with advancing age, small frame, use of medications that cause secondary osteoporosis, low intake of calcium and vitamin D, low testosterone levels, and treatment for prostate cancer. It has been estimated that up to 45% of men in the United States have low bone density (Gaines et al., 2010). The prevalence of vitamin D deficiency/insufficiency in the elder population is estimated to be between 25% and 54%. The wide range, in part, is due to the different cut-off levels that are used to define deficiency. Many researchers use the cut-off of 15 ng/ml, whereas others use 20 ng/ml. The bioassay used to assess vitamin D levels in human sera has been more widely available and more affordable, making assessment of vitamin D status common in clinical practice. The IOM's current recommendation for vitamin D_3 (cholecalciferol) is 600 IU/day for ages 1 to 70 years, and then 800 IU/day, though many clinicians recommend a daily dose of 1,000 to 2,000 IU/day, especially for men with darker skin and/or living at northern latitudes (Kimlin, 2008).

Folic acid and vitamin B_{12} are important for neurological health, especially in those 65 years and older. Deficiency in these nutrients may be associated with depression and cognitive decline. A double-blind, randomized study of 818 men and women aged 50 to 70 years with raised plasma total homocysteine and normal serum vitamin B_{12} at screening were given 800 mcg/day of folic acid for 3 years. Researchers found folic acid supplementation improved cognitive function, memory, and information processing speed and slowed age-related decline in hearing compared to placebo (Durga et al., 2007). But consistent with other studies, even though homocysteine levels were lowered, there was no change in atherosclerotic progression or arterial stiffening. And in contrast with this study, a meta-analysis of nine randomized trials found no benefit of folic acid, with or without other B-vitamins, on cognitive function (Wald et al., 2010). The type of folic acid supplementation may be important. Some forms may be more bioavailable than others in patients with a genetic polymorphism and in those who take particular medications or use alcohol. A review of the literature found that the 5-methyltetrahydrofolate (5-MTHF) formulation indicated efficacy as adjunctive therapy or monotherapy in reducing depressive symptoms in patients with normal and low folate levels, improving cognitive function and reducing depressive symptoms in elderly patients with dementia and folate deficiency, and reducing depressive and somatic symptoms in patients with depression and alcoholism (Fava & Mischoulon, 2009).

Masking of vitamin B_{12} deficiency, with risk of irreversible nerve damage, is a well-known risk associated with folic acid supplementation, especially in the older population; however, questions of folic acid supplementation and cancer risk have been raised. A meta-analysis by Wien et al. of six randomized controlled trials reporting prostate cancer incidence showed an RR of prostate cancer of 1.24 (95% confidence interval [CI] 1.03–1.49) for the men receiving folic acid compared to controls. No significant difference in cancer incidence was shown between groups receiving folic acid and the placebo/control group for any other cancer type. Total cancer mortality was reported in six randomized controlled trials, and a meta-analysis of these did not show any significant difference in cancer mortality in folic acid–supplemented groups compared to controls (Wien et al., 2012).

A review of 43 studies found that vitamin B_{12} levels in the subclinical low-normal range (<250 pmol/L) are associated with Alzheimer's disease, vascular dementia, and Parkinson's disease. Vitamin B_{12} deficiency (<150 pmol/L) is associated with cognitive impairment. Vitamin B_{12} supplements administered orally (1 mg daily) were effective in correcting biochemical deficiency but improved cognition only in patients with pre-existing vitamin B_{12} deficiency (Moore, 2012). As the rates of type 2 diabetes are increasing exponentially, more and more people are being placed on metformin, a drug shown in multiple studies to deplete vitamin B_{12} levels (Kos et al., 2011; Mahajan, 2010). The amount of B_{12} recommended by the IOM (2.4 mcg/day) and the amount available in general multivitamins (6 mcg) may not be enough to correct this deficiency among those with diabetes (Reinstatler et al., 2012). Clinicians should evaluate vitamin B_{12} status in men over the age of 65 years, vegetarians, those taking metformin, and/or patients with signs of cognitive impairment.

Magnesium (Mg) is the second most abundant intracellular cation in the body and may be particularly important in men's health given the morbidity and mortality of cardiovascular disease and diabetes. Mg is required for synthesis of RNA and replication of DNA, as a cofactor for enzymes that require adenosine triphosphate (ATP), and for neuromuscular transmission, and it plays a major role in regulating insulin effect and insulin-mediated glucose uptake. About 60% of adults in the United States do not consume the estimated average requirement for Mg, and research shows that marginal to moderate Mg deficiency through exacerbation of chronic inflammatory stress may contribute to atherosclerosis, hypertension, osteoporosis, diabetes mellitus, and cancer (Nielsen, 2010). Research has shown that magnesium supplementation decreases plasma C-reactive protein in participants with baseline values greater than 3.0 mg/L (Nielsen, et al, 2010). Low serum Mg levels are associated with higher all-cause mortality and cardiovascular mortality, possibly due to increased left ventricular hypertrophy (Reffelmann et al., 2011). A comprehensive analytical review of 44 human studies shows Mg supplements may enhance the blood pressure–lowering effect of antihypertensive medications (medications) in stage 1 hypertensive subjects when given in doses of 230 to 460 mg/day (Rosanoff, 2010). Oral Mg supplementation at doses of 400 to 600 mg/day has been shown to improve insulin sensitivity in normomagnesemic, overweight, nondiabetic subjects (Hadjistavri et al., 2010; Mooren et al., 2011). In March 2011, the U.S. Food and Drug Administration (FDA) notified prescribers that proton pump inhibitors may reduce Mg levels, especially when taken for longer than 1 year, putting patients at risk for cardiac arrhythmias and seizures, and it suggested regular monitoring (Chen et al., 2012). Other drugs associated with hypomagnesemia include cisplatin, cyclosporine, gentamicin, tobramycin, tacrolimus, laxatives, furosemide, and hydrochlorothiazide (Atsmon & Dolev, 2005). Serum Mg may be normal even when intracellular Mg is very low. Magnesium supplementation is quite safe, except in patients with poor renal function. Vitamin D enhances magnesium absorption.

Zinc is important for growth, sexual maturation, and reproduction in men. Zinc concentrations are very high in the male genital organs, particularly in the prostate gland, which is largely responsible for the high zinc content in seminal plasma. Spermatozoa themselves also contain zinc, which is derived from the testis (Ebisch et al., 2007). Zinc deficiency leads to hypogonadism and infertility in men. One study found a 74% increase in normal sperm count and a 3% increase in abnormal morphology in subfertile men after supplementation of folic acid in combination with zinc sulfate (Wong et al., 2002). Zinc, at doses of 30 mg/day, has also been shown to be beneficial in acne vulgaris, a condition many young males struggle with (Dreno et al., 2001). Bioavailability of zinc from highest to lowest is as follows: zinc bisglycinate, organic yeast salts, zinc gluconate, and then zinc oxide (Gandia et al., 2007; Siepmann et al., 2005). The upper tolerable intake level for zinc is 50 mg/day. When zinc is taken at doses of 30 mg/day or higher, 1.0 to 2.0 mg of copper should be taken simultaneously to prevent deficiency.

Omega-3 Fatty Acids

The leading cause of death in American men is cardiovascular disease. A large body of data has demonstrated the beneficial effects of fish and fish oil for maintaining cardiovascular health. Omega-3 fatty acids lower plasma triglycerides, resting heart rate, and blood pressure and may also improve myocardial filling and efficiency, lower inflammation, and improve vascular function. There is consistent evidence that omega-3 fatty acids reduce morbidity and mortality from coronary heart disease (Mozaffarian & Wu, 2011). Numerous cardiac societies recommend the addition of 1 g/day of fish oil, eicosapentae-noic acid (EPA) and docosahexaenoic acid (DHA), for cardiovascular preven-tion, after a myocardial infarction, and for prevention of sudden cardiac death. Fish oil is highly effective for reducing elevated triglycerides. The FDA has approved omega-3 acid ethyl esters for the treatment of hypertriglyceridemia (levels >500 mg/dl) in adults based on placebo-controlled trials showing that 4 g/day reduced median triglyceride levels by approximately 45%.

Epidemiologic data suggest fish consumption might prolong survival in men with prostate cancer by enhancing the response of prostate cancer to ablation therapy and retarding progression to androgen-independent growth (Chavarro et al., 2008; Fradet et al., 2009; McEntee et al., 2008). A phase II trial of men undergoing radical prostatectomy randomly assigned them to either a low-fat diet with 5 g of fish oil daily (dietary omega-6:omega-3 ratio of 2:1) or a control Western diet (omega-6:omega-3 ratio of 15:1) for 4 to 6 weeks prior to surgery. The low-fat diet and fish oil had no effect on serum insulin-like growth factor 1 (IGF-1) levels, though in secondary analyses, the intervention resulted in decreased prostate cancer proliferation and decreased prostate tis-sue omega-6:omega-3 ratios (Aronson et al., 2011). In contrast, DHA was pos-itively associated with high-grade disease in the Prostate Cancer Prevention Trial (Brasky, 2011). A systematic review evaluated the role of omega-3 fatty acids in advanced cancer (Ries et al., 2011). A total of 38 studies were included in the analysis. The authors noted that although smaller trials, often unrandom-ized and without a control group, reported a beneficial effect of omega-3 fatty acids in patients with advanced cancer and cachexia, the results of the larger randomized controlled trials failed to support the positive results. No signifi-cant adverse effects were noted in any of the studies.

Clinical trial evidence has not supported increased bleeding with omega-3 fatty acid intake, even when combined with other agents that might also increase bleeding such as aspirin and warfarin (Bays, 2007; Watson et al., 2009). Fish oil supplements available in the United States are relatively free of detectable levels of mercury, polychlorinated biphenyls, and organochlorine pesticides (Melanson et al., 2005).

Key Supplements for Benign Prostatic Hyperplasia

A review of DS for men's health would not be complete without an in-depth discussion of supplements for benign prostatic hypertrophy and prostate cancer prevention and treatment. In vitro, in vivo, and clinical studies exist to various degrees for *Serenoa repens* (saw palmetto), *Pygeum africanum*, selenium, *Camellia sinensis* (green tea), soy foods and supplements, lycopene, *Actaea racemosa* (black cohosh), and others. These topics are reviewed in the chapters on urology and oncology.

Key Supplements for Erectile Dysfunction

DSs are a common alternative or adjunctive approach to erectile dysfunction (ED), addressing such symptoms as decreased libido or erectile quality or duration. A thorough integrative health approach to ED would include a full history and physical, searching for and correcting any physiological, psychological, or iatrogenic causes or factors involved (Heidelbaugh, 2010). That said, there might be a role for DSs in this condition, although there are varying levels of evidence for their efficacy.

One such DS is made from the inner bark of yohimbe (*Pausinystalia yohimbe)*, a tree native to central Africa. It has been used as an aphrodisiac and treatment for impotence for centuries. Yohimbe bark contains the alkaloid yohimbine; purified yohimbine hydrochloride, an FDA-approved drug for ED, is the primary form of yohimbe that has been studied for ED (Aung et al., 2004). Yohimbine is thought to act as an α_2 receptor antagonist, which would explain its beneficial effects on penile blood flow (Aung et al., 2004). Clinical trial results on yohimbine are contradictory. For example, in 85 men 10 mg of yohimbine three times daily for 8 weeks improved numerous objective and subjective ED parameters compared to placebo, although there were more adverse effects (none serious) in the yohimbine group (Vogt et al., 1997). However, another study failed to find a benefit for 36 mg of yohimbine daily versus placebo for mixed-type ED (Kunelius et al., 1997). In systematic reviews (Ernst & Pittler, 1998; Ernst et al., 2011), the scales are tipped slightly in favor of yohimbine efficacy in ED compared to placebo; adverse effects were noted but thought to either be rare or mild and reversible. These include hypertension, anxiety, manic symptoms, and undesirable interactions with commonly used medications such as antidepressants, antihypertensives, and anticoagulants (Drewers et al., 2003).

There may be additive effects when yohimbine is combined with L-arginine, a nitric oxide precursor and, therefore, penile smooth muscle relaxant (Moyad et al., 2004). One clinical trial compared 6 g of L-arginine plus 6 mg of yohimbine 1 to 2 hours prior to sexual intercourse to 6 g of L-arginine or placebo and found statistically significant benefits for the combination treatment (Lebret et al., 2002). In addition, L-arginine by itself has been used for ED in the dosages of 1.5 to 5 g daily with benefits in some, but not all, clinical trials (Chen et al., 1999; Moyad et al., 2004).

Another plant used for ED is *Panax ginseng* (family Araliaceae), also known as Asian ginseng and Korean ginseng. Korean red ginseng is *Panax ginseng*; the red refers to the fact that the root is steamed as part of the preparation, and it is commonly used in ED (Jang et al., 2008). The proposed mechanisms for *Panax ginseng* include increased nitric oxide in the penile corporal sinusoids (Hong et al., 2002; Jang et al., 2008; Moyad et al., 2004) and central neurotransmitter effects (Moyad et al., 2004). A meta-analysis of seven randomized controlled trials found an overall benefit for ginseng in ED (risk ratio of 2.40, CI 1.65–3.51), though the methodology of some of the studies and total number of patients involved was less than ideal to draw definitive conclusions. In the meta-analysis, the highest quality clinical trial involved 900 mg of Korean red ginseng three times daily for 8 weeks versus placebo in 45 men with ED, finding that the ginseng group had statistically significant improvements in numerous symptom scores (Hong et al., 2002). Side effects mentioned in some clinical trials include headache, insomnia, and gastrointestinal upset (Jang et al., 2008; Moyad et al., 2004).

Dehydroepiandrosterone, or DHEA, has a structure and mechanism of action similar to testosterone, which includes nitric oxide penile vasodilation effects, and, possibly, central nervous system effects (Morales et al., 2009; Moyad et al., 2004; Reiter et al., 1999); it has also been studied for ED. In one clinical trial in men with low serum DHEA but normal serum testosterone, 50 mg of DHEA daily over 6 months improved standardized erectile function scores compared to a placebo group (Reiter et al., 1999). Another randomized controlled trial compared 4 months of 80 mg of oral testosterone twice daily, 50 mg of DHEA twice daily, or placebo in 106 men with sexual dysfunction and low serum testosterone and DHEA (Morales et al., 2009). No differences in global questionnaire scores and ED-related scoring systems were found for any of the three groups. Of note, significant increases in serum DHEA and slight increases in serum testosterone were noted in the DHEA treatment group.

Maca (*Lepidium meyenii, L. peruvianum*) is a root vegetable belonging to the Brassica family (looks like a giant radish) that is cultivated in the central Peruvian Andes and used for both food and medicine. Maca grows in the most inhospitable of climates and thus has been treasured as a nutrient-dense food for indigenous populations for at least two millennia. Traditionally, maca was highly valued for its purported aphrodisiac and/or fertility-enhancing properties (Rowland & Tai, 2003). A small number of clinical trials suggest that maca root, at doses of 1.5 to 3.0 g/day, leads to a small but statistically significant improvement in sexual well-being, as evidenced by the International Index of Erectile Function (IIEF-5) (Gonzales et al., 2002; Zenico et al., 2009). Maca does not appear to significantly affect serum concentrations of reproductive hormones including testosterone, estradiol, and 17-hydroxyprogesterone in healthy men (Gonzales et al.,, 2002). There are no known safety concerns with maca.

Finally, for ED there is also preliminary evidence for the use of other DSs such as damiana (*Turnera diffusa* and *Turnera aphrodisiaca*) via its progestin-binding mechanism (Aung et al., 2004); the antioxidant extract from French maritime pine bark (*Pinus pinaster*), pycnogenol (Stanislavov & Nikolova, 2003); and the well-known ginkgo leaf (*Ginkgo biloba*), used for dementia and vascular pathology of different types (Moyad et al., 2004). The clinical use of these DSs for ED needs to be refined with further research before definitive clinical recommendations can be provided.

Key Supplements for Energy/Physical Performance

Improving energy and physical performance are topics of interest to many men, and DSs may have a role. Assuming a thorough medical evaluation, establishing an accurate diagnosis, and correcting any relevant factors, DSs may address issues of poor energy or fatigue and suboptimal physical performance. There are many DSs used for these issues (see Table 3.1); this section will review the evidence behind an important category of DSs, adaptogens, for which there may be a role for these symptoms.

Tonics, also known as adaptogens, are one widely used class of botanical medicines, being a part of the pharmacopoeia of many cultures (Davydov & Krikorian, 2000). As per Table 3.1, men use adaptogens to address both fatigue and exercise performance. One definition of an adaptogen is that it is "an agent that increases resistance to physical, chemical, and biological stress and builds up general vitality, including the physical and mental capacity for work" (Tyler, 1994). It may be difficult to determine how to use a substance with such diverse effects in clinical practice, though in vitro and in vivo research provide some guidance. The first step for a clinician interested in this topic is to consider the research separately for each

Table 3.1: Commonly Used Supplements by Men for Poor Energy or Fatigue and Suboptimal Physical Performance

Poor Energy or Fatigue	Physical Performance
Adaptogens ("tonics")	Adaptogens ("tonics")
Vitamin D_3 or D_2	Creatine
Vitamin B_{12}	Taurine
"Energy" drinks	DHEA
	Antioxidants (vitamins, herbal medicines)
	Amino acids

adaptogenic plant. For example, for ED, as noted earlier, *Panax ginseng* has been studied for more generalized medical effects. Relevant to its tonic effects, there is a beneficial stress-protecting effect on the hypothalamus-pituitary-adrenal axis, as well as on immune system parameters (Kiefer & Pantuso, 2003). There are some clinical trials for *Panax ginseng*, often using the extract G115 standardized to 4% ginsenosides at a dose of 100 to 200 mg daily, showing improvements in immune system parameters and for mood or psychological effects but little, if any, effects on physical performance (Kiefer & Pantuso, 2003).

The research on physical performance is slightly more convincing for the adaptogen *Eleutherococcus senticosus*, or "Eleuthero," sometimes referred to also as Siberian ginseng (Huang et al., 2011). One clinical trial using 800 mg of Eleuthero root or rhizome daily for 8 weeks in nine athletes found an improvement in endurance capacity and cardiovascular function compared to a crossover placebo period (Kuo et al., 2010). The positive ergogenic effects in this trial fit with the conclusions from other experts (Davydov & Krikorian, 2000), though other researchers doubt significant effects on physical performance (Goulet & Dionne, 2005).

Another species of "ginseng," *Panax quinquefolius*, or North American ginseng, also has its own unique proven clinical effects. Research results have been mixed, from no change in postexercise immune system effects to some improvements in incidence or severity of upper respiratory infections (Biondo et al., 2008), neurocognitive function (Scholey et al., 2010) and postprandial glucose in diabetes (Vuksan et al., 2000). In contrast, the effects of another adaptogen, *Rhodiola rosea*, or Arctic roseroot, seem to be primarily on psychological function. Clinical trials on *Rhodiola rosea* seem to document an antifatigue effect that helps to increase mental performance, perhaps even having an antianxiety effect (Olsson et al., 2009; Panossian et al., 2010). Some clinical trials have been done on the standardized extract SHR-5, dosed four tablets daily (a total of 576 mg of the extract daily).

There are numerous other botanical adaptogens available in the herbal marketplace, and, as for the few described here, they each have their own nuance of physiological effect and clinical use. There may, indeed, be a role for adaptogens in the male patient with fatigue or concerns about physical performance; the use of these interesting plants will surely be guided by future clinical trials, blended with the traditional knowledge of herbal medicine experts from the cultures where the use of these plants originated.

Conclusions

Dietary supplements are routinely used by men as means of prevention and treatment for a variety of conditions. First and foremost, it is important to assess the safety and efficacy of dietary supplements being used, as quality is variable. Often, it is as important to guide the male patient on what products to avoid as it is to recommend what to take. Still, there is usefulness for vitamin and herbal preparations for the conditions important in men's health such as cardiovascular disease prevention, sexual health, prostate health, and optimization of physical activity.

Resources

NONSUBSCRIPTION SERVICES AVAILABLE AT NO CHARGE
Dietary Supplements Labels Database

The Dietary Supplements Labels Database offers information about label ingredients in more than 6,000 selected brands of dietary supplements. It enables users to compare label ingredients in different brands and information is provided on the manufacturers' "structure/function" claims. Ingredients of dietary supplements in this database are linked to other National Library of Medicine databases such as MedlinePlus and PubMed to allow users to understand the characteristics of ingredients and view the results of research pertaining to them. http://www.nlm.nih.gov/medlineplus/dietarysupplements.html

National Institutes of Health Office of Dietary Supplements

The Office of Dietary Supplements (ODS) fact sheets give a current overview of individual vitamins, minerals, and other dietary supplements. ODS has fact sheets in two versions—Health Professional and Quick Facts. Quick Facts is also available in Spanish. http://ods.od.nih.gov/

MedlinePlus—Dietary Supplements

This is the consumer health database from the National Library of Medicine where you can find extensive information on DSs regarding their effectiveness, usual dosage, and drug interactions. http://www.nlm.nih.gov/medlineplus/druginformation.html

SUBSCRIPTION SERVICES
Natural Medicines Comprehensive Database

From the publishers of the Pharmacist's Letter, this database contains extensive information about common DS uses, evidence of efficacy and safety, mechanisms, interactions, and dosage. This website also provides continuing medical education courses, information by medical condition, a listserv, and a section on supplement–drug interactions. http://www.naturaldatabase.com

Natural Standard

This is an independent collaboration of international clinicians and researchers who have created a database that can be searched by complementary and alternative medicine subject or by medical condition. The quality of evidence is ranked for each supplement. http://www.natural-standard.com

REFERENCES

Allen NE, Key TJ, Appleby PN, et al. Animal foods, protein, calcium and prostate cancer risk: the European Prospective Investigation into Cancer and Nutrition. Br J Cancer. 2008;98(9):1574–1581.

Aronson WJ, Kobayashi N, Barnard RJ, et al. Phase II prospective randomized trial of a low-fat diet with fish oil supplementation in men undergoing radical prostatectomy. Cancer Res Rev. 2011;4(12):2062–2071.

Atsmon J, Dolev E. Drug-induced hypomagnesaemia: scope and management. Drug Saf. 2005;28(9):763–788.

Aung HH, Dey L, Rand V, Yuan CS. Alternative therapies for male and female sexual dysfunction. Am J Chin Med. 2004;32(2):161–173.

Bacon CJ, Bolland MJ, Ames RW, et al. Prevalent dietary supplement use in older New Zealand men. N Z Med J. 2011;124(1337):55–62.

Baron JA, Beach M, Wallace K, Grau MV, Sandler RS, Mandel JS, Heber D, Greenberg ER. Risk of prostate cancer in a randomized clinical trial of calcium supplementation. Cancer Epidemiol Biomarkers Prev. 2005;14(3):586–589.

Bays HE. Safety considerations with omega-3 fatty acid therapy. Am J Cardiol. 2007;99(6A):35C–43C.

Biondo PD, Robbins SJ, Walsh JD, McCargar LJ, Harber VJ, Field CJ. A randomized controlled crossover trial of the effect of ginseng consumption on the immune response to moderate exercise in healthy sedentary men. Appl Physiol Nutr Metab. 2008;33(5):966–975.

Brasky TM, Till C, White E, et.al. Serum phospholipid fatty acids and prostate cancer risk: results from the prostate cancer prevention trial. Am J Epidemiol. 2011;173(12):1429–1439.

Chavarro JE, Stampfer MJ, Hall MN, Sesso HD, Ma J. A 22-y prospective study of fish intake in relation to prostate cancer incidence and mortality. Am J Clin Nutr. 2008;88(5):1297–1303.

Chen J, Wollman Y, Chernichovsky T, et al. Effect of oral administration of high-dose nitric oxide donor L-arginine in men with organic erectile dysfunction: results of a double-blind, randomized, placebo-controlled study. BJU Int. 1999;83:269–273.

Chen J, Yuan YC, Leontiadis GI, Howden CW. Recent safety concerns with proton pump inhibitors. J Clin Gastroenterol. 2012;46(2):93–114.

Chen Y, Zhao L, Lu F, Yu Y, Chai Y, Wu Y. Determination of synthetic drugs used to adulterate botanical dietary supplements using QTRAP LC-MS/MS. Food Addit Contam Part A Chem Anal Control Expo Risk Assess. 2009;26(5):595–603.

Clark LC, Combs GF Jr, Turnbull BW, et al. Effects of selenium supplementation for cancer prevention in patients with carcinoma of the skin. A randomized controlled trial. Nutritional Prevention of Cancer Study Group. JAMA. 1996;276(24):1957–1963.

Davydov M, Krikorian AD. Eleutherococcus senticosus (Rupr. & Maxim.) Maxim. (Arialaceae) as an adaptogen: a closer look. J Ethnopharmacol. 2000;72:345–393.

Dreno B, Moyse D, Alirezai M, et al. Multicenter randomized comparative double-blind controlled clinical trial of the safety and efficacy of zinc gluconate versus minocycline hydrochloride in the treatment of inflammatory acne vulgaris. Dermatology. 2001;203(2):135–140.

Drewers SE, George J, Khan F. Recent findings on natural products with erectile-dysfunction activity. Phytochemistry. 2003;62(7):1019–1025.

Durga J, van Boxtel MP, Schouten EG, Kok FJ, Jolles J, Katan MB, Verhoef P. Effect of 3-year folic acid supplementation on cognitive function in older adults in the FACIT trial: a randomised, double blind, controlled trial. Lancet 2007;369(9557):208–216.

Ebisch IM, Thomas CM, Peters WH, Braat DD, Steegers-Theunissen RP. The importance of folate, zinc and antioxidants in the pathogenesis and prevention of subfertility. Hum Reprod Update. 2007;13(2):163–174.

Ernst E, Pittler MH. Yohimbine for erectile dysfunction: a systematic review and meta-analysis of randomized clinical trials. J Urol. 1998;159:433–436.

Ernst E, Posadzki P, Lee MS. Complementary and alternative medicine (CAM) for sexual dysfunction and erectile dysfunction in older men and women: an overview of systematic reviews. Maturitas. 2011;70(1):37–41.

Fava M, Mischoulon D. Folate in depression: efficacy, safety, differences in formulations, and clinical issues. J Clin Psychiatry. 2009;70(Suppl 5):12–17.

Fradet V, Cheng I, Casey G, Witte JS. Dietary omega-3 fatty acids, cyclooxygenase-2 genetic variation, and aggressive prostate cancer risk. Clin Cancer Res. 2009;15(7):2559–2566.

Gaines JM, Marx KA, Caudill J, Parrish S, Landsman J, Narrett M, Parrish JM. Older men's knowledge of osteoporosis and the prevalence of risk factors. J Clin Densitom. 2010;13(2):204–209.

Gandia P, Bour D, Maurette JM, Donazzolo Y, Duchène P, Béjot M, Houin G. A bioavailability study comparing two oral formulations containing zinc

(Zn bis-glycinate vs. Zn gluconate) after a single administration to twelve healthy female volunteers. Int J Vitam Nutr Res. 2007;77(4):243–248.

Gardiner P, Graham R, Legedza AT, Ahn AC, Eisenberg DM, Phillips RS. Factors associated with herbal therapy use by adults in the United States. Altern Ther Health Med. 2007;13(2):22–29.

Gonzales GF, Córdova A, Vega K, Chung A, Villena A, Góñez C, Castillo S. Effect of Lepidium meyenii (MACA) on sexual desire and its absent relationship with serum testosterone levels in adult healthy men. Andrologia. 2002;34(6):367–372.

Goulet ED, Dionne IJ. Assessment of the effects of Eleutherococcus senticosus on endurance performance. Int J Sport Nutr Exerc Metab. 2005;15(1):75–83.

Hadjistavri LS, Sarafidis PA, Georgianos PI, et al. Beneficial effects of oral magnesium supplementation on insulin sensitivity and serum lipid profile. Med Sci Monit. 2010;16(6):CR307–312.

Heidelbaugh JJ. Management of erectile dysfunction. Am Fam Physician. 2010;81(3):305–312.

Heinonen OP, Albanes D, Virtamo J, et al. Prostate cancer and supplementation with alpha-tocopherol and beta-carotene: incidence and mortality in a controlled trial. J Natl Cancer Inst. 1998;90(6):440–446.

Hong B, Ji YH, Hong JH, et al. A double-blind crossover study evaluating the efficacy of Korean red ginseng in patients with erectile dysfunction: a preliminary report. J Urol. 2002;168:2070–2073.

Huang L, Zhao H, Huang B, Zheng C, Peng W, Qin L. Acanthopanax senticosus: review of botany, chemistry and pharmacology. Pharmazie. 2011;66(2):83–97.

Huncharek M, Muscat J, Kupelnick B. Dairy products, dietary calcium and vitamin D intake as risk factors for prostate cancer: a meta-analysis of 26,769 cases from 45 observational studies. Nutr Cancer. 2008;60(4):421–441.

Jang DJ, Lee MS, Shin BC, Lee YC, Ernst E. Red ginseng for treating erectile dysfunction: a systematic review. Br J Clin Pharmacol. 2008;66(4):444–450.

Kiefer D, Pantuso T. Herbal medicines: Panax ginseng. Am Fam Physician. 2003;68:1539–1542.

Kimlin MG. Geographic location and vitamin D synthesis. Mol Aspects Med. 2008;29(6):453–461.

Klein EA, Thompson IM Jr, Tangen CM, et al. Vitamin E and the risk of prostate cancer: the Selenium and Vitamin E Cancer Prevention Trial (SELECT). JAMA. 2011;306(14):1549–1556.

Kos E, Liszek MJ, Emanuele MA, Durazo-Arvizu R, Camacho P. The effect of metformin therapy on vitamin D and B12 levels in patients with diabetes mellitus type 2. Endocr Pract. 2011 Sep 22:1–16.

Kunelius P, Häkkinen J, Lukkarinen O. Is high-dose yohimbine hydrochloride effective in the treatment of mixed-type impotence? A prospective, randomized, controlled double-blind crossover study. Urology. 1997;49(3): 441–444.

Kuo GM, Hawley ST, Weiss LT, Balkrishnan R, Volk RJ. Factors associated with herbal use among urban multiethnic primary care patients: a cross-sectional survey. BMC Complement Altern Med. 2004;4:18.

Kuo J, Chen KW, Cheng IS, Tsai PH, Lu YJ, Lee NY. The effect of eight weeks of supplementation with Eleutherococcus senticosus on endurance capacity and metabolism in human. Chin J Physiol. 2010;53(2):105–111.

Lebret T, Hervé JM, Gorny P, Worcel M, Botto H. Efficacy and safety of a novel combination of L-arginine glutamate and yohimbine hydrochloride: a new oral therapy for erectile dysfunction. Eur Urol. 2002;41(6):608–613.

Ledesma MC, Jung-Hynes B, Schmit TL, Kumar R, Mukhtar H, Ahmad N. Selenium and vitamin E for prostate cancer: post-SELECT (Selenium and Vitamin E Cancer Prevention Trial) status. Mol Med. 2011;17(1–2): 134–143.

Lippman SM, et al. Effect of selenium and vitamin E on risk of prostate cancer and other cancers: the Selenium and Vitamin E Cancer Prevention Trial (SELECT). JAMA. 2009;301:39–51.

Lun V, Erdman KA, Fung TS, Reimer RA. Dietary supplementation practices in Canadian high-performance athletes. Int J Sport Nutr Exerc Metab. 2012;22(1):31–37.

Mahajan R, Gupta K. Revisiting metformin: annual vitamin B12 supplementation may become mandatory with long-term metformin use. J Young Pharm. 2010;2(4):428–429.

McEntee MF, Ziegler C, Reel D, Tomer K, Shoieb A, Ray M, Li X, Neilsen N, Lih FB, O'Rourke D, Whelan J. Dietary n-3 polyunsaturated fatty acids enhance hormone ablation therapy in androgen-dependent prostate cancer. Am J Pathol. 2008;173(1):229–241.

Melanson SF, Lewandrowski EL, Flood JG, Lewandrowski KB. Measurement of organochlorines in commercial over-the-counter fish oil preparations: implications for dietary and therapeutic recommendations for omega-3 fatty acids and a review of the literature. Arch Pathol Lab Med. 2005;129(1):74–77.

Miller GM, Stripp R. A study of western pharmaceuticals contained within samples of Chinese herbal/patent medicines collected from New York City's Chinatown. Legal Med (Tokyo, Japan). 2007;9(5):258–264.

Moore E, Mander A, Ames D, Carne R, Sanders K, Watters D. Cognitive impairment and vitamin B12: a review. Int Psychgeriatr. 2012;24(4):541–556.

Mooren FC, Krüger K, Völker K, Golf SW, Wadepuhl M, Kraus A. Oral magnesium supplementation reduces insulin resistance in non-diabetic subjects—a double-blind, placebo-controlled, randomized trial. Diabetes Obes Metab. 2011;13(3):281–284.

Morales A, Black A, Emerson L, Barkin J, Kuzmarov I, Day A. Androgens and sexual function: a placebo-controlled, randomized, double-blind study of testosterone vs. dehydroepiandrosterone in men with sexual dysfunction and androgen deficiency. Aging Male. 2009;12(4):104–112.

Moyad MA, Barada JH, Lue TF, Mulhall JP, Goldstein I, Fawzy A; Sexual Medicine Society Nutraceutical Committee. Prevention and treatment of erectile dysfunction using lifestyle changes and dietary supplements: what works and what is worthless, part II. Urol Clin North Am. 2004;31(2): 259–257.

Mozaffarian D, Wu JH. Omega-3 fatty acids and cardiovascular disease: effects on risk factors, molecular pathways, and clinical events. J Am Coll Cardiol. 2011;58(20):2047–2067.

Nielsen FH. Magnesium, inflammation, and obesity in chronic disease. Nutr Rev. 2010;68(6):333–340.

Nielsen FH, Johnson LK, Zeng H. Magnesium supplementation improves indicators of low magnesium status and inflammatory stress in adults older than 51 years with poor quality sleep. Magnes Res. 2010;23(4):158–168.

Olsson EM, von Schéele B, Panossian AG. A randomised, double-blind, placebo-controlled, parallel-group study of the standardised extract shr-5 of the roots of Rhodiola rosea in the treatment of subjects with stress-related fatigue. Planta Med. 2009;75(2):105–112.

Panossian A, Wikman G, Sarris J. Rosenroot (Rhodiola rosea): traditional use, chemical composition, pharmacology and clinical efficacy. Phytomedicine. 2010;17(7):481–493.

Post-White J, Ladas EJ, Kelly KM. Advances in the use of milk thistle (Silybum marianum). Integrative Cancer Ther. 2007;6(2):104–109.

Qato DM, Alexander GC, Conti RM, Johnson M, Schumm P, Lindau ST. Use of prescription and over-the-counter medications and dietary supplements among older adults in the United States. JAMA. 2008;300(24):2867–2878.

Reffelmann T, Ittermann T, Dörr M, Völzke H, Reinthaler M, Petersmann A, Felix SB. Low serum magnesium concentrations predict cardiovascular and all-cause mortality. Atherosclerosis. 2011;219(1):280–284.

Reinstatler L, Qi YP, Williamson RS, Garn JV, Oakley GP Jr. Association of biochemical B12 deficiency with metformin therapy and vitamin B12 supplements: the national health and nutrition examination survey, 1999–2006. Diabetes Care. 2012;35(2):327–333.

Reiter WJ, Pycha A, Schatzl G, et al. Dehydroepiandosterone in the treatment of erectile dysfunction: a prospective, double-blind, randomized, placebo-controlled study. Urology. 1999;53:590–595.

Ries A, Trottenberg P, Elsner F, Stiel S, Haugen D, Kaasa S, Radbruch L. A systematic review on the role of fish oil for the treatment of cachexia in advanced cancer: An EPCRC cachexia guidelines project. Palliat Med. 2012;26(4):294–304.

Rosanoff A. Magnesium supplements may enhance the effect of antihypertensive medications in stage 1 hypertensive subjects. Magnes Res. 2010;23(1):27–40.

Rowland DL, Tai W. A review of plant-derived and herbal approaches to the treatment of sexual dysfunctions. J Sex Marital Ther. 2003;29(3):185–205.

Saper RB, Phillips RS, Sehgal A, Khouri N, Davis RB, Paquin J, Thuppil V, Kales SN. Lead, mercury, and arsenic in US- and Indian-manufactured Ayurvedic medicines sold via the Internet. JAMA. 2008;300(8):915–923.

Scholey A, Ossoukhova A, Owen L, Ibarra A, Pipingas A, He K, Roller M, Stough C. Effects of American ginseng (Panax quinquefolius) on neurocognitive function: an acute, randomised, double-blind, placebo-controlled, crossover study. Psychopharmacology (Berl). 2010;212(3):345–356.

Siepmann M, Spank S, Kluge A, Schappach A, Kirch W. The pharmacokinetics of zinc from zinc gluconate: a comparison with zinc oxide in healthy men. Int J Clin Pharmacol Ther. 2005;43(12):562–565.

Stanislavov R, Nikolova V. Treatment of erectile dysfunction with pycnogenol and L-arginine. J Sex Marital Ther. 2003;29:207–213.

Timbo BB, Ross MP, McCarthy PV, Lin CT. Dietary supplements in a national survey: prevalence of use and reports of adverse events. J Am Diet Assoc. 2006;106(12):1966–1974

Tyler VE. *Herbs of Choice: The Therapeutic Use of Phytomedicinals*. New York, NY: Pharmaceutical Products Press, 1994

Vaysse J, Balayssac S, Gilard V, Desoubdzanne D, Malet-Martino M, Martino R. Analysis of adulterated herbal medicines and dietary supplements marketed for weight loss by DOSY 1H-NMR. Food Addit Contam Part A Chem Anal Control Expo Risk Assess. 2010;27(7):903–916.

Vogt HJ, Brandl P, Kockott G, Schmitz JR, Wiegand MH, Schadrack J, Gierend M. Double-blind, placebo-controlled safety and efficacy trial with yohimbine hydrochloride in the treatment of nonorganic erectile dysfunction. Int J Impot Res. 1997;9(3):155–161.

Vuksan V, Stavro MP, Sievenpiper JL, Beljan-Zdravkovic U, Leiter LA, Josse RG, Xu Z. Similar postprandial glycemic reductions with escalation of dose and administration time of American ginseng in type 2 diabetes. Diabetes Care. 2000;23(9):1221–1226.

Wald DS, Kasturiratne A, Simmonds M. Effect of folic acid, with or without other B vitamins, on cognitive decline: meta-analysis of randomized trials. Am J Med. 2010;123(6):522–527.e2.

Watson PD, Joy PS, Nkonde C, Hessen SE, Karalis DG. Comparison of bleeding complications with omega-3 fatty acids + aspirin + clopidogrel—versus—aspirin + clopidogrel in patients with cardiovascular disease. Am J Cardiol. 2009;104(8):1052–1054.

Wien TN, Pike E, Wisløff T, Staff A, Smeland S, Klemp M. Cancer risk with folic acid supplements: a systematic review and meta-analysis. BMJ Open. 2012;2(1):e000653.

Wiygul JB, Evans BR, Peterson BL, et al. Supplement use among men with prostate cancer. Urology. 2005;66:161–166.

Wong WY, Merkus HM, Thomas CM, Menkveld R, Zielhuis GA, Steegers-Theunissen RP. Effects of folic acid and zinc sulfate on male factor subfertility: a double-blind, randomized, placebo-controlled trial. Fertil Steril. 2002;77:491–498.

Zenico T, Cicero AF, Valmorri L, Mercuriali M, Bercovich E. Subjective effects of Lepidium meyenii (Maca) extract on well-being and sexual performances in patients with mild erectile dysfunction: a randomised, double-blind clinical trial. Andrologia. 2009;41(2):95–99.

4

Mind–Body Medicine and Men's Health

BRAD S. LICHTENSTEIN

Introduction

I took my first yoga class with my mother in the basement of our synagogue in Pittsburgh, Pennsylvania, at 7 years of age. From then on, I was hooked. Almost 40 years later, I can still recall the instructor's final meditation as we rested on our backs in Savasana (Corpse Pose) at the end of the hour-long class. My body having moved in interesting and unique ways, I was ready to settle into the floor and allow my mind to become still and quiet. "Imagine lying by a gently flowing river," the instructor said. "Whenever a thought arises, simply place it on a log and allow it to drift away down the river. If a new thought comes up, continue the process. It is not about having...." This image, whether she actually said it or not, has stayed with me.

While my experience may have been unique for a 7-year-old growing up in suburban Pennsylvania in the early 1970s, such mind–body disciplines as yoga and meditation are gaining credibility and recognition as important and powerful healing modalities across the country. In fact, according to the 2007 National Health Statistics Reports on Complementary and Alternative Medicine Use Among Adults and Children in United States, about 19.2% of adults use some form of mind–body practices, a number that may be underreported. When prayer is included as a healing modality, the percentage of Americans who practice a form of mind–body medicine increases to 45%.

This goal of this chapter is to provide a working definition of mind–body medicine, explain the theoretical mechanisms of action, discuss stress and its impact on the mind and body, and explore various mind–body practices as they impact various disease states.

Description of Mind–Body Medicine

The National Institutes of Health (NIH) define mind–body therapies as "interventions that use a variety of techniques designed to facilitate the mind's capacity to affect bodily function and symptoms." However, a broader and more inclusive definition from the National Center for Complementary and Alternative Medicine (NCCAM) defines mind–body medicine as any approach that enhances the "interactions among the brain, mind, body and behavior, and on the powerful ways in which emotional, mental, social, spiritual, and behavioral factors can directly affect health." The techniques and practices that fall into this category are any "intervention strategies believed to promote health; [such as] relaxation, hypnosis, visual imagery, meditation, yoga, biofeedback, tai chi, qi gong, cognitive-behavioral therapies, group support, autogenic training, and spirituality." Some authors have included a variety of other practices such as journaling, exercise, and dance under this heading. Regardless, whatever the practice, several key factors are important.

- Mind–body medicine focus on quality of life and creating self-awareness, self-knowledge, and personal growth.
- Mind–body medicine emphasizes one's innate capacity to grow and heal.
- Mind–body medicine views illness as a means of transformation versus something that needs to be cured and eradicated.
- Practitioners who teach mind–body medicine techniques consider themselves trainers and catalysts, and individuals learning the techniques are viewed as empowered, rather than patients who are sick or diseased.

Theoretical Mechanism of Action and Stress Response

Imagine this: It's Friday night, and you are about to head home for the weekend. You have managed to meet all your deadlines for the week, and the projects have been sent to all the appropriate people. With your annual review in a few weeks, you are feeling satisfied and content. Just as you are about to shut off your computer, you check your e-mail one final time. There in your inbox is a message from your boss marked high priority. As you click on the message it simply reads: "Can you meet me in my office Monday morning at 8 AM? Must talk." Your heart stops, then finds itself up in your throat. Your mind races— *what did I do wrong?* you think.

As Wahbeh et al. (2009) discussed in their recent systematic review of mind–body medicine and immune system outcomes, identifying the specific mechanisms of action and immune system changes in mind–body medicine is challenging, especially when one is confronted by the myriad techniques that make up the field. However, mind–body medicine emphasizes the reduction of stress. Pioneers in the field, such as Edmund Jacobson, developer of progressive muscle relaxation, and Johannes Heinrich Schultz, developer of autogenic training, were adamant about focusing on relaxation versus treating particular pathology, despite the fact that both techniques have been shown to lead to improvement for a multitude of illnesses and symptoms.

Ask most people whether they have stress, and invariably your question is met with a resounding, YES! Equally as frequent you probably hear someone, at some time during the day, admonishing someone, perhaps yourself, to RELAX! We use these words so frequently, but what do they actually mean? Because the main argument for the benefits of mind–body medicine is its effect on the stress response, let's explore the meaning of that term.

The word *stress* first appeared around the 14th century in Middle French from the word *destresse* ("distress"), which had its roots from the Latin word *strictus*, which meant "to compress." By the 1500s the word *stress* was used when describing a force exerted on a system (or person) to the point of strain, stress, or fatigue. Therefore, stress occurs whenever we feel a disruption in our normal balance and homeostasis. The agent of that change, that which causes a disruption in our balance, is commonly referred to as a stressor. Keep in mind that a stressor can impact us on all levels, such as environmental (e.g., excessive temperatures, pollution, natural disasters), social (e.g., crowding, traffic, war), physiological (e.g., disease, broken bones, allergens), and psychological (e.g., guilt, shame, humiliation, worry, rumination). So although you may think of bills, marital squabbles, and unhappy bosses as stressors, there is more to it than that. The mind–body's attempt to restore balance after exposure to a stressor is considered our stress response.

The first two forms of stressors are easier to identify and manage, provided you have the means. If it is excessively cold, you can put on another layer of clothing or seek shelter. If it is excessively hot and you live in the city without air conditioning, for those who are more compromised, the stress may be too much on the body. Psychological stressors tend to be more insidious and difficult to manage, because most of us don't have a framework for thinking about and handling our psychological stressors. One of the most common models of stress is called the *cognitive appraisal model* that suggests that it is not the actual event, or external stimulus, that is the issue, but rather our way of perceiving and interpreting it, and our subsequent response. For instance, my boss may request a meeting with me for tomorrow. This request and the meeting itself have no charge, are not stressful. My reactions, both cognitively and behaviorally, generate the stress response.

If my immediate response is to assume (cognitive) that my boss wants to fire me, and I wish to keep my job (followed by a stream of other catastrophic thoughts), I will experience stress. The ability to shift focus and learn new ways to respond and change thinking can minimize the stress reaction.

So what is happening when we experience stress? The nervous system is a complicated system and not as simplistic as I will outline here. That said, stress begins with a perception. When a threat to our safety is perceived, whether immediate and physical, such as an angry lion crossing our path ready to pounce, or more existential, such as a fight with your spouse, the limbic system, and particularly the amygdala, gets activated. One of the main jobs of the amygdala is to determine safety. When a situation is deemed unsafe, the amygdala calls the troops into action and the body goes into fight-or-flight mode. For simplicity's sake, two types of fight-or-flight responses exist— the short-term (sympathetic adrenomedullary axis) and the long-term (hypothalamic-pituitary-adrenocortical axis [HPAC]) response. Immediately following the perception of stress, the sympathetic nervous system becomes activated and the brain sends a signal to the adrenal medulla to release epinephrine (adrenaline) and norepinephrine, which allow us to run like mad away from the lion or give us the strength to fight. In acute situations, this response is functional and adequate. We flee or fight; in either way, after a brief duration the stressor is over and we can return to balance.

However, most of our stressors in the modern world are not of the short-duration type. In long-term situations, the HPAC kicks in several minutes later and is longer acting. The hypothalamus within 15 seconds sends corticotropin-releasing hormone (CRH) to the anterior pituitary, and from here a signal is sent to the adrenal cortex and cortisol is released. Cortisol can potentiate the action of adrenaline, allowing the body to shift its focus away from activities of rest, relaxation, and repair, such as digesting food, wound healing, or fighting infection. Instead, cortisol dampens our pain response and decreases the inflammatory response in order for us to focus on the task at hand—fighting or fleeing. If we are preparing for battle day in and day out, this suggests our sympathetic nervous system remains on high alert nonstop. See Figure 4.1 for an outline of what the stress response might look like.

Hans Seyle researched the long-term consequences of stress on the body and proposed his **general adaptation syndrome** with three general phases of stress, which provides a working construct for mind–body medicine.

- Phase 1—Alarm Reaction—*fight-or-flight response*
  - Initial exposure to stressor; balance is disrupted; release of epinephrine and norepinephrine (adrenomedullary response to threat/emergency)

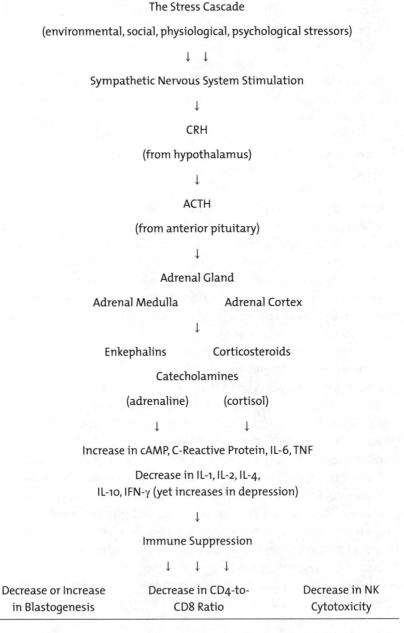

FIGURE 4.1. The stress cascade. CRH = corticotropin-releasing hormone; cAMP = cyclic adenosine monophosphate; IL = interleukin; TNF = tumor necrosis factor; IFN = interferon; NK = natural killer.

- Phase 2—Resistance
  - Adaptation from prolonged exposure to stressor; body returns to previous state of arousal; energy is available; constant glucocorticoid production (adrenocortical response)
- Phase 3—Exhaustion/Burnout
  - Adrenal glands become depleted and compromised from chronic activation; body unable to mount resistance; permanent damage → illness/death

This model is an oversimplification of the complexity of the stress response, yet it does provide a framework from which to work. Again, Seyle identified that when a stressor is first presented, the body secretes hormones, mainly epinephrine and norepinephrine, to prepare us to flee from or fight an attacker. Unfortunately, for most of us, this attacker can never be directly identified and we are left with a pervasive sense of unease and unrest, and our nervous system stays on alert. According to Dickerson and Kemeny (2004), the types of stressors that lead to the greatest hormonal response (cortisol and adrenocorticotropic hormone [ACTH]) were those that were *uncontrollable or performance tasks* where we were *evaluated by others*. Left unchecked, excessive stress hormone production damages the body and causes physical symptoms.

Some estimate that 75% to 90% of all illnesses have a stress component. By managing stress, disengaging from the constant barrage of sympathetic nervous system activity, and stimulating the parasympathetic response (rest and digest), we are better equipped to manage our symptoms, if not reduce or eliminate them entirely. Some consequences of a prolonged stress response include cardiovascular disease, recurrent colds and flus, poor wound healing and tissue destruction, weight gain, insomnia, fatigue and exhaustion (because the body constantly has to be on guard and mobilized), and disruption of memory. Learning to remain calm and relaxed and cultivating a state of equanimity and peace are hallmarks of all mind–body techniques. Although researchers and physicians are reluctant to make the broad, sweeping claim that stress is a major factor in the causation of disease, the mounting evidence clearly indicates that stress does nothing to improve illness or disease. Rather than search for the specific mind–body technique for a particular disease, focusing on the reduction of stress may be the more appropriate, all-around approach to care.

Take weight gain, for instance. Reports often implicate stress in the rise of obesity, but what might be the link? One aspect might just be sleep, or lack thereof. First of all, sleep disruption increases glucocorticoid production, which can negatively impact the immune system. However, lack of sleep also disrupts the production of ghrelin and leptin—two peripheral hormones that directly stimulate appetite regulation centers in the hypothalamus. Ghrelin, an orexigenic hormone, is produced in the stomach and stimulates appetite in response to hunger, mainly for energy-dense foods with high carbohydrate content (sweet, salty, and starchy foods). Leptin, on the other hand, is an anorexigenic hormone produced in adipocytes (fat cells) that suppresses appetite in response to satiety. Research consistently demonstrates an increase in both hunger and appetite for those who are sleep deprived, corresponding to a decrease in leptin and an increase in ghrelin. Rather than emphasize weight loss through caloric control, diets, and exercise, treating the cause, the disruption of sleep due to the stress response, may prove more efficacious.

Gender Experience of Stress

When it comes to stress, men and women tend to differ in how they responses to stress, both psychologically and biologically. Various coping strategies have been identified that emphasize these differences. Men, who tend to be more independent thinkers, whether due to genetics or socialization, generally demonstrate problem-focused coping skills, whereas women employ more emotion-focused strategies. Emotion processing may lead to excessive rumination without much action, and this has been proposed to be one potential reason women report depression and anxiety twice as often as men.

On the other hand, it has been posited that women "tend and befriend" when under stress, where they seek out connection and become more nurturing. This may be related to the hormone oxytocin secreted at times of stress. Men secrete oxytocin as well, but testosterone interferes with its action. This leaves men secreting more testosterone and cortisol, which, when elevated over time, are implicated in decreased immunity and increased cardiovascular disease.

However, statistics on prevalence of stress and mental illness and gender may be questionable. Some research suggests that doctors diagnose depression in women more often than men because men may not exhibit the most easily recognized symptoms of depression as much as women. For example, women may present more with depressed mood, whereas men may present more with anhedonia, fatigue, or changes in sleep or eating habits. When standardized depression measures taking into account all aspects of depression are used, the prevalence of depression is similar between men and women.

Case Study

Kevin, an affable, 54-year-old fellow, was a self-described typical American—hardworking and married with a teenage son, with little time for self-care, whether it be in the form of exercise, changing his eating habits, or adopting any other practices that would take time out of his already packed schedule. With a constant self-deprecating smile, he repeatedly interrupted his own story to interject, "I know, I know, I really should do something about that" when discussing his being overweight (230 lbs) and hypertensive (blood pressure: 140/85 mm Hg) and having symptoms of fatigue, headaches (two to three times per week), and insomnia (5 hours of sleep per night). Like a majority of men providers see in private practice, Kevin's wife scheduled this appointment, and he reluctantly agreed after his traditional doctor told Kevin that if he doesn't make some significant changes immediately, he was headed for diabetes, stroke, or heart attack. Despite the fact that Kevin had met with a naturopathic physician, nutritionist, and personal trainer a few times during the past 6 months, he had failed to implement any changes.

My first step was to identify Kevin's personal goals, motivations, and concerns. His wife and providers believed that if Kevin cared *enough* about his family or health or was scared enough about having a heart attack or stroke, he would change. But this fails to take into account that his current lifestyle/behaviors provide him with some benefit. His overeating sugary snacks, working 16-hour days without meals, isolating himself from his family in his study, and waking up at 2 AM and composing endless lists of tasks to complete all, in some way, decreased Kevin's anxiety, if only momentarily. As I told Kevin, unless he finds other ways to address his anxiety, he will continue these activities.

After this conversation, which took an entire session, Kevin returned the following week to learn slow diaphragmatic breathing at a rate of six breaths per minute, followed by a technique called autogenic training. After 40 minutes, Kevin's blood pressure dropped from 148/100 mm Hg at the onset of the appointment to 110/80 mm Hg. Within 1 month, his blood pressure was stable, he was able to discontinue his hypertension medication, and he began sleeping through the night, which significantly helped with his fatigue.

Stress and Cardiovascular Disease

One of the biggest challenges with research in the field of mind–body medicine centers around terminology, criteria, and measurement. Take the word *stress,* for example. With individual patients, it must be clarified where that person experiences the stressor—at home, at work, within his community, during leisure activities? Who is involved—family, friends, coworkers, bosses? What is the duration of the stressor—brief or protracted over time? How are the impacts on the body measured? If perception is the key element in deeming any situation a stressor, then by its very nature, the experience is highly individualized.

That said, several studies have indeed demonstrated a mind–body connection between "psychological" stress and health and disease. For example, depression and continual external locus of control are two significant risk factors for developing myocardial infarction. Those with a low locus of control tend to feel victimized by life circumstances, perceiving they have little influence over their lives and their reactions. They believe events happen *to* them and feel helpless and unable to shape their future. This is frequently seen in studies of work satisfaction, where individuals with less freedom to adjust their work environment, with fixed schedules, who work in confined spaces, and who have time and activities monitored experience greater stress and hence poorer health outcomes. The main ingredient here is the perception of choice and influence and a feeling of helplessness, regardless of setting or situation.

The association between low locus of control and increased risk for myocardial infarction seems to hold across cultures. The same seems to hold true for depression as well.

HYPERTENSION

As Astin et al. and Pelletier point out, in cases of essential hypertension, mind–body techniques not only are cost-effective but also have been proven in some cases to be curative. Breath retraining, breath meditation, respiration biofeedback, and at-home breath-pacing devices, such as the Resperate, all of which either result in or emphasize slow, diaphragmatic breathing, have been shown to reduce systolic blood pressure in cases of noncomplicated hypertension. Physiologically, the baroreceptors, located in the lungs and chest wall, have great influence over the breathing drive and sympathetic nervous system activity. When in a perpetual state of stress, and due to poor posture, functional breathing is often compromised; people tend to breathe faster and more shallowly. Without the mechanical stimulation of slow movement through breathing, the baroreceptors do not get significant stimulation, and hence become desensitized. Less baroreceptor activity leads to an increase in cardiac output and peripheral resistance and can result in sustained elevated blood pressure. Furthermore, the heart rate slows down during exhalation due to vagal efferent stimulation to the sinoatrial node, which is absent during inspiration. Hence, prolonged expiration at a ratio approximately double that of the length of inspiration can stimulate a relaxation response.

Paced, slow breathing (approximately six breaths per minute) therefore has a calming and relaxing effect because it directly results in a decrease in sympathetic nervous system stimulation. The goal, however, is to "generalize" this pattern of breathing into daily life. It is not enough to practice once or twice a week; one must train oneself to breathe in this manner consistently throughout the day.

MYOCARDIAL INFARCTION

Breathwork is also implicated in decreasing the risk and recurrence of myocardial infarction. The work of van Dixhoorn demonstrated that cardiac patients who learned to breathe by expanding the total circumference of the lower ribcage/diaphragm area were less likely to suffer from recurrent myocardial infarctions than controls. Additionally, they decreased their medication usage and visited their health care providers less frequently. What is fascinating is that the process of teaching breathwork is relatively simple, yet does require some dedicated practice. With the practitioner sitting behind the patient, the first step is to assess the back and spine, noting asymmetries, curvatures, and muscle bulking indicating any dysfunction. Structural integrity must first be assessed, because the inability to sit in an upright position without stress or strain is foundational. Barring any gross physical abnormalities, the practitioner rests his or her palms on the lower ribs, around the T_{11}–T_{12} area, and advises the patient to breathe into his or her hands. The sensation of touch and pressure better allow the patient to sense into this area of the body and learn through touch to expand the ribcage/torso sideways during inhalation. One to two sessions of instruction with a practitioner, along with consistent home practice, was enough to significantly reduce the risk of recurrent heart attack. Again, when the patient breathes slowly and diaphragmatically, the nervous system shifts to a more relaxed, parasympathetic state, and the heart rate becomes more variable and blood pressure is reduced.

EMOTIONS AND CARDIOVASCULAR DISEASE

Pelletier has noted that much has been studied on the connection between so-called negative emotions and the onset of cardiovascular events, namely, depression, anxiety, and hostility or anger. Researchers spend an inordinate amount of time and money arguing over the criteria of these emotional states/traits, but the evidence supports the notion that prolonged expression of these emotions is a risk factor for the development of atherosclerosis and other cardiovascular events. Chronic states of these emotions are linked to increased stimulation of the sympathetic nervous system and the hypothalamic-pituitary-adrenomedullary axis, which leads to a reduction in the production of growth and sex hormones. When plasma levels remain elevated in emotional states of depression, anxiety, and anger, several symptoms that lead to cardiovascular disease become present, such as increased truncal obesity, increased resting heart rate, reduced heart rate variability, diminished baroreceptor reflexes, increased platelet aggregation, and so forth.

Stress and the Prostate

If we agree that the neurological, hormonal, and immunological systems are all interrelated, it stands to reason that there is a significant impact of stress on all organ systems. Researchers are now offering basic physiological and biochemical explanations.

Several studies show a correlation between prostate health and stress as measured by increased activity of both the hypothalamic-pituitary-adrenal axis and the sympathetic nervous system. In healthy subjects, elevated levels of prostate-specific antigens were found in those with greater stress, and in men with benign prostatic hyperplasia (BPH), both prostate volume and postvoid residual bladder volume were associated with prolonged, lifelong stress. The sympathetic nervous system and its resultant hormones, epinephrine and norepinephrine, have been implicated in both the increase in the size of the prostate and worsening of symptoms. Both hormones bind to α receptors and appear to prevent apoptosis, thereby leading to an increase in the size of the prostate. Furthermore, both epinephrine and norepinephrine lead to increased contraction of the pelvic floor as well as the prostate itself, thus stimulating the need to urinate. Furthermore, those with BPH have more concomitant signs and symptoms of excessive sympathetic nervous system activation, such as obesity, hypertension and other cardiovascular diseases, and increased insulin and risk of type 2 diabetes.

Various Mind–Body Modalities

Table 4.1 highlights several mind–body modalities that can be used to help decrease the stress response(Astin et al., 2003; Pelletier, 2004). Practitioners must be trained in particular approaches to teach patients how to best incorporate these modalities into their lives. One approach that is especially well

Table 4.1: Various Mind-Body Techniques

Mind–Body Technique	Description
Relaxation and progressive muscle relaxation	Originally developed by Edmund Jacobson; goal to induce deep relaxation and hence reduce sympathetic arousal by relaxing all muscles; when muscle contraction can be reduced to zero, ruminating thinking can stop or be greatly reduced.
Hypnosis	Process of creating an enhanced state of consciousness (trance-like state) where one is attentive and focused, yet more open to suggestion. Being in a trance-like state involves heavy concentration and dissociation from current objective experience. It may involve suggestibility, meaning the state of being especially open to others' suggestions; however, this is not an essential aspect of a hypnotic state.
Autogenic training	Form of self-hypnosis developed by Johannes Heinrich Schultz; practice a series of phrases or "formulas" to induce a state of relaxation and nervous system balance (warmth, limb heaviness, cardiac regularity, slow and deep breathing, abdominal warmth, forehead cooling).
Biofeedback	Developed from multiple streams of thought during the 1960s and 1970s; utilizes instruments that will detect and amplify basic physiological signals (such as sweating, temperature, heart rate, breathing, muscle tension, and brain waves) coupled with relaxation techniques to train the individual to perceive the minute changes and control and modulate them, thereby reducing symptoms of stress. Example: thermal biofeedback where individual is trained to raise the temperature of fingers, useful in cardiovascular disease, in hypertension, after stroke and heart attack, and in headaches
Breathwork and heart rate variability	Based on Eastern and Western techniques of breathing; focus is to change the location, depth, and rate of breathing, thereby changing biochemistry, which impacts nervous system and reduces stress and symptomatology.
Cognitive-behavioral therapies	Based on the theory that affective experience is based on irrational and faulty cognition.
Meditation, mindfulness-based stress reduction	Meditation takes many forms, from spiritual practice to transcendental meditation (when one mantra is focused on) to mindfulness and Vipassana meditation. All include some attempt to quiet or to focus the brain on some inner or outer experience, such as the breath, or a sound, smell, or verbalization such as a mantra. The goal is to quiet or be less controlled by the constant brain chatter, or ordinary stream of internal dialogue without judgment. Mindfulness meditation focuses on the ability to observe thoughts without judgment, projection, or attachment.

studied, mindfulness-based stress reduction (MBSR), will be described in more detail.

Stress Reduction Programs

MINDFULNESS-BASED STRESS REDUCTION

In the area of stress reduction, one of the most researched approaches is MBSR, developed over 30 years ago by Jon Kabat-Zinn. Although research tends to examine specific populations or particular diseases that would benefit from MBSR training, such as prostate cancer, hypertension, and social anxiety, the primary goal of this program is mindfulness instruction. Mindfulness is the nonjudgmental awareness of the present moment, and is not so much a technique for health but more a way of being and an engagement with life. However, research has demonstrated several neurological, hormonal, and immunological changes that result from the program.

Designed to be led in groups, MBSR consists of eight 2.5-hour weekly sessions, as well as an additional 1-day intensive retreat. Participants are encouraged to engage in daily mindfulness exercises and keep track of their experiences. No matter what exercises are practiced during the session or at home, the focus is the same—the cultivation of mindfulness. When yoga postures, or asanas, are introduced during the group session, the emphasis is not to increase flexibility or strength, but to build awareness of the present moment. *How do you feel, in your body, when you move this way? What thoughts arise as you breathe, twist, turn, stand, or sit? What moods are present right now?* Quickly, people confront the realization that most of our lives are spent somewhere other than the present. Instead of feeling the sensations and remaining present to them, most often we judge, evaluate, compare, or try to change. Although these are necessary skills to help complete our tasks of daily life, they are time and place dependent. The premise of MBSR is that by learning to embrace the moment without running away from it, we can reduce stress and therefore the subsequent deleterious physiological, immunological, and psychological impacts. When we learn to cultivate mindfulness, we are, in essence, cultivating our self-regulation capacity. Attending to the moment allows us to become nonreactive self-observers who learn that we are able to choose our mental focus rather than be victim to our thoughts. Some claim that the stress reduction witnessed in MBSR trainees is a direct result of the reduction of intrusive worrisome and troubling thoughts, which leads to a reduction in emotional distress, thereby causing a decrease in autonomic arousal. Learning this mindfulness, then, can increase a sense of agency and self-mastery, where you recognize you do not have to follow every sensation or thought that arises, but merely can witness it like a gentle observer.

Imaging studies, such as functional magnetic resonance imaging, reveal that mindfulness can positively impact brain structures. The practice of mindfulness has been shown to increase activation of the left prefrontal cortex, which is associated with greater adaptive responses to negative or stressful life events and significant reductions in anxiety and negative affect. Interestingly, the prefrontal cortex seems to be involved in self-referential processing, or interoception, which is the awareness of momentary self-reference or attending to internal states, feeling states, and emotion appraisal. This area receives connections from all systems of the body and integrates these external and internal stimuli with judgments about their emotional relevance to self. Moreover, the prefrontal cortex seems to exert an inhibitory influence over the amygdala, quieting our generalized conditioned fear response.

What does all this mean? When we learn to be mindful, we learn, in essence, to pay attention to what is rather than allow our mind to run off in a stream of ruminating chatter, or what some call narrative focus. Experiential focus, or attending broadly to physical sensation, emotions, and thoughts without selecting any one as a particular object, inhibits cognitive rumination that perpetuates the stress response. For instance, when we have pain, rather than sit and be present to the sensations of pain, we often judge and fixate on the cessation of pain. This distances us from the actual experience and leads to a contraction, both mentally and physically, around the pain itself, which only heightens the sensation we are desperately trying to minimize or extinguish. Studies on pain in cancer show that when subjects learn to meditate on the actual pain itself, the severity and intensity decreased, although it did not go away altogether for several subjects.

Conclusion

Through hormonal systems designed for survival, the mind and emotions exert powerful influences over physical health. Cardiovascular health, immune function, sexual function, and even prostate health are all impacted when the perception of stress or feelings of anxiety become constant. There are many proven modalities to help elicit a more healthy and adaptive relaxation response, countering the negative impact of constant stress. Modalities such as progressive muscle relaxation, mindfulness-based stress reduction, and autogenic training can be powerful therapeutic techniques but must be taught thoroughly and practiced on a regular basis to have a positive and lasting impact on health.

REFERENCES

Astin JA, Shapiro SL, Eisenberg DM, Forys KL. Mind-body medicine: state of the science, implications for practice. *J Am Board Fam Pract.* 2003;16: 131–147.

Dickerson SS, Kemeny ME. Acute stressors and cortisol responses: a theoretical integration and synthesis of laboratory research *Psychol Bull.* 2004 May;130(3):355–391.

Kessler RC, Berglund PA, Demler O, Jin R, Walters EE. Lifetime prevalence and age-of-onset distributions of DSM-IV disorders in the National Comorbidity Survey Replication (NCS-R). *Arch Gen Psychiatry.* 2005;62(6):593–602.

Pelletier KR. Mind-body medicine in ambulatory care: an evidence-based approach. *J Ambul Care Manage.* 2004;27(1):25–42.

Wahbeh H, Haywood A, Kaufman K, Harling N, Zwickey H. Mind-body medicine and immune system outcomes: a systematic review. *Open Complement Med J.* 2009;1:25–34.

5

Spirituality

FREDERIC C. CRAIGIE, JR.

A 22-year-old young man sits with his 35-week-pregnant partner, wondering what it will be like to be a father. A 42-year-old bank manager has gone without cigarettes for 7 days and struggles with urges to smoke. A 37-year-old disabled man deals with intermittent depression. A 52-year-old construction worker has a massive myocardial infarction and subsequent coronary artery bypass graft surgery and faces significant curtailment of his normal life. A 64-year-old state worker retires after 30 years and thinks about what should occupy the rest of his life.

Their journeys are different, but the challenges these men face touch on common themes. Their journeys and challenges bring into question what "health" means to them. They bring into question what it means to live life well. And not too far into conversations with these men, it would not be surprising to find them wrestling with the question of what it means to be a man.

These are spiritual questions. Neither the questions nor the answers may have specifically spiritual language, but they are "spiritual" in the sense that they bring these men to the big questions of wholeness and living well that spirituality subsumes.

The young man says that he hopes to be a good father by sharing in the care of his child, loving his wife, and "being there for her." The bank manager makes his way through urges to smoke by "turning it over to God." The disabled man comments that he has realized if there is something causing him to be depressed, he fixes it, and if not, he will "just try to put up with being depressed and do what I need to do." The construction worker says that he is learning to "accept help, talk about what I'm feeling, and spend more time with my family" than he has done before. The retiree says it has always been important to give of himself and "help somebody," although he doesn't know how he might do this.

In this chapter, we will explore three aspects of the subject of spirituality in integrative men's health. First, we will address background questions, including: What is "spirituality?" Why is it important? What is "spiritual care" and who provides this? Second, we will look at some practical and concrete approaches to making spiritually part of the process of health care, healing, and wellness. Finally, we will look at some of the literature about specifically *men's* spirituality, with some reflections about how these ideas may be incorporated into health care and well-being.

Background: What Is "Spirituality"?

Although the conversation about spirituality in health and health care has grown exponentially over the years, there is really no consensus definition of what "spirituality" means. Your definition is likely to be as rich and meaningful as mine.

VITAL AND SACRED

A fine, succinct definition of spirituality comes from former Surgeon General Dr. C. Everett Koop (Koop, 1994): "The vital center of a person; that which is held sacred." The ideas of "vitality" and "sacredness" can be profoundly helpful in the work of caring for patients and promoting men's health. What is "the vital center" for a middle-aged man who has had a serious heart attack? What sustains a grade school teacher who feels overwhelmed and depressed? What is sacred enough for an overweight man to engage in efforts to manage his diabetes better? When are the times when a retired person feels real enthusiasm about life? What keeps a high school student who has had suicidal ideas from carrying them out? For any of us, when do we feel most "vital" and alive, and what sustains us during challenging times?

As we begin to wrestle with these questions, we can begin to see the personal meaning of health and wholeness. We understand better the personal nature of suffering and the personal motivation for change. And we are often in a position of being better able to support the personally understood life force that sustains all of us as people on our life journeys.

OUTER AND INNER

Spirituality is an outer experience and an inner experience. The outer, observable, behavioral aspects of spirituality include spiritual practices such as meditation or reading sacred texts and spiritual connections such as participation in a spiritual or religious community. The inner aspects of spirituality include personal values, passions, and commitments that inform and energize the ways that people live.

A man in a 12-step program to support alcohol abstinence reads the Bible, supports and receives support from his daily meeting, and walks in the woods behind his rural Maine home. These are "outer," behavioral experiences that touch on what is "vital and sacred" for him.

At the same time, he deals with urges to drink by reminding himself that "the body is the temple of the Lord" and by picturing how much he desperately wants to show his young son what it means "to be a man and to face what you need to face." These are "inner" experiences that touch on what is "vital and sacred" for him.

The distinction between outer and inner matters because spirituality in health is often understood and described in terms of practices. To make spirituality a part of your health, you can learn meditation, or go on a pilgrimage, or sign up for a spiritual book group. Although they can often be extraordinarily meaningful, it is limiting to spirituality to think of it only, or primarily, in terms of practices.

Spirituality in health is as much an inner experience as an outer experience. Questions such as those in the following list can help to chart an exploration of what is "vital and sacred":

- What is sacred for you?
- What do you take pride in?
- What matters to you; what do you care about?
- What does it look like for you to live with dignity?
- When do you feel really alive?
- What kind of person do you aspire to be?
- What legacy would you hope to leave for your children?
- What does it mean to you to be a man?

I have suggested elsewhere a framework for elaborating five dimensions of spiritual experience (Craigie, 2010). They are connections with community, spiritual practices and devotions, meaning and purpose, passions, and relationships with transcendent Presence or Spirit.

Why Is Spirituality Important?

Spirituality is important in an integrative approach to health (Craigie, 2010).

ASSOCIATIONS WITH HEALTH

First, spirituality is intimately related to health, wholeness, and well-being. The etymology is revealing. Our modern words *health, whole,* and *holy* all derive from the same Old English word root, "hāl."

Beyond the linguistic connections, there are hundreds of studies that find an overwhelmingly positive association of various spiritual and religious beliefs and practices and measures of coping, quality of life, and health. There are *cross-sectional studies* that show associations of measures like "strength and comfort from religion," "daily spiritual experiences," and "spiritual well-being" with outcomes of quality of life, physical health, and mortality (Maselko & Kubzansky, 2002; Underwood & Terisi, 2002). There are *longitudinal studies* that find associations of spiritual well-being with health and coping measures over a period of time (Morris, 2001). There are *meta-analytic studies* that pool results of individual research projects to reveal trends in the association of spiritual beliefs and practices with physiological processes, such as cardio-vascular, neuroendocrine, and immune function, and with other measures of coping, emotional well-being, and mortality (Powell et al., 2003). There are *intervention studies* that explore the benefits of various spirituality-inclusive interventions on mood, dignity, well-being, quality of life, and connections with others (Moritz et al., 2006).

Increasingly, researchers have been exploring dimensions, or components, of spirituality. A particularly intriguing distinction has been the partitioning of "spiritual well-being" into the methodologically and empirically distinct components of "religious well-being" and "existential well-being." Religious well-being encompasses a variety of religious practices and often pertains to people's perceived relationships with God. Existential well-being pertains to a sense of satisfaction and life purpose. Although both of these components are typically associated with health, existential well-being tends to be more robust (Tsuang et al., 2007).

SPIRITUALITY MEDIATES CHOICES IN HEALTH BEHAVIORS

Why *should* someone stop smoking, anyway? If you are diabetic, why *should* you care what your A1c is? I believe that health really does not have inherent value for people; it is meaningful only insofar as our health allows us to live meaningfully, in concert with what is "vital and sacred."

Psychologist David Waters from the University of Virginia has developed a framework in which he emphasizes the relationship of "health goals" and "life goals." "Health goals" are the choices and lifestyle behaviors that people can pursue to address their most important health issues, such as exercising, stopping smoking, and developing a good nutritional plan. "Life goals" touch on the things that are most important to people in their lives, along the lines of what we are calling "vital and sacred."

Waters proposes that focusing on patients' health goals without understanding their life goals will result in mutual frustration and thwart progress toward patients' health and wellness. He argues that it is essential to first understand patients' life values, then to present a menu of choices in health goals that would potentially serve the life goals that patients are identifying. The formula is: "What is really important in my life is _____; therefore, my health goals are _____."

Spiritual Care

Specialty spiritual care is provided by spiritual care professionals. Chaplains, clergy, and spiritual directors have special training and expertise in ministering to human suffering and can be extraordinarily valuable colleagues in supporting people's health and healing. Spiritual care, however, is not limited to spiritual care professionals, in the same way that the promotion of heart health is not limited to cardiologists, and the promotion of behavioral health is not limited to psychologists and psychiatrists. Working in a palliative care setting, for instance, Daaleman and colleagues (2008) found that patients and family members identified a broad collection of people providing spiritual care, the largest group being family and friends, followed by clinicians and other health care workers, followed by clergy. Nor is spiritual care limited to professional practices or settings at all. Men's groups, fraternal organizations, 12-step programs, and meaningful friendships offer opportunities for men to relate to one another with caring and purpose and to support one another on their journeys.

What, then, is "spiritual care"? A perspective that particularly resonates with me comes from palliative care and hospice consultant J. S. Lunn (2003, p. 154): "Meeting people where they are and assisting them in connecting or reconnecting to things, practices, ideas, and principles that are at their core of their being...the breath of their life, making a connection between yourself and that person."

You will note the relationship of this perspective with Koop's view of spirituality, in terms of "the vital center" and sacredness. I suspect Lunn might just as well have said "assisting people to connect with what is 'vital and sacred' in their lives." My own, more elemental way of framing these ideas is that spiritual care has to do with *helping people to connect with the things that really matter to them.*

This perspective emphasizes the role that anyone may have in helping people to define and give expression to the values and passions that are deeply meaningful for them. Framed this way, spiritual care is less oriented to helping people make their way through anguished spiritual issues that our spiritual specialist colleagues would work with ("Why do little children get cancer?"), and more oriented to helping people to live with meaning and dignity in whatever situations they may find themselves.

The former owner of a concrete business suffers an incapacitating injury in a fall. He loses his business, subsists on a modest disability income, and sits at home feeling bored and depressed. He laments that he feels "useless" and lacks any sense of "pride." A spiritual care conversation might explore what he still cares about. What matters to him? What have been qualities of his life in which he has taken pride in the past? What would he do if he had more energy, or optimism? How would he hope to make his way through the darkness that might show his children something about resilience and, perhaps, about being a man?

As we think about spiritual care, I also want to emphasize Lunn's ideas of "meeting people where they are" and "making a connection between yourself and that person." The foundation of spiritual care rests with our ability to be present to people, to genuinely care about them, to be able to hear their stories, and to partner with them as they face the challenges of life (Puchalski & McSkimming, 2006). In fact, our compassionate presence with people may often be powerful and sufficient spiritual care in and of itself.

A colleague of mine who had been dealing with a variety of health problems recently visited a physician in our community who is a practitioner of traditional Chinese medicine and acupuncture (Craigie, 2012). She tells the story:

> You go in the door and a golden retriever greets you. It's this really soft and peaceful environment. The doctor welcomed me, holding both of my hands in his, looking into my eyes with gentleness and caring. As we did the acupuncture treatment, we had this quiet conversation where he was so clearly interested in who I am and what my life is like. As I left, I thought that the acupuncture had been helpful, but mainly, I just felt so loved. (p. 68)

As a faculty member at a teaching program in integrative medicine, I have no doubt that the acupuncture had active therapeutic benefits. But, clearly, the spirit and energy of love in the presence of this practitioner was profoundly important. Sometimes, moreover, this is enough.

Arenas of Spirituality in Integrative Men's Health

Whether you are a spiritual care professional, a health care clinician, or a human being in friendship relationships with men, working with or "bringing forth" spirituality takes place in three arenas (Craigie, 2010). The preponderance of literature about spirituality in health care addresses clinical issues and approaches. The "clinical arena" of spirituality pertains to the ways in which clinicians support patients in giving expression to the things they care about and living with meaning and dignity. In friendship relationships, we might call this the arena that focuses on approaches to helping or caring.

There are, however, two other arenas that are vitally important in the larger picture of spirituality in integrative men's health. First, if the foundation of spiritual care lies in the compassionate presence that clinicians or friends extend to men, then the groundedness and centeredness of clinicians/friends—their spiritual well-being—is vitally important in undergirding the ability to be compassionately present. It is hard to be genuinely present to people if your attention, focus, and heart are somewhere else. This is the "personal arena" of spiritual care.

Second, there is (perhaps surprisingly) a significant amount of literature about the "spirit," "soul," or "culture" of health care organizations and the ways in which qualities of organizational life impact the provision of quality care. While it is beyond the scope of this chapter to explore this arena in detail, I can point out that this literature suggests that qualities like a shared understanding of mission, a sense of community and partnership among caregivers, and aspects of visionary and empowering leadership can make a significant difference with outcomes like staff satisfaction and retention, patient satisfaction, and various process and outcome measures of quality care (Craigie, 2010). Organizations that "have it" with these qualities stand in stark contrast to health care organizations (as most clinicians have experienced at some point) that reflect detached and impersonal leadership, lack of support and teamwork, and loss of sight of any meaningful sense of collective mission.

The three arenas of spirituality in integrative men's health complement each other. Clinicians, for instance, can have wonderful clinical skills and approaches, but if they are personally distracted or dispirited, or if they work in organizations that are demoralizing or disempowering, then the goal of providing good spiritual care will be extraordinarily difficult to sustain. Stated positively, clinicians who are grounded and centered, working in settings that have an energetic spirit of collaboration toward a shared purpose, cultivating good spiritual care skills, can have a remarkable influence in supporting the health and well-being of the patients they serve.

Working With Spirituality in Integrative Men's Health

THE PERSONAL ARENA

How does one cultivate the inner qualities of centeredness, groundedness, and spiritual well-being that undergird our compassionate and healing presence with people? Recent literature on physician wellness provides helpful empirical insights about this question. Drawing on several studies of physician wellness practices, Shanafelt et al. (2003) suggested a number of approaches, including:

- Nurturing personal connections with family and colleagues,
- Creating meaningful and viable work roles,
- Pursuing personal interests and self-awareness and protecting time to follow good health practices, and
- Cultivating spiritual and philosophic approaches to life that emphasize a positive outlook, identifying and acting on values, and stressing balance between personal and professional life.

My own conversations with clinicians and groups about spiritual well-being touch on several areas.

Personal calling and mission. Most clinicians go into health care for honorable and generous reasons. Typically, these reasons have to do with service, helping people, participating in healing, and generally making the world a better place. For physicians, these reasons are often well articulated in admission essays for medical school and residency training (as I'm sure they are for other disciplines as well). My experience is that it is easy, in the midst of the daily bustle, to lose sight of one's personal understanding of calling. However, I also find that there is an almost reverential quality in people remembering what that calling has been. "Why did you become a doctor (or nurse, or counselor)? What was the *story* of your deciding to go into your field?" For many people, reconnecting with the original motivation for doing their work can have a calming and centering effect.

Similarly, developing an understanding of personal mission can have a centering effect, for two reasons. First, personal mission helps to focus one's attention and heart on what is important, and therefore to let go as much as possible of what is not important. Second, the core values that form one's personal mission typically bear energy that more pedantic and conceptual statements lack. The idea of being a good social worker who meets 11 specific performance criteria may be a reasonable vocational goal, but a statement of mission of "I will invite my patients into a better life by speaking the truth as I see it, with dignity and respect" has very different energy.

As a practical matter, I suggest "three Cs" as a guideline for developing a personal mission. Good statements of personal mission are "core," "concise," and under one's personal "control."

Core values and passions. "Calling" focuses attention on the sacred origins of one's vocation. "Mission" focuses attention on the overarching purpose of one's life. Beyond these specific focal points, men can nurture the experiences of centeredness, groundedness, and spiritual-well being by the day-to-day awareness and cultivation of specific core values and passions.

What kind of person do you want to be? What are the personal qualities that are important in your life? How do you wish to be treating other people? What are the particular priorities for you, and how do you wish to be spending your time? Sitting with such questions can help men to be more intentional in how they move through their daily lives.

Two areas of health literature can be helpful in developing these ideas. Literature on *flourishing,* first, highlights aspects of life that are associated with high levels of wellness (Keyes, 2007). Examples are self-acceptance, personal growth, purpose in life, and positive relations with others. A recent popular-press book distills some of the empirical data about flourishing in practical form (Seligman, 2011).

Literature on *positive psychology,* second, particularly emphasizes the understanding and expression of positive qualities of character. Research in this field over many years has identified six virtues that are universally esteemed across time and culture (wisdom and knowledge, courage, humanity, justice, temperance, and transcendence) and 24 strengths of character (qualities such as curiosity, authenticity, kindness, forgiveness, and gratitude) that are instrumental in giving expression to these virtues (Peterson & Seligman, 2004). This literature has also given rise to extensive and readily available resource material (e.g., http://www.authentichappiness.org) that enables people to identify and explore strengths of character that are particularly pertinent to them.

Restoring the soul. There is also substantial literature on approaches to resilience. For purposes of a chapter on spirituality, we'll call this "restoring the soul." Approaches to this take the form of behaviors and attitudes. *Behaviors* include:

- Devotional practices: Reading of sacred texts or other uplifting writing, prayer or meditation, listening to spiritually centering music.
- Energy practices: Tai Chi, yoga.
- Breathing practices: There are good Internet descriptions of "yoga breathing" or "4-7-8 breathing."
- Mini-meditation: Islam has the tradition of *Salah,* the five-times-daily ritual of prayer. Similarly, many religious traditions have the custom

of grace (etymology: *gratia*, "gratitude") as a blessing before meals. A family physician friend comments that she pauses before entering a room, "feet flat on the floor, to remember how I want to be there for this person."

- Reflective practices: Many people find that journaling helps to get emotions and points of uncertainty "out there" and helps them to find a greater sense of coherence and direction.
- Physical exercise: Walking, jogging, swimming, elliptical training, basketball, and so forth.
- Joy: Partaking of places and activities that bring a smile to your face and cause you to lose track of time.

Practices like these, set amid the daily rhythms of life, provide regular opportunities to become refocused and spiritually centered.

In my professional life, I find that I can't always count on having more than a minute or two of "down time," so I gravitate to the shorter practices. As an example, a variety of mini-meditation that I follow is the "stairway ritual." When I walk up a flight of stairs from my office to meet patients in our waiting room, I deliberately take the last six or seven steps a little more slowly, one at a time, and use this opportunity to let go of distractions and toxic energy and to open my heart to be present to the person I am about to see. This makes a difference for me. It is a way of grounding myself in intention and healing presence that brings a little of the Sacred into my daily routine and takes virtually no additional time.

Attitudes are equally important in fostering resilience, centeredness, and spiritual well-being. The premise, as cognitive therapists have pointed out for years, is that emotional travail or emotional well-being result not from the events of life, but from our assumptions, beliefs, and appraisals of those events.

If a Maine paper mill closes and a man is laid off, his reaction and state of well-being will depend significantly on his beliefs about what being laid off means to him. An appraisal of "This is terribly unfair and it's the only thing I can do and the future is hopeless" will undermine a successful adaptation to being laid off. An appraisal of "Whether or not this is fair doesn't really matter; I have to make the best of this and maybe there are some other possibilities out there" will more likely promote a successful adaptation.

Of course, in the real world, functioning in the midst of genuine suffering demands more than an exercise of wordsmithing rational and optimistic interpretations of events. But it is a start, and often the *recognition* that beliefs mediate emotions and levels of wellness can help people to begin to move in adaptive directions.

If spirituality has to do with the "vital" and "sacred," then attitudes that refocus attention on overarching values for living will be particularly meaningful. In the previous paragraphs, I used the phrase "core values and passions." The 12-step community articulates a wonderful series of "aphorisms," such as "One day at a time" and "Let go and let God."

A colleague of mine, Dr. Howard Silverman, speaks of "affirmations" that articulate meaningful values or principles about people's professional work and personal lives. Examples are:

- I will treat my patients who struggle with alcohol use with dignity, caring, and respect, but I will not take responsibility for their choices.
- Judging myself on whether I have more or less stuff than my neighbors is folly. My worth has to do with what is inside me and how I treat people.
- It is OK for men to cry. It is not a sign of weakness or inadequacy.

For many men with experience in sports, the language and rubric of "ground rules" captures well the idea of personal values and principles.

Finally, as we consider behaviors and attitudes that support inner qualities of centeredness, groundedness, and spiritual well-being, I would make a special case for the practice of mindfulness. Popularized and pioneered in America by Dr. Jon Kabat-Zinn, mindfulness consists of being aware (or mindful) of present moments, without categorizing, processing, or judging (Kabat-Zinn, 2005). Mindfulness draws energy and attention away from the past and the future, cultivating a rich and nonevaluative experience of present events *externally* (such as the physical environment and interactions with other people) and *internally* (such as somatic sensations, emotions, thoughts, and beliefs).

Mindfulness belongs in the conversation about spirituality for three reasons. First, mindfulness has its origins in Eastern (particularly, Buddhist) spiritual traditions and overlaps substantially with contemplative practices in a variety of spiritual traditions worldwide. Second, the notion of nonjudgmental perception of present moments overlaps with spiritual ideas and practices of nonattachment, transcendence, and gratefulness. And third, mindful awareness in practice is often paired with emphasis on intentional living in faithfulness to personally meaningful values.

THE CLINICAL ARENA

What I have called the "clinical arena" of spirituality has to do with the ways in which any of us can support men in giving expression to the things they care about and living with meaning and dignity. What is "vital and sacred" for *this* man (your patient, your friend, your colleague) at *this* point in his life, and how can he be supported in pursuing and expressing that?

Organizational consultant Margaret Wheatley (2002) comments that "real change begins with the simple act of people talking about what they care about" (p. 22) The first perspective in spiritual care conversations, then, is not giving advice; not fixing people's problems; not offering erudite theological commentary; not, for that matter, endlessly reflecting what people say in a "nondirective" way. It is, rather, being able to hear people's stories and honor their suffering, and then to invite them to move beyond their suffering by giving a voice to what matters to them. Having people talk about what they care about brings into the room a very different energy.

There are countless ways of introducing this conversation:

- What do you care about? What matters to you?
- What do you hope for?
- What does it mean to you to "live life well?"
- How would you put into words the kind of person you wish to be?
- How do you want to be handling the things that you're facing right now? If you felt like you were doing pretty well handling the things that you're facing, what would that look like?
- What are you like when you are at your best?
- When have you felt really "alive?"
- What does "success" mean to you?
- What do you take pride in?
- What keeps you going?
- What would you hope your friends would say that they admire in you? What do you think they do admire in you?
- When has there been a time when you have been handling some challenges in your life pretty well?

This is a conversation about what matters to people—to men—in general in life. And it is about what matters to men in the circumstances in which they find themselves. As my Maine colleague Ken Hamilton, MD (2008), asks, "This is what life is giving you. Now, what are you going to do with your life?"

There are a number of frameworks, with acronyms, for spiritual care conversations. The most prominent of these is FICA, from Christina Puchalski (1999).

Structuring spiritual care conversations. Let's look in more detail at some practical approaches to structuring these conversations.

Possibilities and exceptions. Conversations that emphasize possibilities and forward directions that arise out of an understanding of what people care about can be powerful ways to motivate positive change. The conversation is less about how depressed a man is and more about how he would wish to be instead of being depressed, what that would look like, and how he might begin to go there. The conversation is less about how poorly a couple communicates and more about what draws them together, what they value in each other, and how they can begin to renew some positive interactions.

The idea of exceptions to problem states can often be helpful. A man complains that he has a "short fuse and flips out." When has there been a time when he had a longer fuse, and what was happening then? When has he faced some emotional challenge and handled it with a little more patience, and how did he do that?

FICA Spiritual History Tool

F—Faith and Belief

"Do you consider yourself spiritual or religious?" or "Do you have spiritual beliefs that help you cope with stress?" If the patient responds "No," the health care provider might ask, "What gives your life meaning?" Sometimes patients respond with answers such as family, career, or nature.

I—Importance

"What importance does your faith or belief have in our life? Have your beliefs influenced how you take care of yourself in this illness? What role do your beliefs play in regaining your health?"

C—Community

"Are you part of a spiritual or religious community? Is this of support to you and how? Is there a group of people you really love or who are important to you?" Communities such as churches, temples, and mosques, or a group of like-minded friends can serve as strong support systems for some patients.

A—Address in Care

"How would you like me, your healthcare provider, to address these issues in your healthcare?"

These conversations involve being alert to what people are saying about what matters to them and pursuing that. In the wake of an illness and hospitalization, a man says that he feels "useless." When has he felt useful, and what went into that? What elements of usefulness remain for him, even if the ability to carry a bundle of shingles up a step ladder is presently out of the question? Struggling with a bitter separation, a man says he feels "lost." What would it mean to feel "found"? When has he felt more of a sense of direction, and what might he learn from that?

Individual language. My practice (which differs from that of many colleagues who write about spirituality and health) is that I very rarely introduce spiritual language in conversations. I find that asking the plain-English questions we have considered (like "What keeps you going? What sustains you through this?") invariably results in people supplying their own language. It is very common for people to introduce language like "God," "my faith," "my spirituality," "my Higher Power," or "the Man Upstairs." I want to anchor conversations in the other person's language because it is meaningful to him, and because he has ownership of the terms of how we speak about these things.

Three steps. A template for structuring these conversations that I generally follow has three parts, as shown in the sidebar.

The first step invites people to define what they want. In professional relationships and often in friendship relationships, people present descriptions of what is wrong, or how they are suffering, or the ways in which their lives pose challenges. As we have discussed, it is important to hear people's stories and to honor their suffering and challenges, but the first step in moving beyond their suffering is to define how they would want to be, *instead.* For a man who is depressed, how would he wish to be, instead? For a man who is struggling with a chronic illness, how would he describe how he wants to make his way through? For a man who says that he is "lonely and lost," how would he want his life to be different?

What people want can be defined in two ways, in terms of goals and in terms of qualities. "Goals" are fixed endpoints like deciding on a new career, saving money for retirement, losing 30 pounds, or remaining abstinent. "Qualities" are elements of character and qualities of daily living, like being more patient, generous, understanding, or courageous.

In either case, a definition of what people want is important because meaningful visions for the future provide direction and provide energy. Being "less depressed" is an understandable wish, but "building back my relationship with my son" provides direction (i.e., how a man might become less depressed) and energy inherent in something that is "vital and sacred."

The sidebar gives some examples of questions that can promote conversation about what people want. I often find that the questions "What do you want?" and "How would you put into words what you're trying to figure out?" promote this conversation as well.

A temple for collaborative spiritual care conversation

Three elements and some examples of conversation

Presuming a background of trust and patients feeling valued and understood...

1. Where do you want to go?
   What do you care about?
   What is your goal?
   What do you wish to accomplish?
   How would you like to be different?
   How would you like to be handling this?
   What kind of person do you want to be as you move through this?
2. How are you going to get there?
   a. Your (patient's) wisdom
      What is your sense about what you do now?
      When are the times when you feel like you are moving forward?
      What have you learned in your life that applies to this?
   b. My (clinician's) wisdom
      That is what the data say.
      That is what my patients have said.
      That is what I have learned from my experience.
3. What is the next step?
   What will you do to follow up at this point?
   What do you see yourself putting energy into now?
   When we next meet, what would you hope to report?

Having defined where people want to go, the second step is to explore possible approaches to getting there. I think of this as a collaborative process that brings together the wisdom of the patient (or friend) with the wisdom of the clinician (or helper). The people we are supporting have ideas about how they can make changes, based on their own wisdom and life experiences: "Maybe I can be more patient with Allison if I start each day with a short moment to remember that I love her." And we, the clinicians/helpers, have ideas about how people make changes, arising out of empirical literature, out of our experience supporting other people, and out of our own experience as human beings: "My experience from working with couples is that thinking about what it means to love each other is a pretty good priority right now."

The final step is to encourage people to plan specific ways to follow up on the conversation. The most exquisite and illuminating spiritual care conversation won't amount to much unless people experiment with doing something to live differently as a result.

Spiritual care conversations across the life cycle. Clinicians and friends/helpers can join the conversation about how they can "connect with the things that really matter to them" at any time. In health care, the conversation arises at any number of particular points, such as:

- Well-person visits: What does this man hope for at this point in his life? Where does he see himself investing energy?
- Lifestyle change: For movement toward more healthful practices (stopping smoking, beginning an exercise program, attending more carefully to diabetic monitoring, etc.), why does this man want to make this change? How does he hope his life will be different or richer as a result?
- Life transitions: Changes like commitment to a partner, birth of a child, starting a new job, retirement, or deaths of parents transform the landscape of life and present opportunities to envision the kind of person you want to be in your newly configured roles.
- Bad news: In the setting of painful uncertainty or diagnoses, what are the priorities for men? What remains sacred for them? How would they wish to live their lives in the midst of this suffering?

Transcendence and valued directions. Finally, a recurring theme in spiritual care has to do with the complementary journeys of transcendence and meaningful living (Craigie, 2010, 2012). In dealing with any of the events and challenges of life, there is a journey of transcending painful elements of the past, the uncertainty of the future, and aspects of life that can't be changed. And there is a journey of moving forward in valued directions.

These journeys are complementary because they are both necessary elements of healing and wholeness. A 38-year-old middle school teacher says that he holds back in developing new relationships because of his history of being emotionally and sexually abused as a child. He will probably have a hard time exploring new relationships until he begins to make peace with his past and, conversely, making peace with his past will be a hollow exercise unless he allows this healing to provide the impetus to explore some new relationships.

There are a number of approaches to transcendence that are rooted in spiritual and psychological traditions. They include:

- Letting go
- Willingness/acceptance
- Nonattachment
- Serenity
- Spiritual surrender

- Gratitude/gratefulness
- Forgiveness

Most men will resonate with some of these approaches and not others. In my practice, I find that "letting go" is a widely understood part of the consciousness of men (although *how* to do this is usually an important topic of conversation) and "serenity" is very familiar to people who have been involved in 12-step programs, and often to other people as well.

The conversation about "valued directions" follows the approaches and templates we have considered having to do with the values that are deeply important to people, and how they might pursue these values.

Spirituality of Men

So far, we have considered spirituality as it applies to all people, with examples drawn from life experiences of men. What about specifically *male* spirituality? Are there gender differences in the expression of spirituality? Are men "spiritual" *at all?* How might ideas and patterns in a male spirituality inform the ways that we work with men, as patients, colleagues, or friends? Modest literature on male spirituality, much of it arising out of work with the men's movement and the psychology of men in the last couple of decades, shows four recurring themes.

FOUR THEMES

First, men are "spiritual." People cannot "not be spiritual." If we think of spirituality in the inclusive ways in which we have been considering it—what is "vital and sacred," what "matters" deeply in people's lives—then all women and men have dimensions of spirituality because there are things that are sacred and that matter deeply to us all. Theologian Matthew Fox (2008), for instance, sees men often having spiritually rich dimensions to their lives, in terms of "giving life one's all" in devotion to family, country, lives of work, artistic pursuits, and social causes.

Second, the experience and expression of spirituality among men is often hidden or unacknowledged. Fox comments that few men would think of "giving life one's all" as "spirituality." He attributes men's shying away from "spirituality" to a number of reasons, such as lack of facility and comfort with spiritual language, lack of experience and recognition for self-awareness and reflection, and lack of mentors and cultural traditions by which spiritual values and beliefs would be handed down across generations.

Third, there are gender differences in the experience and expression of spirituality. Women and men, asserts Franciscan priest Richard Rohr (2005), "pay attention to different things." A key difference, according to Rohr, is that men are more oriented to action and movement than women—fixing, explaining, building, developing, and so forth—and less attuned to their "inner lives."

Much of the empirical literature about gender differences in spirituality follows a paradigm of greater-or-lesser prominence of various measures of spirituality. Bryant (2007), for instance, reports on data from surveys of college students at over 400 schools across the country. She found that women scored higher than men on such constructs as religious commitment and engagement, spiritual quest, charitable involvement, and social activism. Men scored higher on a measure of religious skepticism.

Fourth, men can grow. Writers about male spirituality commonly argue that men need to be engaged in the journey of developing (the spatial metaphors of "broadening" and "deepening" come to mind) their spirituality. This journey is described both as maturing an understanding of male spirituality and as incorporating elements of female spirituality into an overall, balanced whole.

In a classic book about "the mature masculine," Moore and Gillette (1991) present four metaphors of masculinity (King, Warrior, Magician, Lover) and suggest how men may journey from immature to mature forms of these dimensions of male life. In less mature and dysfunctional forms, for instance, the "King" element of masculinity is oriented to norm-less power and even abuse of others. A more mature form of this element is assertive and guided by transcendent principles and values. Similarly, Fox (2008) speaks of the journey from being a "soldier" (doing what one is told even if one's heart leads in the opposite direction) and being a "spiritual warrior" (acting in a definite way on behalf of the leading of the soul).

Rohr (2005), moreover, describes the overall journey of male spirituality as a bringing together of mature elements of masculine and feminine energies. Masculine energies around movement, service, and speaking the truth are brought together with feminine energies around attention to the inner life and relationships.

WORKING WITH MALE SPIRITUALITY

Recognize themes. Working with people in both health care and friendship relationships is helped by the ability to recognize and develop approaches to recurring patterns. We work with patterns like constellations of symptoms that signify disease, and recurring dynamics in substance abuse. To the extent that there are themes and gender differences in spirituality, we as professionals and friends can develop familiarity and facility working with recurring patterns that we see. We may, for instance, recognize and affirm men "giving their all" in family, vocational, or civic settings. Or we may respectfully explore with men some recurring (and self-limiting) themes around worth being tied to productivity, or perhaps around the difficulty of expressing feelings or vulnerability.

Also recognize individuality. Although it can be helpful to understand shared characteristics and values of groups of people, it is also important to recognize individuality. With expressly religious life, for instance, it can be helpful to be aware of Christian Scientists' views of health care, or Jehovah's Witnesses' practices around blood products and dis-fellowshipping. But *this* Christian Scientist, or *this* Witness, may well have personally constructed and individually distinct values about these or other practices. So it is important to explore the particular values and beliefs of this person, in front of you.

With the spirituality of men, similarly, we may recognize recurring cultural themes but also need to understand individual values and practices. What does it mean to *this* man to be a man? What is it that undergirds "success" and human value for *this* man?

Invite men into broader view of spirituality. Finally, working with male spirituality means encouraging men along the journey of broadening and deepening their spirituality. This happens in a number of ways.

Conversation. As professionals, colleagues, and friends, we can engage men in conversation about what matters to them, as men, and how they see themselves moving forward:

- What does it mean to you to be a man?
- What is essential for you to feel "successful" as a man?
- Who is a man whom you have admired? What qualities in his life may be points of growth for you?
- How would you hope to be growing as a person and as a man in the future?

Reflective resources. There are also good resources available for men to provide examples and self-reflective questions about male spirituality. Like Moore and Gillette 20 years ago, Rohr, Fox, and others suggest metaphors and narratives that can challenge men with a new understanding of masculinity. Their collections of metaphors and narratives—Father Sky, the Blue Man, the Green Man, Iron John—introduce men to qualities like gentleness, mysticism, reverence for the earth, creativity, collaboration, sharing, authenticity, and respect for the inner life that may not now be part of the spirituality of men. Fox (2008), in particular, has an excellent appendix of reflective exercises for developing the 10 archetypes he presents.

Community. And for many men, becoming part of a community or fellowship of men can be a vital part of the journey. Men's groups. Faith-based groups organized around the study of sacred texts. Twelve-step programs. Groups like these provide opportunities for non-superficial interaction and mutual support in the journey of moving into fullness of life as men.

Conclusion

Spirituality, taken here to mean the individual's sense of meaning or purpose, is a vitally important aspect to the integrative care for men. The meaning a disease or health challenge holds for a particular patient can impact how health care providers assist in treatment and advise lifestyle changes that are needed. In general, men have ways of relating to their friends and family, their community, and even their own feelings of connectedness that should shape the interaction between patient and provider in order to make this crucial relationship an optimally therapeutic one.

REFERENCES

Bryant AN. Gender differences in spiritual development during the college years. *Sex Roles.* 2007;56(11–12):835–846.

Craigie FC. *Positive spirituality in health care: Nine practical approaches to pursuing wholeness for clinicians, patients, and health care organizations.* Minneapolis: Mill City Press, 2010.

Craigie FC. 3 steps to make life count from here on. *Spirituality Health.* 2012;Jan-Feb:66–71.

Daaleman T, Usher B, Williams S, Rawlings J, Hanson L. An exploratory study of spiritual care at the end of life. *Ann Fam Med.* 2008;6(5):406–411.

Fox M. *The hidden spirituality of men.* Nevato, CA: New World, 2008.

Hamilton KH. HOPE groups and soulcircling. Paper presented at Thomas Nevola, MD, Symposium on Spirituality and Health; June 10, 2008; Waterville, ME.

Kabat-Zinn J. *Wherever you go, there you are: Mindfulness meditation in everyday life.* New York: Hyperion, 2005.

Keyes CLM. Promoting and protecting mental health as flourishing. *Am Psychologist.* 2007;62(2):95–108.

Koop CE. Spirituality and health. Paper presented at Thomas Nevola, MD, Symposium on Spirituality and Health; June 8, 1994; Augusta, ME.

Lunn J. Spiritual care in a multi-religious context. *J Pain Palliat Care Pharmacother.* 2003;17(3–4):153–166.

Maselko J, Kubzansky L. Gender differences in religious practices, spiritual experiences and health: Results from the US General Social Survey. *Soc Sci Med.* 2002;62(11):2848–2860.

Moore R, Gillette D. *King, warrior, magician, lover: Rediscovering the archetypes of the mature masculine.* San Francisco: HarperOne, 1991.

Moritz S, Quan H, Rickhi B, et al. A home study-based spirituality education program decreases emotional distress and increases quality of life—a randomized, controlled trial. *Altern Ther Health Med.* 2006;12(6):26–35.

Morris E. The relationship of spirituality to coronary heart disease. *Alt Therapies.* 2001;7(5):96–98.

Peterson C, Seligman MEP. *Character strengths and virtues: A handbook and classification.* New York: American Psychological Association/Oxford University Press, 2004.

Powell LH, Shahabi L, Thoresen C. Religion and spirituality: Linkages to physical health. *Am Psychologist.* 2003;58(1):36–52.

Puchalski CM. Taking a spiritual history: FICA. *Spirituality Med Connection.* 1999;3(1):1.

Puchalski CM, McSkimming S. Creating healing environments: An initiative seeks to restore "heart and humanity" to depersonalized health care. *Health Progress.* 2006;87(3):30–35.

Rohr R. *From wild man to wise man: Reflections on male spirituality.* Cincinnati: St. Anthony Messenger, 2005.

Seligman MEP. *Flourish.* New York: Free Press, 2011.

Shanafelt TD, Sloan JA, Habermann TM. The well-being of physicians. *Am J Med.* 2003,114:513–519.

Tsuang MT, Simpson JC, Koenen KC, Kremen WS, Lyons MJ. Spiritual well-being and health. *J Nerv Mental Dis.* 2007;195(8):673–680.

Underwood L, Terisi J. The daily spiritual experience scale: Development, theoretical description, reliability, exploratory factor analysis, and preliminary construct validity using health-related data. *Ann Behav Med.* 2002;24(1):22–33.

Wheatley M. *Turning to one another: Simple conversations to restore hope to the future.* San Francisco: Berrett-Koehler, 2002.

6

Physical Activity and Men's Health

BRUCE B. CAMPBELL AND MYLES D. SPAR

Benefits of Physical Activity

In the United States, only 31% of men report regular physical activity, defined as three sessions a week of vigorous activity lasting 20 minutes or more or five sessions of light/moderate physical activity lasting 30 minutes or more. About 40% of adults report no leisure physical activity.

Although it may seem obvious that physical activity confers many health benefits, there are multiple studies specifically detailing just how beneficial regular exercise is for health, particularly when considering the diseases most prevalent in men such as heart disease, metabolic syndrome, obesity, and sexual dysfunction.

Strong Evidence of Benefits of Exercise

- Lower risk of early death
- Lower risk of coronary heart disease
- Lower risk of stroke
- Lower risk of high blood pressure
- Lower risk of adverse blood lipid profile
- Lower risk of type 2 diabetes
- Lower risk of metabolic syndrome
- Lower risk of colon cancer
- Prevention of weight gain
- Weight loss, particularly when combined with reduced calorie intake
- Improved cardiorespiratory and muscular fitness
- Prevention of falls
- Reduced depression
- Better cognitive function

Moderate Evidence of Benefits of Exercise

- Better functional health (for older adults)
- Reduced abdominal obesity
- Lower risk of hip fracture
- Lower risk of lung cancer
- Weight maintenance after weight loss
- Increased bone density

PREMATURE DEATH

People who are active for approximately 7 hours per week have a 40% lower risk of dying early than those who are active for less than 30 minutes a week. Furthermore, a 35-year longitudinal study from Sweden showed that men who were highly physically active at age 50 were 32% less likely to die during the study than the least active men. Even men who started exercising between ages 50 and 60 had a 49% lower death rate than the men who stayed inactive. A Harvard study of 36,500 male graduates showed that sedentary men gained 1.6 years in life expectancy from becoming active(Byberg et al., 2009).

CARDIOVASCULAR DISEASE

Many prospective cohort studies and meta-analyses show inactivity associated with increased risk for cardiovascular disease (CVD), CVD mortality, stroke, diabetes, hypertension, and metabolic syndrome. One meta-analysis showed a relative risk of death from coronary heart disease to be 1.9 (95% confidence interval 1.6–2.2) for sedentary compared to active adults (Berlin and Colditz, 1990).

OBESITY

Low levels of physical activity are a significant risk factor for obesity. Physical activity helps with weight loss and with maintaining healthy weight.

DIABETES AND METABOLIC SYNDROME

Physical activity helps to prevent type 2 diabetes, with the risk for fit adults of developing the disease being 30% lower than inactive people (Tuomilehto et al., 2001). This was seen with both moderate and vigorous activity.

COLON AND LUNG CANCER

Colon cancer is the third most common cause of cancer death in men. Physical activity is associated with a 40% lower risk of colon cancer, based on a systematic review of 48 studies and over 40,000 cases of the disease. Physical activity reduces the risk of lung cancer in men by 20% to 50%, with evidence of a dose-response effect. [54] The mechanism may be from decreased inflammation or enhanced immune function, including enhanced natural killer (NK) cell function among those who exercise regularly.

MUSCULOSKELETAL HEALTH

Regular activity reduces risk of falls among the elderly and is associated with reduced risk of hip fractures. Weight-bearing exercise also improved bone density and risk of osteoporosis (Gutin, 1992).

MOOD

Exercise training programs have shown improvements in depression, anxiety, and hostility. There seems to be a dose-response effect of exercise on symptoms of depression and anxiety (Dunn et al., 2001).

COGNITIVE FUNCTION

Not only does physical activity help to prevent stroke, but it also helps to decrease cognitive decline associated with aging. One study of 1,324 older adults without dementia showed that those who engaged in regular exercise since their 40s or 50s had a 39% lower risk of mild cognitive impairment; those who started exercising in their 60s had a 32% lower risk. Those with mild cognitive impairment at the beginning showed improvement after 6 months of high-intensity aerobic activity (Baker et al., 2009).

ERECTILE DYSFUNCTION

Many of the conditions that are improved with physical activity are risk factors for erectile dysfunction (ED). In addition, there was shown to be an improvement in both erectile and endothelial dysfunction in a review in the *Journal of Andrology,* which looked at multiple studies including both retrospective analyses and prospective trials (La Vignera, 2012).

Overuse Syndromes

Although physical activity carries many health benefits, regular exercise is not without risk of injury. This section reviews the diagnosis and treatment of common overuse syndromes found in men related to physical activity, including tendinopathy, stress fractures, and shin splints.

TENDINOPATHY

Pathophysiology

In overuse tendinopathy, there is typically an absence of inflammatory cells observed on biopsy specimens taken from athletes with chronic tendon pain. Instead, the histopathology of tendinopathy demonstrates fibrosis, calcification, and neovascularization within the tendon (Khan et al., 1999). The resultant tissue consists of a disorganized matrix of tissue that is stiff, painful, and weak. The term *tendinosis* describes these degenerative histopathological findings. In contrast, tendonitis is characterized by an inflammatory reaction, which frequently results from acute injury. Tendinopathy is frequently incorrectly termed *tendonitis*. Given the current understanding of the noninflammatory, degenerative pathology of tendinopathy, a shift in the treatment paradigm from anti-inflammatory modalities toward a rehabilitation-oriented approach is required.

Risk Factors

Significant risk factors for the development of tendinopathy include repetitive loading on the tendon and advancing age (Maffuli et al., 2003). Middle-aged and elderly individuals participating in recreational sporting activities are more prone to overuse tendinopathy than younger athletes. Pre-existing biomechanical abnormalities such as flat foot or high-arched foot, inappropriate footwear, and inadequate rest can contribute to tendinopathy. Fluoroquinolone antibiotic use is also associated with an increased risk of tendinopathy and tendon rupture (Khaliq and Zhanel, 2003).

Clinical Features

Patients complain of pain with activities that cause tendon loading. Joint stiffness and muscle weakness may occur. Common physical findings of tendinopathy include tenderness and thickening over the affected segment of the tendon. The degenerated and weakened state of the tendon can lead to tendon rupture or tear. Acupuncture can be helpful with all tendinopathies. Physical therapeutic techniques aimed at breaking up scar tissue and promoting blood flow into affected areas are especially helpful. Specific tendinopathies with corresponding treatments are described here.

Common Tendinopathies

ACHILLES TENDINOPATHY Achilles tendinopathy is characterized by chronic posterior heel pain and swelling. Pain is aggravated by tendon loading activities, such as walking and running, and external pressure caused by the back of the shoe (Thomas et al., 2010). Common causes include overtraining, exercising on uneven surfaces, poor flexibility of the gastrocnemius muscle, overpronation of the foot, inappropriate footwear, and fluoroquinolone therapy.

Patients often exhibit tenderness 3 to 5 cm above the insertion to the calcaneus, an area that corresponds to the poorest vascularity (Simpson and Thomas, 2010). A prominence may be palpable. Radiographic findings may reveal insertional spurring or intratendinous calcifications.

Treatment includes avoidance of high-impact physical activity, heel lifts, and open-back shoes to reduce stress on the tendon. Eccentric training, characterized by stretching the tendon while under tension, has been shown to be beneficial (Alfredson et al., 1998). Corticosteroid injections are not recommended, as they may increase the risk of tendon rupture. Surgery, which may include tendon debridement or resection of insertional spurring, is reserved for refractory cases (Thomas, 2010).

ROTATOR CUFF TENDINOPATHY The rotator cuff muscles are important for shoulder movements and for stabilizing the shoulder joint; they consist of the supraspinatus, infraspinatus, teres minor, and subscapularis. Pain related to degenerative, age-related atrophy of the rotator cuff tendons is more common than from acute injury (Matsen, 2008). The supraspinatus tendon is most commonly affected, and rotator cuff tendinopathy can lead to tendon tear.

Risk factors for rotator cuff tendinopathy include repetitive overhead activity, such as in tennis, golf, and swimming. Older age and anatomic factors that predispose to rotator cuff impingement, such as osteoarthritis on the undersurface of the acromioclavicular joint, represent other risks. Patients commonly report shoulder pain with overhead activity or while lying on the affected shoulder at night.

Physical findings often include pain and limited range of motion with abduction and internal rotation, and positive signs of impingement (Hawkins-Kennedy and Neer tests) (Burbank et al., 2008). Weakness can be concerning for a tear. Plain radiographs are typically unrevealing but may demonstrate calcification at the insertion of the supraspinatus or an alternative cause of shoulder pain. Ultrasound and magnetic resonance imaging (MRI) are both useful imaging studies if a tear is suspected (Iannotti et al., 2005).

Treatment includes rest and avoidance of overhead activities. Physical therapy that focuses on range of motion and strengthening the rotator cuff muscles can be beneficial. Subacromial glucocorticoid injection may be considered in individuals who fail to improve with conservative measures, although there is limited evidence to indicate a clear benefit (Koester et al., 2007). Surgical repair may be an option in refractory cases, if the quality and quantity of tissue are sufficient for durable repair (Matsen, 2008). In individuals in whom the cuff is not reparable, surgery to remove adhesions and scar tissue may relieve pain and increase range of motion.

PATELLAR TENDINOPATHY Patients with patellar tendinopathy, commonly referred to as "jumper's knee," complain of anterior knee pain (Maffulli et al., 2003). It is caused by activities that involve repetitive loading of the patellar tendon, such as jumping. Pain is often aggravated by walking down stairs, running, and prolonged sitting.

Physical examination often reveals localized tenderness at the tendon insertion at the inferior pole of the patella (Visnes and Bahr, 2007). Pain is reproduced by having the patient resist knee extension or squat on a decline. Patellar tendinopathy is primarily diagnosed clinically. Ultrasonography and MRI may provide additional diagnostic value, although findings may not correlate with clinical symptoms.

Treatment includes avoidance of causative physical activities. Patients may benefit from physical rehabilitation that focuses on eccentric tendon exercises, such as decline squats (Visnes and Bahr, 2007). If conservative management fails, surgery may be considered, although there is limited evidence regarding the effectiveness of surgery (Peers and Lysens, 2005).

ELBOW TENDINOPATHY Two common tendinopathies, lateral and medial elbow tendinopathy, are often referred to as "tennis elbow" and "golfer's elbow," respectively. Lateral elbow tendinopathy is characterized by tendinosis involving the wrist extensor muscles at their insertion at the lateral humeral epicondyle. Conversely, in medial elbow tendinopathy there are degenerative changes involving the wrist flexor tendons at their insertion at the medial humeral epicondyle.

Risk factors for both tendinopathies include repetitive wrist extension, in the case of lateral elbow tendinopathy, and repetitive wrist flexion, in the case of medial elbow tendinopathy. Obesity, smoking, and age over 40 represent other risk factors (Peers and Lysens, 2005).

The diagnosis of elbow tendinopathy is clinical. Patients with lateral elbow tendinopathy report pain and tenderness over the lateral epicondyle. Pain is elicited with resistance to wrist extension with the elbow in full extension. In medial elbow tendinopathy, patients report pain and tenderness over the medial epicondyle. Pain is aggravated with resistance to wrist flexion with the elbow straight.

Treatment includes avoidance of activities that require repetitive wrist extension or flexion and physical therapy that focuses on eccentric training. Instruction on proper stroke mechanics and appropriate racket type can be beneficial to tennis players before returning to play. In lateral elbow tendinopathy, a proximal forearm brace may reduce tendon strain at its insertion (Walther et al., 2002). Glucocorticoid injection for elbow tendinopathy may provide short-term relief of pain but does not prevent recurrence and may lead to worse long-term outcomes (Coombes et al., 2010; Placzek, 2007) A number of other potential therapies, including autologous blood and botulinum toxin injections, may be helpful, though evidence of their benefit is limited (Suresh et al., 2006). Refractory pain despite conservative measures warrants imaging to look for another cause. Patients with persistent symptoms related to lateral epicondylitis may be referred to a surgeon, although there is a lack of consensus on a standard surgical approach.

ILIOTIBIAL BAND FRICTION SYNDROME

Iliotibial band friction syndrome (IBFS) is a frequent cause of lateral knee discomfort in runners. The injury occurs as a result of trauma to the iliotibial band (ITB) as it repeatedly slides over the lateral femoral condyle (Cosca and Navazio, 2007). Individuals often report a burning discomfort involving the lateral knee during activities such as running and cycling, and pain may radiate up the thigh. Risk factors include varus alignment of the knee and repetitive long-distance running, especially on uneven terrain. Hip abduction weakness is also thought to play a role in the development of IBFS (Fredericson, 2000).

Examination elicits tenderness of the ITB over the lateral femoral condyle. Tightness of the ITB may be noted with passive adduction of the leg, with the patient lying on the unaffected side. Imaging studies are usually not indicated.

Treatment includes nonsteroidal anti-inflammatory drugs (NSAIDs), ITB stretching, rest from aggravating activities, avoidance of running on uneven surfaces, and hip abductor strengthening (Ellis et al., 2007). Cyclists may benefit from seat height and pedal adjustments. Corticosteroid injection may be considered in refractory cases (Fredericson and Wolf, 2005).

PLANTAR FASCIITIS

Plantar fasciitis is one of the most common causes of foot pain, especially in runners. It arises as a result of repetitive microtrauma to the plantar fascia from excess mechanical stress and is characterized by pain in the heel or arch of the foot, typically worse with the initial weight bearing after arising from bed or from prolonged sitting (Cosca and Navazio, 2007). The discomfort may diminish with further physical activity, only to intensify thereafter. Risk factors include flat feet, high-arched feet, nonsupportive footwear, and excessive running on hard surfaces.

Physical examination reveals focal tenderness over the origin of the plantar fascia at the medial base of the heel. Pain may be elicited with passive dorsiflexion of the toes. Imaging is typically not indicated if there is a high clinical suspicion but may reveal calcaneal spurring or an alternative cause of pain such as fracture.

Treatment includes rest, shoe inserts to provide arch and heel support, and plantar fascia stretching. Icing and NSAIDs may provide some pain relief, but evidence of their efficacy is limited. Patients should avoid going barefoot or wearing flat shoes. Patients with chronic plantar fasciitis may benefit from dorsiflexion night splints (Powell et al., 1998). Judicious steroid injection may be considered in cases of refractory pain. However, repeated injection may predispose to heel pad atrophy and plantar fascia rupture (Sellman, 1994). Surgical management, which involves fasciotomy, is reserved for those who fail to respond to nonoperative therapy after 6 to 12 months (Thomas, 2010).

STRESS FRACTURES

A stress fracture occurs when a bone is subjected to repeated loadbearing, such as running. During periods of repetitive mechanical stress, there is an imbalance in bone remodeling where bone formation lags behind bone resorption. The weakened bone is vulnerable to microfractures, which can propagate into stress fractures (Patel et al., 2011).

Risk factors for stress fractures include repetitive load-bearing physical activities, a prior history of stress fracture, diminished bone density, and poor biomechanics. The weight-bearing bones of the lower extremity, particularly the tibia and metatarsals, are especially prone to stress fractures (Matheson et al., 1987).

Patients typically report a gradual onset of localized pain, which is worse with load-bearing activities. Physical examination usually elicits focal bone tenderness over the fracture site. For nonpalpable areas, applying a stress over the area of concern may also reproduce the patient's pain.

Plain x-rays may reveal a stress fracture but lack sensitivity, and findings may take weeks to months to appear. Bone scans have high sensitivity but lack specificity, with a large percentage of positive findings occurring at asymptomatic sites. MRI is both sensitive and specific in diagnosing stress fractures and has emerged as the preferred imaging study (Gaeta et al., 2005).

Treatment includes avoidance of activities that place stress on the bone and pain control with ice and analgesics, such as acetaminophen or low-potency opiates. Some studies have reported that anti-inflammatory medications may inhibit fracture healing (Wheeler and Batt, 2005). Crutches, pneumatic splints, and walking boots can be used for lower extremity stress fractures. Patients should be encouraged to cross-train in other physical activities such as cycling and swimming to maintain fitness during recovery. Patients may gradually resume the activity after several weeks of rest and improved symptoms. Certain stress fractures are at risk for fracture progression and nonunion. High-risk stress fractures include the femoral head and neck, patella, anterior tibia, medial malleolus, fifth metatarsal, talus, navicular, and pars interarticularis of the lumbar spine (Patel et al., 2011). These site-specific stress fractures should be referred to an orthopedist.

MEDIAL TIBIAL STRESS SYNDROME (SHIN SPLINTS)

Medial tibial stress syndrome (MTSS), commonly termed *shin splints*, is one of the most common overuse sports injuries, especially in runners. It is caused by repetitive loading on the lower leg. Although the exact pathogenesis remains unclear, recent studies support the view that MTSS is not an inflammatory process of the periosteum but rather a stress reaction of bone that has become painful (Tweed et al., 2008). Patients typically report exercise-related pain, characterized as a dull ache, along the shin. Biomechanical factors such as hyperpronation of the foot can predispose to shin splints (Moen, 2009).

Physical examination often elicits diffuse tenderness over the mid- to distal posteromedial tibial border, in contrast to the focal tenderness over the anterior tibia commonly seen in a stress fracture (Cosca and Navazio, 2007). MTSS can develop into a stress fracture, and distinguishing between the two can be clinically challenging.

The diagnosis of MTSS is primarily clinical. Imaging studies, including MRI and bone scans, may be useful in distinguishing MTSS from a stress fracture (Moen, 2009). Plain radiographs are unremarkable in patients with MTSS, but also may be normal in those with stress fractures.

Treatment includes avoidance of repetitive loading on the lower leg, stretching, and possible orthotics or insoles to correct biomechanical factors. MTSS may be prevented by using shock-absorbing shoe insoles, although the evidence for this intervention is limited (Craig, 2008).

Injury Prevention

Given the numerous health benefits associated with exercise and the current obesity epidemic within the United States, there is a need for increased physical activity in society. However, increased physical activity increases risk of injury and overuse syndromes. Running injuries occur in 40% to 50% of runners on an annual basis (Fields, 2010). Sports injuries are now cited as one of the most common injuries in modern Western societies [35]. Treating athletic injuries is frequently difficult, costly, and time consuming. There is a need for effective prevention strategies to reduce sports-related injury risk.

Stretching is commonly practiced before and after physical activity to prevent injury. However, a meta-analysis by the U.S. Centers for Disease Control and Prevention found that static stretching was not significantly associated with a reduction in sports-related injuries [36]. Dynamic stretching, in which the joint is mobilized in a gentle and continuous movement prior to exercise, may be more beneficial in preventing injury, but this is still being investigated. Further studies are necessary to determine the role of stretching in injury prevention.

In a recent review of 25 studies involving over 30,000 participants evaluating interventions to prevent lower limb running injuries, researchers found no evidence to support that any particular training regimen of exercises to improve strength, flexibility, and coordination reduces injury (Yeung, 2011). There is limited evidence that reducing duration and frequency of running may be effective. Although there is evidence to support the use of a patellofemoral brace for preventing anterior knee pain, very little evidence supports the use of insoles for preventing running-related injuries. Clearly, more studies are needed to determine the efficacy of various interventions for the prevention of running-related injuries.

Appropriately fitting footwear with adequate support may also help prevent running injuries. Recently, barefoot running has become popular. Proponents claim improved performance and decreased injury risk. However, a recent review reports no evidence that either confirms or refutes improved performance or reduced injury risk and concludes that many of the claimed advantages to barefoot running are not supported by the literature (Jenkins and Cauthon, 2011). The authors conclude that barefoot running may be acceptable for individuals who understand and can minimize the risks.

Anabolic Androgenic Steroids and Other Substances to Improve Athletic Performance

Recently, there has been an increase in use of anabolic androgenic steroids, growth hormone, and insulin-like growth factor among recreational athletes to enhance performance and appearance. Surveys have indicated that individuals may take these substances in combination or separately. The use of these substances has spread to involve the adolescent population. A recent study reported that 4.3% of male high school students nationwide had taken anabolic steroids at least once without a doctor's prescription (Eaton et al., 2010).

Anabolic androgenic steroids (AASs), which include all synthetic derivatives of testosterone, increase muscle mass and strength but have many health risks to multiple organ systems. Nearly 100% of individuals using AASs will experience adverse side effects. Given their potentially deleterious effect, AASs are classified as schedule III controlled substances, which require a prescription and are banned in competitive sports (Jenkinson and Harbert, 2008).

Adverse cardiovascular sequelae of AAS use include elevated blood pressure, elevated low-density lipoprotein (LDL) levels, reduced high-density lipoprotein (HDL) levels, myocardial infarction, and stroke. AASs are directly toxic to cardiac muscle, which can result in cardiomyopathy, arrhythmia, and sudden death (Dhar et al., 2005).

Neuropsychiatric side effects associated with AASs include aggressive behavior, depression, mania, psychosis, paranoia, mood swings, and suicide (Buttner and Thieme, 2010). Individuals who use AASs are more likely than nonusers to abuse other drugs and alcohol. AAS users may also develop an abscess at the site of the injection, septic arthritis, hepatitis B and C, and HIV from sharing needles.

AAS use suppresses gonadotropin release, and therefore causes testicular atrophy and infertility. Sperm counts often return to normal 4 months after discontinuation, but may take longer to normalize (Knuth et al., 1989). Gynecomastia occurs as a result of testosterone conversion to estradiol. Other side effects of AASs include acne, alopecia, premature epiphyseal bone closure in adolescents, tendon rupture, and hepatotoxicity. Many of the adverse effects of anabolic steroids are reversible upon discontinuation of the drug (Jenkinson and Harbert, 2008).

Like anabolic steroids, human growth hormone (HGH) has been shown to increase lean body mass. However, most studies have found HGH to not be effective in improving strength or endurance (Meinhardt et al., 2010). HGH has multiple adverse effects and is illegal in competitive sports. Many over-the-counter supplements claim to increase endogenous HGH levels. However, HGH is only available by prescription that is administered as an injection. Adverse cardiovascular effects of HGH include dyslipidemia, hypertension, cardiomegaly, and ventricular hypertrophy (Dhar et al., 2005). Other adverse outcomes related to HGH use include insulin resistance, diabetes, fluid retention, premature epiphyseal closure, arthralgias, and carpal tunnel syndrome (Fernandez and Hosey, 2009).

Insulin-like growth factor 1 (IGF-1) is also purported to increase muscle mass and performance, but no definitive studies support this belief. Cardiovascular toxicities of IGF-1 are similar to those of HGH. IGF-1 may also result in hypoglycemia, acromegaly, edema, myalgias, and dyspnea (Holt and Sonksen, 2008).

Given the widespread use of performance-enhancing agents in society, there is a need for more effective educational campaigns to alert the public about the harmful effects of these substances. Teenagers informed about the adverse effects of AASs have been reported to be less likely to use these substances compared with those uninformed (Radakovich et al, 1993). Because many men are reluctant to stop using these hormones, health care providers need to ask their male patients about the issue.

Supplements that are used to improve athletic performance include those mentioned in the chapter on supplements. Three types of ginsengs were discussed in that chapter as they relate to their use in physical activity and performance. Other supplements commonly used include creatine, taurine, branched-chain amino acids, and dehydroepiandrosterone (DHEA).

Creatine is naturally produced in the human body and taken up preferentially by muscle cells, where it is used for adenosine triphosphate (ATP) production. Creatine does seem to increase the size of muscle cells, theoretically increasing muscle strength. This has not been proven, but extensive research has shown that supplementation at the amounts generally recommended for muscle strength does not cause adverse side effects. Still, those with kidney disease or at risk for kidney disease are generally advised against using it as a precaution (Bizzarini and De Angelis, 2004).

Taurine is an amino acid naturally found in the body that has been touted as an energy booster. Although small studies have shown some improvement in VO$_2$ max after daily use of taurine as a supplement, there have not been consistent findings of benefit from its use (Zhang, 2004).

Branched-chain amino acids (BCAAs) have similarly been used to improve athletic performance. They include leucine, isoleucine, and valine. Supplemental intake of these amino acids is purported to decrease exercise-induced muscle damage, increase muscle recovery, and help to build lean muscle mass in response to strength training. There is some evidence that supplemental BCAAs do have anabolic effects in human muscle (Blomstrand, 2006). When manufactured according to good manufacturing practices, BCAAs seem to be a safe supplement to take, with no serious adverse side effects.

DHEA is a natural androgenic hormone produced in the adrenal gland. DHEA has been recommended in doses ranging from 10 to 100 mg/day for anabolic and antiaging effects. Although DHEA may improve lean muscle mass due to androgenic effects, there is no evidence that it improves athletic performance.

Conclusion

Physical activity is a key component to optimal health in men. This chapter highlighted many of the proven health benefits of regular exercise. There are potential injuries and painful conditions that may be associated with physical activity; thus, intensity of activity should be increased gradually and safely. Some supplements may help to increase energy, recovery, and lean muscle mass.

REFERENCES

Alfredson H, Pietila T, Jonnson P, Lorentzon R. Heavy–load eccentric calf muscle training for the treatment of chronic Achilles tendinosis. Am J Sports Med. 1998;26(3):360–366.

Baker LD, Frank LL, Foster-Schubert K, et al. Effects of aerobic exercise on mild cognitive impairment: a controlled trial. Arch Neurol. 2010;67(1):71–79.

Berlin JA, Colditz GA. A meta-analysis of physical activity in the prevention of coronary heart disease. A Jnl Epi. 1990:132;612–628.

Bisset L, Beller E, Jull G, et al. Mobilization with movement and exercise, corticosteroid injection, or wait and see for tennis elbow: randomized trial. BMJ. 2006;333:939–941.

Bizzarini E, De Angelis L. Is the use of oral creatine supplementation safe? J Sports Med Phys Fitness. 2004;44(4):411–416.

Blomstrand E, Eliasson J, Karlsson HK, et al. Branched-chain amino acids activate key enzymes in protein synthesis after physical exercise. J Nutr. 2006;136(Suppl 1):S269–S273.

Burbank KM, Stevenson JH, Czarnecki GR, Dorfman J. Chronic shoulder pain: part I. Evaluation and diagnosis. Am Fam Physician. 2008;15;77(4): 453–460.

Buttner A, Thieme D. Side effects of anabolic androgenic steroids: pathological findings and structure-activity relationships. Handbook Exper Pharmacol. 2010;195:459–484.

Byberg L, Melhus H, et al. Total mortality after changes in leisure time physical activity in 50 year old men: 35 year follow-up of population based cohort. BMJ. 2009;338:b688.

Coombes BK, Bisset L, Vicenzino B. Efficacy and safety of corticosteroid injections and other injections for treatment of tendinopathy: a systemic review of randomized controlled trials. Lancet 2010;376:1751–1767.

Cosca DD, Navazio F. Common problems in endurance athletes. Am Fam Physician. 2007;76:237–244.

Craig DI. Medial tibial stress syndrome: evidence-based prevention. J Athl Train. 2008;3:316–318.

Dhar R, Stout CW, et al. Cardiovascular toxicities of performance-enhancing substances in sports. Mayo Clin Proc. 2005;80(10):1307–1315.

Dunn AL, Trivedi MH, O'Neal HA. Physical activity dose–response effects on outcomes of depression and anxiety. Medicine and Science in Sports and Exercise. 2001;33(Suppl):S587–S597.

Eaton DK, Kann L, Kinchen S, et al. Youth risk behavior surveillance-United States, 2009. MMWR Surveill Summ. 2010;59:16.

Ellis R, Hing W, Reid, D. Iliotibial band friction syndrome-a systematic review. Manual Therapy. 2007;200–208.

Fernandez MM, Hosey RG. Performance enhancing drugs snare non athletes too. J Fam Pract. 2009;58:16–23.

Fields KB, Sykes JC, et al. Prevention of running injuries. Curr Sports Med Rep. 2010;9(3):176–182.

Fredericson M, Cookingham CL, et al. Hip abductor weakness in distance runners with iliotibial band syndrome. Clin J Sports Med. 2000;3: 169–175.

Fredericson M, Wolf C. Iliotibial band syndrome in runners: innovations in treatment. Sport Med. 2005;35:451–459.

Gaeta M, Minutoli F, Scribano E, et al. CT and MR imaging findings in athletes with early tibial stress injuries: comparison with bone scintigraphy findings and emphasis on cortical abnormalities. Radiology. 2005;235:553–561.

Gutin B, Kasper M. Can vigorous exercise play a role in osteoporosis prevention? A review. Osteoporosis International. 1992;2:55–69.

Holt R, Sonksen PH. Growth hormone, IGF-1 and insulin and their abuse in sport. Brit J Pharm. 2008;154:542–556.

Iannotti JP, Ciccone J, Buss DD, Visotsky JL, Mascha E, Cotman K, Rawool NM. Accuracy of office-based ultrasonography of the shoulder for the diagnosis of rotator cuff tears. J Bone Joint Surg Am. 2005;87(6):1305–1311.

Jenkins DW, Cauthon DJ. Barefoot running claims and controversies: a review of the literature. J Am Podiatr Med Assoc. 2011;101(3):231–246.

Jenkinson DM, Harbert AJ. Supplements and sports. Am Fam Physician. 2008;78(9):1039–1046.

Khaliq Y, Zhanel GG. Fluoroquinolone-associated tendinopathy: a critical review of the literature. Clin Infect Dis. 2003;36(11):1404–1410.

Khan KM, Cook JL, Bonar F, et al. Histopathology of common tendinopathies. Update and implications for clinical management. Sports Med. 1999;27:393–408.

Knuth UA, Maniera H, Nieschlag E. Anabolic steroids and semen parameters in bodybuilders. Fertil Steril. 1989;25:1041–1047.

Koester MC, Dunn WR, Kuhn JE, Spindler KP. The efficacy of subacromial corticosteroid injection in the treatment of rotator cuff disease: a systematic review. J Am Acad Orthop Surg. 2007;15(1):3–11.

La Vignera S, Condorelli RA, Vicari E, et al. Statins and erectile dysfunction: a critical summary of current evidence. J Androl. 2012;33(4):552–558.

Maffulli N, Wong J, Almekinders LC. Types and epidemiology of tendinopathy. Clin Sports Med. 2003;22:675–692.

Matheson GO, Clement DB, Mckenzie DC, et al. Stress fractures in athletes. A study of 320 cases. Am J Sports Med. 1987;15:46–58.

Matsen FA III. Clinical practice. Rotator-cuff failure. N Engl J Med. 2008;358:2138–2147.

Meinhardt U, Nelson AE, Hansen JL, et al. The effects of growth hormone on body composition and physical performance in recreational athletes: a randomized trial. Ann Intern Med. 2010;152:568–577.

Moen MH, Tol JL, et al. Medial tibial stress syndrome; a critical review. Sports Med. 2009;39(7):523–546.

Parkkari J, Kujala UM, Kannus P. Is it possible to prevent sports injuries? Review of controlled clinical trials and recommendations for future work. Sports Med. 2001;31(14):985–995.

Patel DS, Roth M, Kapil N. Stress fractures: diagnosis, treatment, and prevention. Am Fam Physician. 2011;83:39–46.

Peers KH, Lysens RJ. Patellar tendinopathy in athletes: current diagnostic and therapeutic recommendations. Sports Med. 2005;35(1):71–87.

Placzek R, et al. Treatment of chronic radial epicondylitis with botulinum toxin A. A double-blind, placebo-controlled, randomized multicenter study. J Bone Joint Surg Am. 2007;89:255–260.

Powell M, Post WR, Keener J, Wearden S. Effective treatment of chronic plantar fasciitis with dorsiflexion night splints: a crossover prospective randomized outcome study. Foot Ankle Int. 1998;19:10–18.

Radakovich J, Broderick P, Pickell G. Rate of anabolic androgenic steroid use among students in junior high school. J Am Board Fam Pract. 1993;6(4):341–345.

Sellman JR. Plantar fascia rupture associated with corticosteroid injection. Foot Ankle Int. 1994;15:376–381.

Simpson M, Thomas H. Tendinopathies of the foot and ankle. Am Fam Physician. 2009;80:1107–1114.

Suresh SP, Ali KE, Jones H, Connell DA. Medial epicondylitis: is ultrasound guided autologous blood injection an effective treatment? Br J Sports Med. 2006;40:935–939.

Thomas JL, Christensen JC, et al. The diagnosis and treatment of heal pain: a clinical practice guideline–revision 2010. J Foot Ankle Surg. 2010;49:S1–19.

Tuomilehto J, Lindström J, et al. Prevention of type 2 diabetes mellitus by changes in lifestyle among subjects with impaired glucose tolerance. N Engl J Med. 2001 May 3;344(18):1343–50.

Tweed JL, Avil SJ, Campbell JA, Barnes MR. Etiologic factors in the development of medial tibial stress syndrome: a review of the literature. J Am Podiatr Med Assoc. 2008;2:107–111.

Visnes H, Bahr R. The evolution of the eccentric training as treatment for patellar tendinopathy (jumper's knee): a critical review of the exercise programs. Br J Sports Med. 2007;41(4):217–223.

Walther M, Kirschner S, Koenig A, et al. Biomechanical evaluation of braces used for the treatment of epicondylitis. J Shoulder Elbow Surg. 2002;11:265–270.

Wheeler P, Batt ME. Do non-steroidal anti-inflammatory drugs adversely affect stress fracture healing? A short review. Br J Sports Med. 2005;39:65–69.

Wilson JJ, Best TM. Common overuse tendon problems: a review and recommendations for treatment. Am Fam Physician. 2005;72:811–818.

Yeung SS, et al. Interventions for preventing lower limb soft-tissue running injuries. Cochrane Database Syst Rev. 2011;(7):CD001256.

Zhang M, Izumi I, Kagamimori S, et al. Role of taurine supplementation to prevent exercise-induced oxidative stress in healthy young men. Amino Acids. 2004;26(2):203–207.

7

Traditional Chinese Medicine

JANET KONEFAL, EDUARD TIOZZO, AND JOHN E. LEWIS

Introduction

E ver since the introduction of acupuncture in the United States in the early 1970s, professional interest and consumer demand for this form of complementary medicine has been growing steadily and becoming a more relevant component of our country's health care. Today, approximately 3,500 physicians and 15,000 licensed acupuncturists or certified licensed health professionals practice this form of treatment. The most recent reports also estimate that 5% to 10% of adult Americans have had lifetime acupuncture use, with men reporting lower use than women (Burke et al., 2006). Given that men have fewer health care visits, adopt fewer health-promoting behaviors, report fewer symptoms of physical and mental illness, and rate their health better than women, it is not surprising that they also seek acupuncture treatments less than women. Furthermore, clinical research can be a critical aspect of how any medical treatment is accepted by society. In the United States, research on men's health concerns are underfunded, and statistically women have outnumbered men in intramural- and extramural-funded clinical research every year for the past two decades. Additionally, although acupuncture was recognized by the National Health Institute in 1997, the majority of clinical trials are still largely funded and performed outside of the United States. In one recent meta-analysis conducted by a group of American and British scientists, only 15% of the acupuncture trials included in the analysis were conducted in the United States (Manheimer et al., 2005). Furthermore, only a limited number of acupuncture studies have been subjected to rigorous scientific investigation, and specific countries like China and Russia have almost 100% positive results and rarely report acupuncture treatments to be equal or inferior to other treatments

(Vickers et al., 1998). In addition, acupuncture is not a uniform system of treatment and it has developed different styles and procedures throughout the world. For example, traditional Chinese medicine relies greatly on observational skills in the diagnosis, including pulse variations and tongue coatings, whereas German acupuncture greatly enhanced the use of auricular acupuncture, which focuses on points in the ear and relies on electrical measurements of the points to determine diagnosis and treatment. Also, some methods of acupuncture, such as Japanese and Chinese, use the full body for treatment and vary in the diameter of the needles and the direction of the insertions or the intensity of the needling. On the contrary, Korean acupuncture tends to focus on the points on the hands and may use needles or magnets to stimulate points, whereas the general practice of auricular acupuncture focuses on points in the ear and may be used alone or in conjunction with body points.

The most modern theory of the mechanism of acupuncture is that the stimulation activates the fascia network, which has similarities to the accepted meridian or pathway model in acupuncture (Bai et al., 2011). It is only with the newest methods of examining the physiology of the body that we can begin to understand the response to stimulation of the acupuncture points. For example, research has demonstrated that sticking an acupuncture needle into a point in the hand greatly diminishes the amount of brain activity associated with pain impulses (Napadow et al., 2012).

In conclusion, different styles and procedures lead to different training requirements and skills, particularly in the United States. Consequently, all these factors make it difficult to interpret and compare the data from different acupuncture trials. Without consistency among treatment protocols and because different treatments can sometimes be used for the same symptom, it cannot be concluded that acupuncture does not work for a certain condition but rather that the set of points used in the study does not work for the condition.

More importantly, and considering the present limitations of the acupuncture research, what are the practical implications of acceptable findings for men's health?

Acupuncture for Chronic Symptoms and Diseases

In the hands of a competent practitioner, acupuncture is very safe. The most common side effects include local pain from needling and slight bleeding or hematoma. According to a World Health Organization report, the incidence of serious adverse events from acupuncture is 0.024%, which concluded that only in extremely rare cases can acupuncture lead to serious complications such as hospital admission, organ trauma, or death. Furthermore, its proven applications in primary care, pain management, oncology, and community-based HIV care and substance abuse treatments have yielded very promising results (Burke et al., 2006).

According to the American Physical Therapy Association, 61% of Americans experience *lower back pain*, with men being more likely than women to report impaired ability to work because of it. Furthermore, the same musculoskeletal problem is the leading reason for visits to licensed acupuncturists. Compared to standard care, acupuncture treatment can significantly improve chronic back pain and bodily function. Furthermore, the amount of self-reported medications has been reported to decrease during acupuncture therapy and, interestingly, has remained lower 1 year after (Cherkin et al., 2009). Even though the reports have shown no evidence that acupuncture is more effective than other nonsurgical treatments commonly used for low back pain (e.g., spinal manipulation and therapeutic massage), it can be concluded that this complementary therapy is safe and effective treatment for short- and long-term relief of chronic low back pain.

Depression is recognized as a major public health problem affecting close to 10% of American adults. This common mental health disorder is frequently associated with feelings of powerlessness and diminished control, often making men perceive depression as a sign of weakness and failure. For various sociocultural reasons, men are more likely to hide their symptoms and avoid seeking help, making it harder for clinicians to identify and diagnose the presence of their clinical depression. What can men expect if they decide to treat depression with acupuncture alone or in combination with antidepressants? Scientists are still reserved about the evidence and benefits of acupuncture in the management of depression, and they appeal for more full-scale clinical trials. However, several well-designed studies have shown that acupuncture can significantly reduce the symptoms of major depression, making it perhaps more effective in treating major rather than mild to moderate depression (Wang et al., 2008).

Insomnia is estimated to affect 35% to 40% of the American adult population, and women report sleeplessness more frequently than men. However, a recent comparison of stress levels over the last 25 years revealed that stress has increased more among American men than women (24% vs. 18%). In addition, men consistently report experiencing more stress associated with work and finances. Stress and insomnia appear to be pathophysiologically integrated, and finding optimal therapeutic interventions for insomnia in both genders should be equally relevant. Any individual with insomnia can have suppressed nocturnal production of melatonin, a hormone released by the brain, consequently resulting in a disruption of sleep/wake cycles. In a preliminary study, 18 patients with insomnia accompanied by anxiety experienced a nocturnal increase in melatonin secretion and improved sleep time and sleep efficiency after 5 weeks of acupuncture (Spence et al., 2004). Several other studies have confirmed similar findings, suggesting that acupuncture, as a treatment that relies on the release of neurochemicals involved in sleep patterns, can represent a safe and effective therapy for sleep problems.

A growing number of trials have examined the benefits of acupuncture on *male sexual health* such as absent or low sperm count (i.e., azoospermia and oligospermia), nonorganic erectile dysfunction (ED), and premature ejaculation (PE). In these trials and the majority of others, one cycle of acupuncture consisted of two weekly sessions, each usually 30 minutes in duration, for up to 8 weeks. In several studies, as many as 70% of patients with azoospermia or oligospermia had improved their sperm fraction and viability when compared with the numbers before acupuncture, resulting also in a 25% improved fertilization rate after the treatment (Zhang et al., 2002). Nonorganic ED, a condition that affects 15 to 20 million American men, is usually related to psychological problems such as stress, anxiety, depression, and personal issues. In one clinical trial, the curative effect of acupuncture was reported by 68% of the patients, with only 10% not reporting any improvements (Engelhardt et al., 2003). Finally, it is estimated that 20% to 30% of the male population suffers from PE, which represents the most prevalent form of male sexual dysfunction. The effective rate of acupuncture on PE has been reported to be as high as 82%, and in one trial it was more effective than a selective serotonin reuptake inhibitor (SSRI), a class of drugs initially designed to relieve depression and now widely used for other conditions such as migraine headaches, fibromyalgia, and diabetic neuropathy (Sunay et al., 2011). All these numbers suggest that acupuncture can be a valid option, or at least an effective adjuvant treatment, for an array of male sexual problems and perhaps other conditions related to neurotransmitters. Thus, more research is warranted as acupuncture is low risk with almost no negative side effects.

Various *prostate diseases*, such as an infected/inflamed and enlarged prostate gland (i.e., prostatitis and benign prostatic hypertrophy), and prostate cancer are among the biggest health threats in men worldwide. For example, in 2008, more men were diagnosed with this form of cancer than women with breast cancer. In addition, it has been estimated that one in six men will be diagnosed with prostate cancer during his lifetime, making prostate cancer the second leading cause of cancer death among American men. Several studies have shown that acupuncture can be effective in alleviating pain and voiding symptoms and improving quality of life associated with prostatitis. In a study of 360 prostatitis patients treated with acupuncture, 89% of prostatitis cases were cured, 10% improved, and only 1% failed treatment. More interestingly, the marked improvements of acupuncture can be seen posttreatment for the same duration as the treatment itself (Chen and Nickel, 2003). Currently, different types of hormone therapies (e.g., androgen deprivation therapy) are used to fight prostate cancer and their main goal is to reduce the amount of male hormones (e.g., testosterone) to reduce tumor cell growth. However, the same therapy may result in hormone imbalances, often leading to hot flashes, which have been reported in up to 80% of men on androgen therapy. Acupuncture treatments can be very effective in reducing the amount of hot flashes, with a 70% reduction after 10 weeks and a 50% reduction even 3 months after the last treatment being reported (Hammar et al., 1999). In conclusion, the existing literature indicates that acupuncture might be an active nonpharmacological option for patients with prostate diseases and their associated reduced quality of life.

The effect of acupuncture has also been studied in individuals infected with *HIV*, perhaps more frequently before and in the early stages of antiretroviral medications that have now become the standard of care and have greatly improved the prognosis of HIV-infected individuals. The results of the available studies have been inconclusive for the pain measures associated with damage to peripheral nerves (i.e., peripheral neuropathy), a neurological disorder that affects one in three HIV-positive persons. However, it seems that this complementary treatment may have positive effects on general health and well-being in this patient population. More specifically, acupuncture may improve mortality rate, particularly of HIV-infected patients with poorer health (Shiflett and Schwartz, 2011).

Despite a paucity of acupuncture research in the military and veteran population and the fact that its practice in most hospitals—both conventional and military—is yet to be adopted, acupuncture and other related techniques have been gaining a prominent role over the last two decades in military medical practice. As a result, the military has established an acupuncture training program for its physicians to not only treat military personnel at home but also implement this treatment in war zones. A few well-designed acupuncture studies have shown promising results in treating pain and *posttraumatic stress disorder* (PTSD), two of the most prevalent conditions in the military and veteran population (York et al., 2011). Therefore, acupuncture can serve as an effective tool, bridging a whole-person healing approach and conventional medicine in this patient population.

Finally, several national studies on gender-related travel differences have indicated that men still dominate the business travel market. Although men traveled more for business- and work-related reasons, women traveled more for leisure purposes. However, regardless of the travel reasons, one can still experience *jet lag* (i.e., desynchronosis). This physiological condition, as a result of rapid long-distance travel (West–East or East–West) on an airplane, is the most noticeable in the first 24 to 48 hours. Symptoms may include headaches, insomnia, loss of appetite, irritability, diarrhea or constipation, poor coordination, and reduced cognitive skills. Reports suggest that it may take an individual 1 day per one time zone crossed to fully recover. In other words, if a businessman crosses six time zones for a 6-day trip, his body may not fully recover by the time he is boarding his return flight. Over the years dozens of experiments, but not randomized and controlled trials, were conducted on acupuncture and jet lag with a high success rate. More specifically, a recent informal study reported that a control group traveling from the United States to China experienced jet lag symptoms lasting from 3 days to 2 weeks, whereas the experimental group receiving acupuncture did not report any jet lag–related problems and could perform at normal levels immediately.

Acupuncture and Sports Performance

With increased *sports injuries* in recreational and organized sports, there is a high need for their effective rehabilitation. Conventional treatment for musculoskeletal injuries includes ultrasound and manual therapies, such as massage, manipulation, and stretch rehabilitation techniques. Similar to general health, the role of acupuncture in the treatment of sports injuries is not new, but its clinical potential is yet to be fully established.

Generally, men (and women) of all fitness levels experience muscle pain (e.g., delayed-onset muscle soreness [DOMS]). DOMS is accompanied by pain and discomfort 1 to 3 days after exercise following a period of reduced or no activity or involving exercises with increased intensity, longer duration, or novel movements. In many individuals a class of over-the-counter drugs (i.e., nonsteroidal anti-inflammatory drugs), such as aspirin and ibuprofen, represent the first treatment to fight DOMS, risking an array of mild to severe side effects. Athletes undergoing acupuncture treatments can expect reduced perceived pain from exercise-induced muscle soreness, which can consequently facilitate more rapid recovery and reduced risk of sport injuries (Hubscher et al., 2008).

Similar findings, also relevant for rehabilitation programs, have been reported on acupuncture and muscle strength. It appears that even a single acupuncture treatment can be effective in improving muscle strength in recreational athletes by as much as 8% (Hubscher et al., 2010). Future studies should reveal if this complementary therapy as an adjunct to exercise rehabilitation could enhance the recovery process of the patients experiencing long-term bed rest and associated impaired neuromuscular function by helping them regain their strength and quality of life more rapidly.

Furthermore, acupuncture therapy appears to demonstrate positive prognosis in other sports injuries such as femoral adductors syndrome, an injury of the inner thigh muscles that affects athletes whenever there is a sudden change of direction during running; ankle sprains; plantar fasciitis, a painful inflammation of the sole of the foot often induced by running and jumping; rotator cuff tendinitis, irritation, inflammation, and swelling of shoulder tendons that does not spare either active or sedentary individuals; patellofemoral pain syndrome, pain in and around the knee cap; and tibial stress syndrome, also called shin splints, which, similarly to plantar fasciitis, affects individuals in running and jumping sports.

Acupuncture and Addictions

With a few exceptions, acupuncture trials in addictions have not provided a level of evidence sufficient to make firm recommendations based on the study findings. However, even though it is premature to confirm or disconfirm the efficacy of acupuncture in the treatment of addictions, it appears that this form of therapy can still provide significant synergistic benefits. In other words, when integrated with standard psychosocial modalities in addiction treatment such as group and education therapies or pharmacological approaches, acupuncture can enhance the efficacy of the same protocols.

Currently, the United States is experiencing some of the highest rates of *drug addiction* than at any time in its history. Furthermore, men are more likely to use cocaine than women, and nearly half of all drug-related emergency room visits are related to cocaine abuse. Treatment of cocaine addiction is complex and must address a variety of psychobiological, social, and pharmacological aspects. When added to weekly coping skills and methadone treatment, "true" acupuncture can result in less cocaine abuse and a higher percent of cocaine-free urine screens (54%) compared to the same treatment combined with "sham" acupuncture (24%), after a 2-month treatment (Margolin, 2003).

Smoking, another form of addiction, still represents the leading preventable cause of death and, together with physical inactivity and poor eating habits, accounts for one third of all deaths in the country. In addition, men smoke more than women. Similar to cocaine studies, the synergistic effects of acupuncture have been reported in smoking trials. If "true" acupuncture is combined with a smoking cessation education program, it can help more smokers (40%) remain smoke free for 1 month after a 5-week treatment intervention. Conversely, the same education program combined with "sham" acupuncture results in lower abstinence rates (22%) (Margolin, 2003).

Finally, *alcohol* represents the number one drug problem in the country. Robust literature findings suggest that men drink more and have more alcohol-related problems than women. Interestingly, studies also indicate that fewer adults with alcohol abuse and addiction are getting treatments than in the past. However, both individual and synergistic effects of acupuncture on alcoholism have not been well documented. Some argue that standard care in a few well-designed studies was too comprehensive and effective, thus not leaving enough additional impact for improvement with the acupuncture protocols.

Acupuncture and Other Diagnostic Tools

A visit to a licensed acupuncturist includes diagnostic tools often specific to acupuncture to help guide the treatment. The pulse and tongue represent very important assessment tools in Chinese medicine by providing a great deal of information about the human body. Even though pulse can be used to gain a deep understanding of the patient on many levels, pulse diagnosis often takes years of practice to master. Observations of the tongue may be easier to assess because it is less meridian specific and less affected by short-term influences such as nervousness. Tongue diagnosis and clinical examination include geography and meridian correlations, where the tip of the tongue corresponds to the lung and the heart, the middle to the stomach and spleen, the sides to the liver and gallbladder, and the base to the kidney, urinary bladder, and gastrointestinal tract. The additional tongue examination also entails tongue colors, shapes, and coating. The normal tongue in traditional Chinese medicine has a light red or pinkish body with a thin white coating, and any degree or type of deviation can indicate a specific disharmony in the body.

Acupressure

In situations where acupuncture is not accessible or affordable and a treatment for lower back pain, headache, anxiety, cold, or flu is needed quickly, one can find relief in acupressure, an ancient Chinese medicine technique derived from acupuncture. Instead of using needles to stimulate certain points, acupressure utilizes pressure from the fingers, hands, elbows, or manual devices. This self-treatment, which can also be applied by another person, is actually similar to the traditional massage procedure where specific points are pressed and rubbed down in a circular motion continuously for 30 seconds up to 10 minutes. How does acupressure work? Pressing specific points on the body that are sensitive to bioelectrical impulses causes the body to release endorphins, which are neurochemicals that help inhibit the pain signals sent to the brain. At the same time, stimulation of the points causes an increase in blood flow and therefore enhanced availability of nutrients and oxygen and the removal of the by-products in tense and painful areas. As a result of bioelectrical and blood energy circulating more efficiently, acupressure can alleviate pain and help the body fight symptoms and illnesses.

There are hundreds of acupressure points on the body; we are including four commonly used for headache, nausea, abdomen pain, and anxiety.

- The large intestine 4 (LI-4 or "union valley") point is located on the top side of the hand, between the thumb and index finger. LI-4 can alleviate headache or any other problems on the face (rhinitis, acne, allergies, toothache, etc.). However, pregnant women should never use this point without professional guidance.
- The pericardium 6 (P6 or "inner gate") point is located two or three finger widths from the wrist and in the grove between the two large tendons. P6 can be effectively used to control nausea and prevent vomiting.
- The liver 3 (LV3 or "great surge") point is located on the top of the foot, between the first and second metatarsal bones. LV3 can be successfully used to alleviate digestive (constipation, diarrhea, irritable bowel syndrome, etc.) and menstrual issues (cramps and irregular cycles).
- The heart 7 (H7 or "spirit gate") point is located on the most distal crease of the wrist. H7 can help improve emotional issues, especially anxiety and worry.

Conclusion

In the last decades, medical technology has improved diagnostic and therapeutic possibilities dramatically. However, at the same time, a growing number of patients are seeking help outside mainstream biomedicine, choosing complementary and alternative therapies, including acupuncture, to treat a variety of illnesses and to maintain their general health and well-being. Fortunately, more physicians in the United States are following the same trend. Patients also report discussing acupuncture with their conventional medical providers more frequently. Nonetheless, despite its acceptance by the medical establishment, the evidence still suggests that acupuncture has not yet been fully integrated into our health care system (e.g., Germany, a country with four times less population than ours, has 10 times more medical doctors practicing acupuncture). Furthermore, research in acupuncture has increased over the last decade, allowing a consensus that this complementary and alternative medicine therapy may be safe and efficacious treatment, independently or in conjunction with other standard care modalities, for various chronic symptoms and diseases. However, larger randomized and well-designed trials are needed to determine the mechanisms, effectiveness, and durability of acupuncture to provide more evidence for health providers and authorities. Finally, future research should also address and clarify the complex interaction of acupuncture and men's health practices that result in higher injury rates, chronic illnesses, disability, and mortality, when compared to women.

Approved Training Programs for Physicians

The American Board of Medical Acupuncture, established in 2000, currently recognizes six training programs in the United States that meet education and certification standards in acupuncture: University of Miami (Florida), University of Berkley (California), Helms Medical Institute (California), Tri-State College of Acupuncture (New York), SUNY Downstate Medical Center (New York), and Harvard Medical School (Massachusetts).

REFERENCES

Bai Y, Wang J, Wu JP, Dai JX, Sha O, Tai Wai YD, et al. Review of evidence suggesting that the fascia network could be the anatomical basis for acupoints and meridians in the human body. Evid Based Complement Alternat Med. 2011;2011:260510.

Burke A, Upchurch DM, Dye C, Chyu L. Acupuncture use in the United States: findings from the National Health Interview Survey. J Altern Complement Med. 2006;12(7):639–648.

Chen R, Nickel JC. Acupuncture ameliorates symptoms in men with chronic prostatitis/chronic pelvic pain syndrome. Urology. 2003;61(6):1156–1159.

Cherkin DC, Sherman KJ, Avins AL, Erro JH, Ichikawa L, Barlow WE, et al. A randomized trial comparing acupuncture, simulated acupuncture, and usual care for chronic low back pain. Arch Intern Med. 2009;169(9):858–866.

Engelhardt PF, Daha LK, Zils T, Simak R, Konig K, Pfluger H. Acupuncture in the treatment of psychogenic erectile dysfunction: first results of a prospective randomized placebo-controlled study. Int J Impot Res. 2003;15(5):343–46.

Hammar M, Frisk J, Grimas O, Hook M, Spetz AC, Wyon Y. Acupuncture treatment of vasomotor symptoms in men with prostatic carcinoma: a pilot study. J Urol. 1999;161(3):853–856.

Hubscher M, Vogt L, Bernhorster M, Rosenhagen A, Banzer W. Effects of acupuncture on symptoms and muscle function in delayed-onset muscle soreness. J Altern Complement Med. 2008;14(8):1011–1016.

Hubscher M, Vogt L, Ziebart T, Banzer W. Immediate effects of acupuncture on strength performance: a randomized, controlled crossover trial. Eur J Appl Physiol. 2010;110(2):353–358.

Manheimer E, White A, Berman B, Forys K, Ernst E. Meta-analysis: acupuncture for low back pain. Ann Intern Med. 2005;142(8):651–663.

Margolin A. Acupuncture for substance abuse. Curr Psychiatry Rep. 2003;5(5):333–339.

Napadow V, Lee J, Kim J, Cina S, Maeda Y, Barbieri R, et al. Brain correlates of phasic autonomic response to acupuncture stimulation: an event-related fMRI study. Hum Brain Mapp. 2012;34(10)2592–2606.

Shiflett SC, Schwartz GE. Effects of acupuncture in reducing attrition and mortality in HIV-infected men with peripheral neuropathy. Explore (NY). 2011;7(3):148–154.

Spence DW, Kayumov L, Chen A, Lowe A, Jain U, Katzman MA, et al. Acupuncture increases nocturnal melatonin secretion and reduces insomnia and anxiety: a preliminary report. J Neuropsychiatry Clin Neurosci. 2004;16(1):19–28.

Sunay D, Sunay M, Aydogmus Y, Bagbanci S, Arslan H, Karabulut A, et al. Acupuncture versus paroxetine for the treatment of premature ejaculation: a randomized, placebo-controlled clinical trial. Eur Urol. 2011;59(5):765–771.

Vickers A, Goyal N, Harland R, Rees R. Do certain countries produce only positive results? A systematic review of controlled trials. Control Clin Trials. 1998;19(2):159–166.

Wang H, Qi H, Wang BS, Cui YY, Zhu L, Rong ZX, et al. Is acupuncture beneficial in depression: a meta-analysis of 8 randomized controlled trials? J Affect Disord. 2008;111(2–3):125–134.

York A, Crawford C, Walter A, Walter AGJ, Jonas BW, Coeytaux R. Acupuncture research in military and veteran populations: a rapid evidence assessment of the literature. Med Acupuncture. 2011;23(4):229–247.

Zhang M, Huang G, Lu F, Paulus WE, Sterzik K. Influence of acupuncture on idiopathic male infertility in assisted reproductive technology. J Huazhong Univ Sci Technolog Med Sci 2002;22(3):228–230.

8

Ayurveda and Men's Health

WALTER W. MILLS AND RACHEL FREIDMAN

Case Study

"You are having a heart attack. We're going to do an emergency cardiac catheterization in the next 30 minutes."

John was shocked to hear the news from the emergency room physician. Although 56 years old, John thought of himself as health conscious and healthy. He followed a low-fat, mostly vegetarian diet; did 45 minutes of exercise most days; maintained a healthy body mass index of 23; didn't smoke; and moderated his alcohol intake. Moreover, he did not have diabetes, high blood pressure, high cholesterol, or a family history of early heart disease. How could this be happening to him?

Fortunately, after the procedure the doctor told him the good news: "Most of your vessels have only minor cholesterol plaques, and the one that was blocked can be opened with a stent."

John went home a few days later to recuperate and search for answers. His cardiologist and family physician rationalized that "this happens; people like you get heart attacks without good cause," but neither had a good explanation. Both agreed that he should embark on secondary prevention with a statin to reduce cholesterol, an angiotensin-converting enzyme (ACE) inhibitor and a beta blocker for blood pressure, and aspirin for clot prevention. John studied the American Heart Association diet and felt that his current diet was at least as good in terms of the fat, cholesterol, and other recommendations.

looking for answers in ayurveda

Still confused as to how, at his "young age," he had suddenly become a heart patient, John decided to explore a different paradigm of medicine and turned to a doctor who also practiced <u>Ayurveda</u>. After completing a comprehensive lifestyle questionnaire, Dr. Vaidya spent a good deal of time asking John questions that no doctor had ever asked him. John wasn't sure why it was important for the doctor to know what his favorite colors and tastes were, or how he felt and acted under stress. The Ayurvedic doctor then moved on to the physical exam, and John was equally befuddled as to why the doctor spent several minutes just feeling his pulse and closely examined his tongue instead of just asking for the traditional "say ahhh."

"Ayurveda means *Science of Life*," Dr. Vaidya explained. "The most important aspect is to understand who you are, hence the comprehensive evaluation I have just performed. Your constitutional type is predominantly Pitta, or Fire. You are strong, of keen intellect, often with great insight. You are able to use your strong energy, your "fire" to accomplish many things, like becoming the CEO of your business and working endless hours at it. You are passionate and have a warm heart that makes you likeable, but when fatigued you become angry and can even be hostile. You are driven by the clock, and recently have had a fear of 'running out of time' with the economic stress of your company. You have had stressful business relationships, having to fire several influential managers. When you spoke of being fired yourself from a company you were loyal to a decade ago, your face flushed and tightened—you continue to carry what Ayurveda would call 'karma' from that experience. While the event is in the past, your body–mind continue to experience it daily with recurring memories, or 'samscaras.' Your wife and children love you but miss you. In a way you have broken their hearts with your absence working long hours at the office. In fact, with the way you describe your wife, she likely has insomnia and anxiety related to your influence."

John slowly nodded, amazed that this doctor could understand this much from a short interview and an examination of his tongue! Dr. Vaidya concluded: "Your medications will help reduce your chance of a second heart attack, but from an Ayurvedic management perspective we must address the imbalances that birthed the heart disease or you cannot really hope to be healthy."

The Prescription for Perfect Health

After sitting with Dr. Vaidya's assessment for a few moments, John knew there was truth to what he heard. He knew he was very angry, fatigued, and stressed. He couldn't recall when he had last slept 8 hours from 10 PM to 6 AM—a question Dr. Vaidya had specifically asked—nor when he had sat and actually mindfully thought about the food he was eating, nor when he last felt truly happy.

John looked at the evaluation-after-visit summary he had been given by Dr. Vaidya. A lot of it made intuitive sense, which is often the experience of the patient as he or she begins the journey to health using the Ayurvedic paradigm—there is something that feels validating and hopeful about understanding one's place in the world and how to better navigate to a higher state of health and well-being.

John discovered his heart disease before he prematurely died from it. He is fortunate to have embarked on an integrative medicine care plan, adhering to allopathic (Western) medical clinical guidelines while also incorporating the oldest, time-tested model for holistic health: Ayurveda.

Practical Ayurveda

This chapter covers basic Ayurvedic theory and practice for men, aimed at providing usable, evidence-based treatment plans for preventing disease and for common problems. Those wishing for more intensive Ayurvedic interventions should do so with certified Ayurvedic practitioners. We have found that 80% of health benefits can be derived by focusing on 20% of the Ayurvedic technologies—primarily lifestyle and self-awareness. This is available for all at low to no cost, and it is these practices that we will focus on most in this chapter.

History

Most Ayurvedic experts hold it to be the oldest organized system of health, tracing its roots to oral traditions in the Vedic Culture of India about 5,000 years ago. Tibetan medicine, traditional Chinese medicine, even Western Greco-Roman medicine have their roots in Ayurveda. The classical texts of Ayurveda, Charaka Samhita and Sursuta Samhita, are complex and can be overwhelming even to the Ayurvedic medical student. These canonical texts emphasize a *holism* that can form an effective foundation (1) for care avoiding the current pitfalls of our Western, allopathic fragmentary and expeditious symptomatic approach. Ayurveda translates into a 21st-century rational lifestyle intervention approach that can be practiced successfully for men wishing to promote their health.

More than a mere system of treating illness, Ayurveda is a science of life (*Ayur* = "life," *Veda* = "science" or "knowledge"). It offers a body of wisdom designed to help patients stay vital while realizing their full human potential. Providing guidelines on ideal daily and seasonal routines, diet, behavior, and the proper use of the senses, it reminds one that health is the balanced and dynamic integration between our environment, body, mind, and spirit.

Tridosha Theory

According to Ayurveda, there are five master elements or mahabhutas that make up everything within our bodies and everything outside of our bodies: space, air, fire, water, and earth. Space carries all the aspects of pure potentiality—infinite possibilities; air has the qualities of movement and change; fire is hot, direct, and transformational; water is cohesive and protective; and earth is solid, grounded, and stable.

Biological systems weave these five forces into three primary patterns known as doshas. They are most easily thought of as mind–body principles that govern our style of thinking and behaving. Vatadosha, woven from the elements of space and air, regulates movement and change in our minds and bodies. Pittadosha, composed of fire and water, governs digestion and metabolism. Kaphadosha, made from earth and water, maintains and protects the integrity and structure of our mind and body.

All three doshas are present in every cell, tissue, and organ—because movement, metabolism, and protection are essential components of life. What makes life interesting is that although everyone has all three doshas, each of us mixes them together in a unique way, which determines the distinctive qualities of our mind and body.

For each element, there is a balanced (*prakruti*) and imbalanced (*vrikruti*) expression. If Vata is dominant in our system, we tend to be thin, light, enthusiastic, energetic, creative, lively, and changeable. In balance, a Vata person is lively and creative, but when there is too much movement in the system, a person tends to experience anxiety, insomnia, dry skin, constipation, and difficulty focusing. (Dr. Vaidya understood from seeing a photo of John's wife during the interview that she was Vata, and correctly surmised that the stress of living with John had aggravated her constitution, hence his "guess" that insomnia and anxiety were problems for her.)

If Pitta predominates in our nature, we tend to be intense, intelligent, and goal oriented and we have a strong appetite for life. When Pitta is functioning in a balanced manner, a person is warm, friendly, disciplined, a good leader, and a good speaker (hence the gift John has for being a business leader). When

Pitta is out of balance, a person tends to be compulsive and irritable and may suffer from indigestion or an inflammatory condition (Western medicine sees coronary artery disease as more of "fire in the arteries" than mere atherosclerotic inert cholesterol plaque now).

When Kapha prevails, we tend to be easygoing, methodical, and nurturing. Balanced, Kapha people are sweet, supportive, and stable. When Kapha is out of balance, a person may experience sluggishness, weight gain, and sinus congestion (or, as in John's case, depression).

The Ayurvedic Physician's Evaluation

An important goal of Ayurveda is to identify a person's ideal state of balance, determine where the person is out of balance, and offer interventions to re-establish balance. When Dr. Vaidya saw John, the focus was on diagnosing his constitutional type, which was Pitta (Fire). This deep respect for the biological individuality of the patient is a cornerstone for Ayurvedic care. It is important for men to understand that Ayurveda doesn't reject the use of conventional medical treatments. Rather, Ayurveda's central principle is that men should make use of whatever healing modalities will restore health and balance to the body, including herbal remedies, dietary changes, pharmaceutical medications, meditation, exercise, psychotherapy, and so on.

Ayurvedic Approaches to Men's Health Concerns

KEY CONCEPT #1: CONSTITUTIONAL TYPES

Regardless of any man's current health status, the first step in adopting an Ayurvedic plan is to become familiar with one's specific constitutional type (called mind–body type or prakriti). Just as John did during his Ayurvedic consultation, one can easily complete the Dosha Questionnaire and accurately derive a general sense of one's own constitution. Answer the questions in Table 8.1 as honestly as possible and see which element receives the highest score.

This part of the Dosha Questionnaire (Part I, Table 8.1) gathers information about one's basic nature—the way one was as a child or the basic patterns that have been true most of one's life. If you developed an illness in childhood or as

Table 8.1: Part I of the Dosha Questionnaire

Frame	I am thin, lanky, and slender with prominent joints and thin muscles	I have a medium, symmetrical build with good muscle development	I have a large, round, or stocky build. My frame is broad, stout, or thick.
Weight	Low; I may forget to eat or have tendency to lose weight.	Moderate; it is easy for me to gain or lose weight if I put my mind to it.	Heavy; I gain weight easily and have difficulty losing it.
Eyes	My eyes are small and active.	I have a penetrating gaze	I have large pleasant eyes.
Complexion	My skin is dry, rough, or thin.	My skin is warm, reddish in color, and prone to irritation.	My skin is thick, moist, and smooth.
Hair	My hair is dry, brittle, or frizzy.	My hair is fine with a tendency toward early thinning or graying.	I have abundant, thick, and oily hair.
Joints	My joints are thin and prominent and have a tendency to crack.	My joints are loose and flexible.	My joints are large, well knit, and padded.
Sleep Pattern	I am a light sleeper with a tendency to awaken easily.	I am a moderately sound sleeper, usually needing less then 8 hours to feel rested.	My sleep is deep and long. I tend to awaken slowly in the morning.
Body Temperature	My hands are usually cold and I prefer warm environments.	I am usually warm, regardless of the season, and prefer cooler environments.	I am adaptable to most temperatures but do not like cold, wet days.
Temperament	I am lively and enthusiastic by nature. I like to change.	I am purposeful and intense. I like to convince.	I am easygoing and accepting. I like to support.
Under Stress	I become anxious and/or worried.	I become irritable and/or aggressive.	I become withdrawn and/or reclusive.
Your Dosha Type	Vata Score:	Pitta Score:	Kapha Score:

an adult, think of how things were before that illness. If more than one quality is applicable in each characteristic, choose the one that applies most.

For fairly objective physical traits, your choice will usually be obvious. For mental traits and behavior, which are more subjective, you should answer according to how you have felt and acted most of your life, or at least in the past few years.

Now that you have identified your dosha type (Part I), determine whether your current lifestyle sustains and nurtures a balanced mind–body state (Part II, Table 8.2). To achieve and maintain a vibrant and joyful state of health you must live to nurture the dynamic state of balance between mind, body, and environment. These questions are intended to assess your current life situation, including any stresses, illnesses, or life changes.

For Part II of the Dosha Questionnaire (Table 8.2), use the scale to indicate how well each statement applies to your life experiences over the past few months. Answer these questions according to what is most true for you now or since this new stress or pattern has occurred.

Summary of the Dosha Questionnaire

The Dosha Questionnaire gives one an inquiry into the proportion of each of the three principles—Vata, Pitta, and Kapha—within one's unique mind–body constitution. The score in Part I of the Dosha Questionnaire reflects one's basic nature. These characteristics tend to change slowly over our lifetime.

The principle that received the highest number of checks is the most predominant force in one's overall mind–body makeup. The principle that received the next highest number of checks is the secondary force. The lowest scoring principle, while still an active force in the mind–body physiology, is the least dominant in one's particular constitution.

KEY CONCEPT #2: AYURVEDIC PERSPECTIVE ON PATHOPHYSIOLOGY OF DISEASE

The guiding principle of Ayurveda is the interconnection of all things. We aren't simply an isolated collection of atoms and molecules, but an inseparable part of the infinite field of intelligence. From this holistic perspective, health isn't merely the absence of illness or symptoms—it is a higher state of consciousness that allows vitality, well-being, creativity, and joy to flow into our experience.

In contrast, illness is a disruption—a blockage in the flow of energy and information (Sanskrit, *prana*) that creates a sense of separation or alienation

Table 8.2: Part II of the Dosha Questionnaire

Scale: 1 (not at all); 2 (slightly), 3 (somewhat), 4 (moderately), 5 (very)

1	I've been feeling worried or anxious.	1	2	3	4	5
2	I've been having difficulty falling asleep or have been awakening easily.	1	2	3	4	5
3	I've been feeling restless or uneasy.	1	2	3	4	5
4	I've been acting impulsively or inconsistently.	1	2	3	4	5
5	I've been more forgetful than usual.	1	2	3	4	5
Vata Mind Score:						
6	My daily schedule of eating meals, going to sleep, or awakening has been inconsistent from day to day.	1	2	3	4	5
7	My digestion has been irregular with gas or bloating.	1	2	3	4	5
8	My bowel movements have been hard, dry, or occurring less than once per day.	1	2	3	4	5
9	My skin has been dry or flaky.	1	2	3	4	5
10	I've been having a number of physical concerns.	1	2	3	4	5
Vata Body Score:						
11	I've been feeling irritable or impatient.	1	2	3	4	5
12	I've been feeling critical and intolerant.	1	2	3	4	5
13	I've been behaving compulsively with difficulty stopping once I've started a project.	1	2	3	4	5
14	I've been strongly opinionated, freely sharing my point of view without being asked.	1	2	3	4	5
15	I've been feely frustrated with other people.	1	2	3	4	5
Pitta Mind Score:						
16	My skin has felt hot and irritable, or has been breaking out easily.	1	2	3	4	5
17	Spicy foods, while I might enjoy them, have not been agreeing with me.	1	2	3	4	5
18	I've been having acid indigestion or heartburn.	1	2	3	4	5
19	I've been feeling overheated, have had a low-grade fever, or have been having hot flashes.	1	2	3	4	5
20	My bowels have been loose or moving more than twice per day.	1	2	3	4	5
Pitta Body Score:						
21	I've been dealing with conflict by withdrawing.	1	2	3	4	5
22	I've been accumulating more clutter than usual in my life.	1	2	3	4	5

(continued)

Table 8.2: (continued)

Scale: 1 (not at all); 2 (slightly), 3 (somewhat), 4 (moderately), 5 (very)						
23	I've been maintaining my routine and feeling resistant to changing my pace.	1	2	3	4	5
24	I've been having difficulty leaving a relationship, job, or situation even though it is no longer nourishing me.	1	2	3	4	5
25	I've been spending more time watching than participating in athletic activities.	1	2	3	4	5
Kapha Mind Score:						
26	I've been holding on to extra pounds.	1	2	3	4	5
27	I've been having difficult getting going in the morning.	1	2	3	4	5
28	My digestion has been slow, or I've been feeling heavy after a meal.	1	2	3	4	5
29	I've had sinus congestion or excessive phlegm in my respiratory tract.	1	2	3	4	5
30	I've been feeling drowsy or sluggish after meals.	1	2	3	4	5
Kapha Body Score:						

from the field. *Ama*, the toxic residue of undigested experiences, blocks the flow of *prana* in the *srotas* (channels of energy flow). Symptoms and sickness are the body's signal that we need to restore balance, eliminate whatever is causing the blockages, and re-establish the healthy flow of energy and information.

Ayurveda teaches that the seeds of disease are usually sown long before there are physical manifestations the patient and doctor can detect. John's heart attack was years, even decades in development. Western medicine can now detect fatty streaks, plaque, and even more subtle aspects of endothelial dysfunction long before there is a coronary thrombosis/ heart attack. Ayurveda's language describes a process where the doshas (Sanskrit, "impurity") are aggravated, then accumulate, and eventually disrupt one's psychophysiology into a recognized disease. The prevention and health-promoting programs of Ayurveda focus on eliminating the aggravated state and thus avoiding disease. This speaks to the subjective experience of patients who aren't diagnosed with a specific disease state, but don't report feeling well and vital. If John had seen Dr. Vaidya prior to the heart attack all his Western tests would have been "normal," but from an Ayurvedic diagnostic perspective the imbalances and prescription would have been obvious, as the "seeds" of the "dis-ease" would have been appreciated already.

Beyond the scope of this chapter are more complete descriptions of Ayurveda anatomy and physiology, which include the Agnis (digestive fires), Datus (various tissues), marmas (local junction points between anatomy and physiology closely corresponding to the meridian points of acupuncture), srotas (channels that transport energy in the body that when blocked can cause dysfunction), and 15 subdoshas (which give rise to increasingly interesting mind–body typologies).

KEY CONCEPT #3: AYURVEDA GUIDING PRINCIPLES

Ayurveda teaches that the mind has the greatest influence in directing the body toward sickness and health. Thousands of years before modern medicine "discovered" the mind–body connection, the ancient sages had mastered it. They developed Ayurveda as a system for contacting our own inner intelligence (or mind), bringing it into balance, and then extending that balance to the body.

Practical Ayurveda: Design Your Own Unique Self-Care Plan

With a little ayurvedic theory, one is able to engage in lifestyle programs that are more accurately tailored to one's constitution (Part I) and current state of balance (Part II). In contrast with conventional biomedical models, which focus on difference among disease, ayurveda is interested in the unique qualities of individuals, respecting that disease differs because people are unique. There may be 10 to 15 types of hypertension in ayurveda based on the specific imbalances in one's physiology that are causing the elevated blood pressure; similarly, there are numerous "types" of diabetes, asthma, heart disease, and so forth based on the individual constitutional type and specific state of imbalance.

Ayurveda teaches that all health-related measures—whether an exercise program, dietary plan, or herbal supplement—should be based on an understanding of an individual's unique mind–body constitution or *dosha*. By knowing a patient's dosha, an Ayurvedic doctor can tell which diet, physical activities, and medical therapies are most likely to help, and which might do no good or even cause harm.

Thus, Dr. Vaidya's prescription for John focused on his Pitta (Fire) constitution and predominately Pitta imbalance. Had John's constitutional diagnosis been Kapha (Earth) or Vata (Air), Dr. Vaidya's treatment plan would have been different.

Here is what John's evaluation's-after-visit summary said:

Your Ayurvedic After-Visit Summary and Care Plan

John, your mind–body type is Pitta-Kapha. This constitutional diagnosis should inform your choices in the future. We will talk more specifics next visit.

Your imbalance show scores of Physical Vata 6; Pitta 9; Kapha 11; your Mental Vata is 6, Pitta 15, Kapha 14. This tells us where to focus, with the high Mental imbalance in Pitta being the most important. Many men experience depression after a heart attack, and the high Kapha means that you already have major risk for this.

For the next 2 weeks I recommend:

Pitta/fire needs to be reduced in your system as it is out of balance and the leading dosha for the inflammation that generated your most pressing health problems

Kapha/earth is aggravated, mostly as a result of your dealing with increased Pitta (and Vata/air) over the past years. Since your heart attack there has been more Kapha accumulation, experienced as lack of energy and depression.

Invoke Your Inner Pharmacy

The first step in regaining balance is to recognize that the environment around you has a profound influence on how you feel. Paying conscious attention to what you hear, touch, see, taste, and smell can help create peace, balance, and vitality in your mind and body. A harmonized daily routine that engages the five senses with nourishing impressions is one of the most important steps toward achieving Perfect Health.

Accumulated Pitta

Out-of-balance Pitta leads to irritability, aggravation, and inflammation. Balancing Pitta requires opening up some space during your day so you are not perpetually generating friction. Think soothing and cooling. Here are some tips to maximize balance and well-being:

Mind

Meditate twice a day to calm the mind and soothe the body.
Find time each day to unplug and relax.

Wear soothing fragrances.
Listen to medium-tempo melodies.
Minimize heavy reading, eating, or watching TV right before bed.
Diffuse soothing fragrances into your environment.
Favor cool and soft colors—blues, greens, and white.
Spend time each day communing with nature.

Accumulated Kapha

Out-of-balance Kapha leads to heaviness, sluggishness, and congestion. Stimulation and movement help overcome the resistance of accumulated Kapha. Think activation and invigoration. Here are some tips to maximize balance and well-being:

Body

Take a yoga class to connect to your body and invoke your natural energy.
Perform a vigorous daily self-massage with invigorating herbalized oil.
Take deep breaths throughout the day.
Favor spicy foods with a predominance of pungent, bitter, and astringent tastes.
Walk 5 to 15 minutes after eating to aid digestion.
Drink invigorating tea.
Put your full attention on your meals when eating.
See me in 2 weeks for further follow-up.

Basic Ayurvedic Preventive Care Toolbox for Men

These basic recommendations are relevant for men at all stages of health and form a basic lifestyle prescription.

HONOR YOUR DAILY BIORHYTHMS

Ayurveda appreciated the daily and seasonal influences on our physiology long before modern science described chronobiology (e.g., circadian rhythm, the daily rise and fall of cortisol, etc.). Vata is more pronounced in the environment and, by extension, in our physiology between 2 and 6 o'clock in the morning and afternoon; Pitta between 10 and 2 o'clock, midday and midnight; Kapha from 6 to 10 o'clock each morning and evening. Respecting this rhythm can have profound positive effects on our physiology. Disruption of this rhythm, as occurs with shiftwork and night workers, can have profound negative effects; studies suggest that shift workers have increased risk of high blood pressure, heart disease, and even cancer.

GET ENOUGH SLEEP

The general recommendation for ideal health is to sleep by 10 PM and arise by 6 AM (Vata may need less sleep; Kapha may need more). Often one notices a natural drowsiness by 9 or 10 PM and, if not asleep, may have a "second" wind and be stimulated to stay awake as a result of the increased quality of Pitta (activity).

EAT YOUR LARGEST MEAL AT LUNCH

Taking time to mindfully consume the larger meal of the day at midday respects the increased Pitta/fire and metabolic principle, enhancing digestion and increasing energy. If still awake at midnight, the "midnight snack" urge would be predicted by Pitta influence at that time of night.

EXERCISE EARLY AND WITH JOY

Five thousand years ago, the master Ayurvedic physician Charaka wrote, "From physical exercise, one gets lightness, a capacity for work, firmness, tolerance of difficulties, elimination of impurities, and stimulation of digestion." Exercise is best in the morning when the Kapha principle dominates (Kapha benefits from movement that balances its natural tendency for inertia, being of "earth"). Exercising should be mild (walking, yoga) or avoided in the late afternoon (by stirring the already movement-oriented Vata qualities) or evening (when Kapha is settling and preparing for sleep). Physical exercise, "Vyayama," is aimed at reducing stress and imbalance. Therapeutic movement can include yoga (asanas), walking, tai chi, swimming, dance, "play," and so forth. The intent of exercise is to generate a feeling of lightness and joy. Fundamental to the Ayurveda exercise prescription is that the amount and intensity be "half of a man's capacity (ardashaktivyayama) and not stressful."

LEARN YOGA AND BREATHWORK FOR MIND–BODY BALANCE

HathaYoga (postures), Pranayama, and meditation are some of the best Ayurvedic techniques for improving mind–body coordination. Daily practice is best, especially for Vata. Gentle yoga for Vata and more vigorous for Kapha is recommended.

Pranayama, the ayurvedic science of breathing, is easy to learn and practice. Three to five minutes of deep "belly" breathing can benefit any dosha. Alternate-nostril breathing is relaxing and balancing. Some techniques are directed at specific doshas and/or areas of the body (marmas, localized areas of energy networks in the body–mind). *Measured breathing is one of the simplest techniques to start.*

Measured breathing: (a) sit quietly, preferably with eyes closed if comfortable; (b) breath in through the nose counting to 4 silently (about one count per second); (c) hold the breath to a count of 7; (d) exhale to a count of 8; (e) repeat for three to 10 cycles; (f) sit quietly for another minute before returning to your activity.

SENSORY MODULATION

Ayurveda sees us metabolizing our environmental experience through our five senses.

Hearing: sounds should be pleasant with specific recommendations for Ghandarva Veda music. "Stirring music" would be good for Kapha, soothing/calm music wise for Vata, and a mix for Pitta.

Touch: Self-massage done with appropriately prepared oils is called Abyanga and can be done in a few minutes. Classic oils are sesame for Vata, coconut for Pitta, dry for Kapha (or ayurvedic massage done during *panchakarma*, a more advanced form of "physical therapy" not addressed in this chapter).

Sight: colors should fit with our dosha: blue for Vata, green for Pitta, red for Kapha.

Taste: There are five tastes, sweet, sour, salty, bitter, pungent, astringent. Each taste affects the doshas. Sweet, sour, salty tastes tend to bring aggravated Vata into balance, whereas they will aggravate Kapha. Pitta is best balanced with bitter, sweet, and astringent tastes. Kapha balance prefers pungent, bitter, and astringent.

Smell: aromatherapies are made to specifically influence the doshas.

LET FOOD BE YOUR MEDICINE

Entire volumes are written about the ayurvedic diet, as in Ayurveda there is the belief that we are what we eat. Tastes largely guide dosha-specific recommendations along with other food qualities. Vata would prefer warm or hot, more oily, heavier foods to complement/balance Vata's lighter, colder qualities of air/space; Pitta prefers cooler, milder foods (think, spicy/hot foods would aggravate "fire"); Kapha would benefit from light, dryer, hot foods (earth being heavy, moist, cool qualities of Kapha and balanced by opposites).

SIMPLIFIED DAILY ROUTINE

Ayurvedic recommendations can become so complex that it's stressful just to try to follow them! Yet Ayurveda should feel natural, simple, and easy. The following are seven simple pearls that capture the power of a simple daily routine.

1. Take time each day to quiet your mind (meditate).
2. Eat a colorful, flavorful diet.
3. Engage in daily exercise that enhances flexibility, strength, and cardiovascular fitness.
4. Sleep soundly at night.
5. Eliminate what is not serving you.
6. Cultivate loving, nurturing relationships.
7. Perform work that awakens your passion.

Topics Specific to Men

Remember that for all men's issues, Ayurveda emphasizes holistic medicine, treating men not as isolated individuals but as an inextricable part of the whole universe. Derived from India's ancient Vedic tradition, Ayurveda sees an underlying intelligence that flows through and connects everyone and everything in the universe. It sees life as the exchange of energy and information between individuals and their extended body—the environment. If a man's environment is nourishing, he will thrive; if his environment is toxic, he may become sick. Therefore, learning how to eliminate toxicity (*ama*) and surround one with a healing environment is a key to health.

PROSTATE HEALTH

About 90% of men over the age of 85 have evidence of benign prostatic hypertrophy (BPH), manifested by symptoms such as weak stream, hesitancy, and increased frequency of urination, especially at night. Because these problems occur during the phase of life when Vata is dominant, Ayurveda views prostate problems as largely related to excess Vata. Other factors that the classic Ayurvedic scriptures implicate in an enlarged prostate include habitually ignoring the urge to urinate, consuming too much meat or wine, and overindulging in sex (Khalsa & Tierra, 2009). Recent observations support the caution around meat; epidemiological studies of men in Japan show increased risk for BPH with increased consumption of meat and dairy products.

As with most disease conditions, Ayurvedic treatment of BPH addresses the underlying root cause rather than just treating the symptoms. As such, the treatment approach usually includes herbs and other treatments to balance disordered Vata. Warming foods like barley and soup are nourishing. Ensuring proper bowel function, whether with diet, herbal suppositories, or medicated enemas, will support the proper downward direction of Vata movement.

BPH may involve imbalances of the other doshas as well; Kapha excess might lead to a boggy, wet, swollen prostate, and Pitta excess would manifest as inflamed prostate tissue. Treatment should therefore be designed around the specific underlying imbalance.

ERECTILE DYSFUNCTION

One in four men over the age of 50 and up to half of all men by age 80 will experience some form of impotence. Caused by chronic conditions like diabetes, hypertension, and atherosclerosis, erectile dysfunction (ED) can also be caused by stress, fatigue, or prescription medication. Like prostate issues, erectile dysfunction is seen in Ayurveda as disorder of Vata, a misdirected movement of energy upward instead of downward in the pelvis; therefore, relieving any associated constipation is similarly critical.

Khalsa and Tierra cite garlic as the top aphrodisiac herb (2009), said to increase desire, circulation, and erectile force in large doses—up to 10 g/day. Other foods that exert similar effects at tempering Vata while increasing Pitta include onions, asparagus, okra, and ginger.

Ashwaganda root (Withaniasomniferum), also called Indian ginseng, is one of the most used herbs in Ayurveda; while used for a variety of Vata-aggravated conditions, it may be helpful as a sexual tonic in the case of decreased libido or erectile dysfunction. Some studies suggest a mild testosterone-like effect.

More than any specific herb or tonic, however, the most important treatment for erectile dysfunction or low libido is overall lifestyle balancing:

1. Get sufficient sleep (at least 8 hours a night).
2. Practice yoga and do daily exercise to manage stress.
3. Avoid alcohol, tobacco, and drugs.
4. Avoid hot, pungent, and bitter foods.
5. Massage with an herbal oil, ideally one infused with aphrodisiac or relaxing herbs.

MENTAL HEALTH: DEPRESSION/ANXIETY

Suicide kills 2.2% of men. Although suicide is attempted more by women, men are more likely to succeed. A man's suicide risk peaks in his 20s, and then later in his 60s and 70s, and is even greater if he is unemployed, socially isolated, or chronically ill.

Western medicine has tended to treat the symptoms of disease, whereas Ayurveda seeks to eliminate illness by treating the underlying cause. For example, for a patient suffering from depression, an allopathic physician would likely prescribe a standard course of antidepressants and, perhaps, therapy.

Using Ayurvedic skill to complement treatment, a physician would search for root imbalances contributing to the patient's depression, seeing the patient as a whole, taking into consideration his lifestyle, activities, diet, recent stressful events, beliefs, and mind–body constitution. For example, usually major depression has significant Kapha (earth) imbalances, though Vata (air) can be quite aggravated as well, hence causing the agitation/anxiety often seen in depression. The Ayurvedic practitioner takes all of these factors into account when developing the treatment plan.

Ayurvedic Herbs Traditionally Used in Men's Health

Ayurveda has thousands of rasayanas (i.e., herbs and supplements) that are prescribed. The past few decades have provided some early scientific research that allows evidence-based recommendations. Science has also demonstrated that safety when using herbs is required. Some Ayurvedic herbs have been found to have significant amounts of lead. Reputable sources for Ayurvedic herbs are available. There are thousands of herbs in the Ayurvedic pharmacopeia. Some of the more popular, which we will not be able to detail, include *Boswellia, ginger, Gota Kola, Guddichi, Guggala,* and *Shatavari.* Excellent resources that provide evidence for these and other herbs are the Natural Medicine Database and the references in the following sections.

The following six herbs account for some of the most commonly used and best studied for men.

ASHWAGANDHA

The name of the Ashwagandha (*Withania somnifera*) shrub roughly translates as "strength of a horse." Its roots have been medicinally used for thousands of years. In classical Ayurveda, the described properties of Ashwagandha include Medhya (promotes intellect and cognitive development), Balya (increases strength and recovery), Rasayana (rejuvenator or life-extending substance), and Nidrajanana (promoter of sleep).

Ashwagandha is used in men to promote energy and stamina without stimulating the heart. As a body-balancing herb, it also addresses insomnia.

Preliminary research suggests Ashwagandha may suppress stress-induced changes of dopamine receptors in the corpus striatum, which may play a role in the development of chronic anxious behaviors (Upton, 2000). Ashwagandha may also have a γ-aminobutyric acid (GABA) mimetic action, which could account for some of its sedating and anticonvulsive properties. This would be in accord with its historical use for insomnia and anxious neurosis (Kulkarni et al., 2008).

Ashwagandha has also been shown to increase production of thyroid hormones T_4 and T_3 while simultaneously increasing hepatic glucose-6-phosphatase activity and reducing hepatic lipid peroxidation in animal models (Panda and Kar, 1998). As we learn more about the comorbidities between hypothyroidism, hypercholesterolemia, and diabetes, Ashwagandha may one day play an important role in the management of these interrelated conditions.

Most commonly, Ashwagandha is dispensed in doses of 500 mg once or twice daily, before meals. Maximal responses are generally seen within 2 to 4 weeks of regular use.

BITTER MELON

Men with prediabetes and diabetes may benefit from bitter melon (*Momordica charantia*). Preliminary evidence suggests bitter melon's hypoglycemic action can be explained through several independent mechanisms: for one, it has been shown to increase peripheral glucose oxidation as well as glucose tolerance and insulin signaling in induced insulin resistance models (Basch et al.,

2003; Sridhar and Vinayagamoorthi, 2008). It also decreases hepatic gluconeogenesis while increasing glycogen synthesis.

Bitter melon increases insulin output from the pancreas, and it also provides a unique compound called polypeptide P, which is an insulin mimetic with a similar structure to bovine insulin (Krawinkel and Keding, 2006).

Bitter melon reduces triglyceride levels in a dose-dependent manner in animal trials (Jayasooriya et al., 2000). Though we don't yet have human data corroborating this effect, animal studies suggest that bitter melon may have a role in reducing cardiovascular risk, particularly in men with diabetes or metabolic syndrome.

Bitter melon products are typically standardized to their constituents, momordicosides and charantin, and usually dispensed in 500- to 600-mg doses, twice daily, following meals. As it does have an insulin mimetic action, it may be necessary to adjust the dose of concurrently prescribed hypoglycemic drugs.

Holy Basil

Also known as Tulsi, holy basil (*Ocimum sanctum*) is actually considered sacred by many people in India. Holy basil's key compounds, including eugenol and caryophyllene, are similar to those found in oregano (*Origanum vulgare*), and it shares the anti-inflammatory, antipyretic, and analgesic actions typical of the oregano family (Godhwani and Vyas, 1987; Padalia and Verma, 2011 and).

In classical Ayurveda, holy basil was used as an antitussive (cough) to clear "excess dampness in the lungs." Recent human trials have validated this, with data showing that this herb can increase lung capacity as well as reduce labored breathing.

It has also been shown to significantly reduce several measures of stress in generalized anxiety disorder (GAD) patients.

Holy basil can be taken in capsule, tea, and liquid forms. It is dispensed in 600- to 700-mg doses, twice daily, before meals. Allow 2 to 4 weeks for optimal results.

Turmeric

Turmeric (*Curcuma longa*) is one of Ayurveda's true treasures, being used by yogis for millennia for men's health. Research has shown it may improve brain function, have high antioxidant activity, and regulate inflammation in conditions like rheumatoid arthritis, and may be useful for cancer prevention.

Recent research has shown that turmeric may suppress inflammatory pathways at multiple sites. Turmeric-derived compounds seem to have anti-inflammatory activity by inhibiting cyclooxygenase-2 (COX-2) and prostaglandins while preserving the protective cyclooxygenase-1 (COX-1). This means turmeric may provide an anti-inflammatory effect without the stomach complications sometimes seen with other anti-inflammatory agents.

Turmeric also reduces thromboxane synthesis, meaning it can reduce vasoconstriction as well as platelet aggregation. Turmeric has shown unparalleled antioxidant activity. Although much more data are needed to corroborate the suggestion that turmeric is a cancer preventive, early-stage studies have shown extensive chemopreventive value. It is also a potent growth inhibitor in several tumor cell line studies.

Due to poor bioavailability, it is best to use standardized turmeric extracts, which are available at 95% curcumin content. Conservative dosing starts at 600 to 700 mg once or twice daily, after meals. Some trials have used doses as high as 2 to 3 g/day in chronic conditions.

Triphala

A common element in many Ayurvedic protocols for men, triphala is not one plant, but three. The Sanskrit word actually means "three fruits," (*tri* = "three," *phala* = "fruit"). It represents the combination of *Emblica officinalis,* Belleric myrobalan, and Chebulic myrobalan.

Use of triphala is based on a key tenet of Ayurvedic theory, that disease is most able to take hold when digestion is compromised. As such, two major formulas were created to normalize digestion and prepare the groundwork for overall wellness: triphala and trikatu (see later).

Triphala provides detoxification and digestive correction by promoting peristalsis and providing organ-specific anti-inflammatory action in the lower gastrointestinal (GI) tract. Triphala is most commonly used for men with GI complaints such as bloating, sluggish digestion, food sensitivities, fatigue after meals, or chronic constipation.

Triphala is best used in capsules, standardized to 50% tannins, and at a dose of 500 to 600 mg before each meal (15 to 20 minutes prior is sufficient). Taken consistently, results are generally seen in as little as 2 weeks. However, it may take as long as 4 to 6 weeks to obtain the full therapeutic effect.

Trikatu

A complementary formula to triphala, trikatu means "three peppers" or "three pungents." It is a combination of black pepper (*Piper nigrum*), Indian long pepper (*Piper longum*), and ginger (*Zingiber officinale*). Whereas Triphala treats the lower GI tract, trikatu treats the upper GI tract, where it enhances the "digestive fire" (Agni) necessary for the breakdown of food and absorption of nutrients. Trikatu in Ayurveda is a "warming formula," used to awaken Agni (digestion) and destroy Ama (accumulated waste and toxins).

Trikatu may enhance bioavailability of nutrients, drugs, and supplements, possibly through increasing the production of digestive enzymes and/or enhancement of first-pass hepatic metabolism. Trikatu also seems to promote the assimilation of food through the intestines and normalizes gastric emptying, thereby reducing the tendency toward flatulence and distention while improving overall energy levels and nutritional status.

Trikatu was shown to reduce low-density lipoprotein (LDL) and triglyceride levels in rabbits fed high-fat diets. It also increased cardioprotective high-density lipoprotein (HDL) levels.

Trikatu is best taken in capsule form and is standardized to gingerols and piperine. Similar to triphala, trikatu is usually taken with meals. If used consistently, it gives results in as little as 2 weeks, though the most significant therapeutic results may take 4 to 6 weeks.

Take-Home Action Plan

The ancient roots and modern branches of Ayurveda span the very corners of time itself and are a driving force in the world of natural health care for men. Men who are open to Ayurveda's complementary focus on the mental, physical, emotional, and spiritual dimensions of human experience will find this ancient system of medicine and its well-documented treatments to be profoundly effective. Any man can use this chapter to start his Ayurvedic journey by taking the Dosha Questionnaire (Tables 8.1 and 8.2) and engaging in the dosha-specific lifestyle guidelines and perhaps some of the herbal treatments. The references provide further advice as well as information on how to connect with Ayurvedic practitioners. Whether you are a man like our patient, John, who was spurred by a serious health threat to investigate the uses of Ayurveda or you want to prevent disease, Ayurveda can support your quest for health and healing.

Foolish the doctor who despises the knowledge acquired by the ancients.

—*Hippocrates*

REFERENCES

Basch E, Gabardi S, et al. Bitter melon (Momordica charantia): a review of efficacy and safety. Am J Health Syst Pharm. 2003;60:356–359.

Godhwani S, Vyas DS, et al. Ocimum sanctum: An experimental study evaluating its anti-inflammatory, analgesic and antipyretic activity in animals. J Ethnopharmacol. 1987;21:153–163.

Jayasooriya AP, Sakono M, et al. Effects of Momordica charantia powder on serum glucose levels and various lipid parameters in rats fed with cholesterol-free and cholesterol-enriched diets. J Ethnopharmacol. 2000;72:331–336.

Khalsa KPS and Tierra M. *The Way of Ayurvedic Herbs: The Most Complete Guide to Natural Healing and Health with Traditional Ayurvedic Herbalism.* Twin Lakes, WI: Lotus Press, 2009.

Krawinkel MB and Keding GB. Bitter gourd (Mormordica Charantia): A Sietary approach to hyperglycemia. Nutr Rev. 2006;64(7 Pt 1):331–337.

Kulkarni SK, Akula KK, et al. Effect of Withania somnifera Dunal root extract against pentylenetetrazol seizure threshold in mice: possible involvement of GABAergic system. Indian J Exp Biol. 2008 Jun;46(6):465–469.

Padalia RC and Verma RS. Comparative volatile oil composition of four Ocimum species from northern India. Nat Prod Res. 2011;25(6):569–575.

Panda S and Kar A. Changes in thyroid hormone concentrations after administration of ashwaganda root extract to adult male mice. J Pharm Pharmacol. 1998;50(9):1065–1068.

Sridhar MG Vinayagamoorthi R, et al. Bitter gourd (Momordica charantia) improves insulin sensitivity by increasing skeletal muscle insulin-stimulated IRS-1 tyrosine phosphorylation in high-fat-fed rats. Br J Nutr. 2008;99(4):806–812.

Upton R, ed. *Amer Herbal Pharmacopoeia 2000.* New York, NY: Wiley and Sons, 2000:1–25.

RESOURCES

Chopra, D. *Perfect Health.* New York: Three Rivers Press, 2000.

Frawley D, Lad V. *The Yoga of Herbs: An Ayurvedic Guide to Herbal Medicine.* 2nd ed. Twin Lakes: Lotus Press, 2001.

Lad V. *Textbook of Ayurveda: A Complete Guide to Clinical Assessment.* Albuquerque: The Ayurvedic Press, 2006.

Miller L. *Ayurvedic Remedies for the Whole Family.* Twin Lakes: Lotus Press, 1999.

Schensul, et al. Healing traditions and men's sexual health in Mumbai, India. Social Science and Medicine 2006;62: 2774–2285.

9

Homeopathy for Men's Health

RONALD BOYER

Homeopathy: An Introduction

Homeopathy is a therapeutic method consisting of prescribing infinitesimal doses of pharmacologically active substances to stimulate, modulate, or trigger an individual and adaptive reaction by the patient.

Homeopathy is considered as one of the most prevalent therapies prescribed by hundreds of thousands of physicians worldwide. Millions of patients have taken, and are still taking, homeopathic medicines. It is a recognized medical specialty in many countries and taught in allopathic medical schools in France, Poland, Bulgaria, Hungary, and Spain, among others, with homeopathic consultations regularly taking place in those university hospitals with complementary and alternative medicine centers.

In the United States, homeopathic medicines are considered as drugs under the law, regulated as such by the U.S. Food and Drug Administration (FDA).[1] The initials "HPUS" on the label of a drug product ensures that legal standards of strength, quality, purity, and packaging exist for the drug product within the package. The active ingredients are official homeopathic drug products and are found in the current Homeopathic Pharmacopeia of the United States. Homeopathy can be used as first-line treatment for a large number of acute or chronic conditions, either alone or in conjunction with conventional medicines.

It is a German doctor, Samuel Hahnemann (1755–1843), who discovered the homeopathic method. Unhappy about the way medicine was practiced

---

1 U.S. Food and Drug Administration. Sec. 400.400 Conditions Under Which Homeopathic Drugs May be Marketed (CPG7132.15).

at his time (purging, bloodletting, etc.), he decided to stop his practice and earn a living by translating medical books. While working on the translation of a book written by a Scottish surgeon, Cullen, he saw that the author was mentioning that quinine was effective against malaria because of its bitterness. Hahnemann knew other bitter substances that had no curative effect on malaria, so he became intrigued. He went to buy quinine and started to ingest relatively high quantities of it. This made him sick with symptoms resembling those of malaria, the very disease quinine was supposed to treat. He wondered if other substances were capable of giving the same inversion phenomenon effect and was surprised to see they were.

He named his method homeopathy, from the Greek *homeo*, meaning "similar," and *pathos*, meaning "disease." The aim was therefore to give patients small doses of the substance capable of creating the same symptoms in healthy individuals.

For that he collated all the signs and symptoms caused by pharmacologically active substances in healthy individuals and capable of treating these signs and symptoms in ill individuals and wrote about this collected knowledge in a book called *Materia Medica*. This collection of knowledge continues to be collated and incorporated into this definitive text on homeopathy.

The aim of homeopathic physicians is therefore to mirror the symptoms of the patient they have in front of them to those displayed by a healthy individual during experimentation.

Once the picture of the patient, in his disease, is similar to the one described in the *Materia Medica*, the homeopathic physician will prescribe infinitesimal quantities of that substance to stimulate the healing process.

This explains the two fundamental laws of homeopathy: similimum (or similitude of the two pictures) and infinitesimal dose.

It also explains why we do not have the luxury of having one disease equal one homeopathic medicine. For several individuals suffering from the same nosological disease, we can have multiple different scenarios. We do not all have the same symptoms of flu. One might have a sudden high oscillating fever, whereas another might have a more progressive one. One might sweat, or be thirsty, or suffer from body aches, whereas another does not. It is therefore absolutely mandatory to individualize the treatment. In other words, each patient needs a "tailor-made" prescription.

The Materia Medica

The *Materia Medica* is based on three sources: toxicology, experimentation, and clinical experience. For a substance to have an effect on an organism, it has to be pharmacologically active and contain substances (alkaloids, enzymes, peptides, etc.) capable of inducing these symptoms:

- If the substance is toxic, the reaction to a toxic dose would create lesions and, sometimes, even cause death. These toxic effects are well known and would give the practitioner the possibility of knowing the "target" of that substance. For example, mercury toxicity presents with kidney lesions and could therefore be prescribed, in homeopathic dilutions, for kidney pathologies.
- If the substance is not toxic, or if it is a toxic one given in nontoxic quantity, the symptoms that the tester will present will be much different. What is noted is personal reactions to the substance. In this case we will get more individualized symptoms. The subject will present with a physiological or, if you prefer, a pathophysiological response such as fever, sweat, pain, discomfort, anxiety, and so forth. These symptoms are the body's personal reaction to the substance.
- Finally, we come to clinical verification. We have seen that this substance is capable of inducing these symptoms in a healthy individual. Can we verify this in practice? Is there clinical evidence that it works?

This explains the great role of pharmacology in homeopathy.

We now examine and interview our patient and ask ourselves again, "What substance in nature is capable of inducing the same lesions or functional or behavioral symptoms?"

The most convenient way to determine this, in acute or localized situations, is to get help with what we call the "Hering Cross," divided in four quadrants.

- Quadrant number 1—Location: Where is the lesion, the tissue, or the function that is affected? This is a very important first step because it is indispensable for the substance that you want to prescribe to have this location as a target. This quadrant is objective; we see or know where it is.
- Quadrant number 2—Sensation: What does it feel like? What are the sensations the patient is feeling? This quadrant is more subjective; we are already in personal, individualized reactions.
- Quadrant 3—Modalities: This defines the evolution of a symptom or of a patient toward an improvement or an aggravation under the influence of outside or physiological circumstances: temperature, position, rest, pressure, eliminations, and so forth. This quadrant is also subjective and individualized.
- Quadrant 4—Concomitant symptoms: Here we note symptoms displayed by the patient that do not seem to have any pathophysiological link to the nosological diagnosis, such as food cravings or aversions, sleep disorders, and so forth.

Once we have filled out these four quadrants, we should start having a pretty clear idea of which substance to look up. How to go from here? If we were to give that substance in measurable doses to our patient, we would add to his pathological symptoms the harmful effect of the substance. Hahnemann was confronted with this problem, so he started diluting more and more to see how far he could go and still get the therapeutic power while avoiding the toxic ones.

His experimentation showed that, even when diluting to incredible lengths (over the Avogadro number), he continued to have that therapeutic effect and, strangely enough, the more he diluted the deeper the curative action.

The dilution process is rather straightforward. You take the raw substance (called *mother tincture*) that, for many substances, can be toxic. You place 1 drop of that mother tincture in a vial containing 99 drops of alcohol and, very importantly, you vigorously shake the vial. You now have a dilution of 1/100, also called 1 C. Again, you place 1 drop of this 1 C in a vial containing 99 drops of alcohol and shake. You now have a 2 C or 10^{-4}. You can continue until you get to the desired dilution, usually between 6 C (10^{-12}) and 30 C (10^{-60}).

What do those dilutions mean?

- First, from a 4 C (10^{-8}) and higher, all toxicity and all side effects of any substance have disappeared, making homeopathy a totally safe therapy.
- Second, from a 12 C (10^{-24}) and higher, we have passed the Avogadro number. The therapeutic effect of the medicine is therefore not based on a chemical level but on a different one.

These infinitesimal dilutions have led detractors to say, and reasonably so, that there is nothing in the medicine. If it is true that there are no molecules or measurable substances to be found, what is happening? For a long time we had no real answer except to mention simply that it worked. More recent scientific techniques have been able to show that the original substance leaves an "imprint" in the solvent, possible to find either by thermoluminescence in a 12 C $(10-24)^2$ and, lately, by Pr. Luc Montagnier, winner of the Nobel Prize in Medicine in 2008, through electromagnetic signals.[3]

So, to summarize, we ask ourselves what substance in nature is capable of inducing such symptoms in a healthy individual. Once we are certain of our choice (through the *Materia Medica*), we prescribe the same substance, in

2 Thermoluminescence of ultra-high dilutions of lithium chloride and sodium chloride: Pr. Louis Rey: *Physica A: Statistical Mechanics and Its Applications,* Volume 323, May 15, 2003, Pages 67–74.

3 Electromagnetic Signals Are Produced by Aqueous Nanostructures Derived from Bacterial DNA Sequences: Luc Montagnier: *Interdiscip Sci Comput Sci* (2009) 1: 81–90.

homeopathic dilutions. This homeopathic medicine will trigger a therapeutic response in the patient.

Finally, we have to differentiate between acute and chronic pathologies. The therapeutic choice for the latter will need a much deeper interview of the patient. This chapter will focus mostly on medicines for the acute, or accidental, situations but will sometimes mention the most frequently indicated medicines for chronic conditions. Also, it goes without saying that homeopathy, being simply a therapeutic method, is in no way a panacea. There are things we can treat and others we cannot. It is our responsibility as physicians to make a medical diagnosis and prognosis and choose if a homeopathic treatment alone is suited, if it would be better for us to associate it with conventional therapy, or if homeopathy is not to be used in that case.

Why Should We Prescribe Homeopathy?

Notwithstanding the fact that homeopathy has been clinically proven for more than 200 years, the main points could be summarized as follows: it is effective, has no side effects, has no toxicity, has no interaction with any other medicines, has no addiction potential, and is cost effective.

Homeopathic Treatments for Men's Health

We have seen that we do not have medicines for "conditions" but for patients suffering "from the condition." It is therefore extremely difficult to say, "What is the treatment for the prostate?" for example. What we can do is give a list of the most frequently prescribed medicines for that condition, give some salient points for each, and with that information trust that the reader will go back to the *Materia Medica* to give, as mentioned, the "tailor-made" prescription to his or her patient.

A list of homeopathic medicines will be given for each pathology with the particular signs and symptoms displayed by the patient as found in the *Materia Medica*.

For acute conditions the prescription will usually be, unless otherwise indicated, in 9 C, 5 pellets two to three times daily, depending on the severity or the discomfort.

I have voluntarily chosen to give the most frequently prescribed homeopathic medicines for each condition with a small number of notable symptoms helping to choose between them. This method has the advantage of giving the reader an understanding of each medicine and helps him or her know where to look in the *Materia Medica*.

Arteriosclerosis and Atherosclerosis

The homeopathic *Materia Medica* proposes some medicines for loss of elasticity and sclerosis of the blood vessels. Taking into account family and/or individual medical history is essential to start a chronic preventive treatment as early as possible.

Homeopathy will be more often prescribed in association with classic treatments, optimizing their prescription and decreasing their potential adverse side effects.

Homeopathy will propose medicines acting on the vascular walls and medicines to treat the patient's pathological tendencies and associated risk factors (obesity, metabolic disorders, smoking, stress, etc.)

ARSENICUM ALBUM 9 C

- Mostly prescribed in thin, pale, and cold-sensitive individuals
- Those presenting with alternation of stamina and weakness
- Lesions of vascular sclerosis

ARSENICUM IODATUM 9 C

- Systematically indicated to prevent arterial sclerosis

BARYTA CARBONICA 9 C

- Slow individuals with memory disorders; they "get lost in their own street"
- Prone to high blood pressure

CALCAREA FLUORICA 9 C

- Early onset of arteriosclerosis with rigidity of the arteries and tendency to have high blood pressure
- Hypermobility of the ligaments
- Tendency to have bone growths (exostosis)

Arteritis of the Lower Limbs

The homeopathic treatment will have the effect of slowing down the evolution of the arteritis and to help increase walking distances.

As prevention and at the beginning stages—stage 1: pulse absent but no pain; stage 2: intermittent limping—we can use the medicines we already mentioned for arteriosclerosis and add the following:

SECALE CORNUTUM 9 C

Secale is a homeopathic dilution of ergotamine, well known for its vasoconstrictive effect in measurable doses. In homeopathic dilutions it will have the role of vasodilation:

- Violent cramps, followed by intense coldness with paleness and cyanosis of the extremities accompanied by burning pain
- Despite the coldness of the skin to touch, the pains are improved by cold

ARSENICUM ALBUM 9 C

- Painful cramps, mainly during the night around 1 AM
- Burning pain improved by heat
- Commonly prescribed in alternation with *Secale cornutum*

PLUMBUM METALLICUM 9 C

- Arteritis in smokers
- Cold and thin limbs with collateral circulation

Arthritis and Rheumatic Pains

Homeopathy is a very useful therapy, or adjunct therapy, for these pathologies because of the frequency of the classic prescriptions having no real therapeutic efficacy while often responsible for iatrogenic pathologies. Also, homeopathic approaches for these conditions are especially useful in the elderly who take multiple treatments and are especially sensitive and exposed to adverse side effects.

Homeopathy will be able to act on the progression of arthritis and limit the frequency and severity of the inflammatory flare-ups. This treatment will be safe, without any side effects or drug interactions. The therapeutic objective is to optimize analgesic, anti-inflammatory, and allopathic long-term treatments, as well as to limit the progression of the disease.

Medicines with a local action for acute conditions are as follows:

MEDICINES FOR INFLAMMATION

Apis mellifica 15 C

- Exudation of the serous membranes (hydrarthrosis)
- Pinkish edema
- Acute, stinging, and burning pain aggravated by touch and pressure
- The pain is improved by cold applications

Ferrum phosphoricum 9 C

- Moderate inflammation, mainly of the shoulders
- The pain is improved by cold

Bryonia alba 9 C

- Elective action on the serous membranes (joint synovia) where it leads to irritation and oozing
- The joints are red and hot
- Throbbing, acute, and stinging pain
  - o Aggravated by the slightest movement
  - o Improved by staying completely still
  - o Improved by large pressure
  - o Improved by local heat

Sulphur iodatum 9 C

- Action on joint synovia
- Subacute inflammatory flare-ups
- Sensation of local burning
- Accompanied by fatigue, nervousness, and weight loss
- The patient is aggravated by efforts, fatigue, and heat

MEDICINES ACTING ON THE FIBROCONJUNCTIVE TISSUES SURROUNDING THE JOINTS

Rhus toxicodendron 9 C

- Painful joint stiffness, lingering at the beginning of movement then fading away with ongoing movement
- Aggravated by dampness, cold, and rest
- Improved by changing position and hot and dry weather

Ruta graveolens 9 C

- Action on periosteum and tendons
- The pains are aggravated by rest and improved by the first movements
- Tendonitis at insertion point

Dulcamara 9 C

- Joint pains triggered or increased by dampness
- Sometimes alternation between joint pains and digestive disorders (diarrhea)

MEDICINES WITH AN ELECTIVE ACTION ON MUSCLES

Arnica 9 C

- Aching and bruising sensation
- The patient is tired; physical burnout
- Jolts and movement aggravate the pains

Lachnantes 9 C

- Medicine of torticollis with contracture of neck muscles
- The patient needs to bend his head on the corresponding side
- Medicine of cervical arthritis

Benign Prostatic Hyperplasia

Homeopathic treatment will help to reduce the size of the prostate, therefore improving urinary flow and discomfort. It has no effect whatsoever on prostatic cancer. In that instance it could be used as a complementary therapy to the classic treatment.

CHIMAPHILA UMBELLATA 9 C

Clinical observation has shown an elective action on the urogenital organs, especially the prostate.

- Urination is difficult; the patient must force to urinate
- He urinates standing, bending forward, legs open, leaning with hand on the wall in front of him
- Recurrent urinary infections
- Chronic cystitis with sensation of a ball in the perineum
- The urine contains mucus

CONIUM MACULATUM 9 C

- The prostate is hard upon examination
- The flow is intermittent
- The patient has the sensation of heaviness in the perineum

LYCOPODIUM 9 C

- Benign prostatic adenoma in a patient suffering with recurrent urinary infections and lithiasis
- The patient often presents with high levels of cholesterol and uric acid

SABAL SERRULATA 6 X

Saw palmetto is also used in measurable doses along with this remedy.
- This is the first-line treatment of functional disturbances linked to prostate hypertrophy
- The patient often suffers from genital pains during intercourse
- Dysuria and discharges of prostatic fluid
- The patient has the sensation that his genital organs are cold

Sabal serrulata is to be prescribed in 6 X (diluted 1 in 10 instead of 1 in 100 for C dilutions), 5 pellets twice daily.

SELENIUM 9 C

- Seminal losses at night without erection
- Main medicine for patients who lose urine after having a bowel movement
- Erectile dysfunction despite maintained libido
- Premature ejaculation

SEPIA OFFICINALIS 9 C

- Recurring urinary infections with fatigue, paleness, and dark circles around the eyes
- Sensation of having a ball in the perineum; sensation as if he was sitting on a ball

STAPHYSAGRIA 9 C

- Imperious urge to urinate
- Urethral burning pains that disappear while he urinates

Prostatitis

ACUTE PROSTATITIS

Mercurius dulcis 9 C

- Increase in volume of the prostate
- Dysuria
- Halitosis
- Hypersalivation

LINGERING PROSTATITIS

Pulsatilla 9 C

- The prostatitis is painful
- Sensation of heat in the perineum
- Frequent urination

Silicea 15 C

- The prostate is hard upon examination
- Possibility of urethral suppuration

Thuja occidentalis 15 C

- After effects of gonorrhea

Gout

Homeopathic treatment will take into account the acute symptoms of the patient but must necessarily be complemented by a chronic homeopathic treatment and lifestyle changes.

ANTIMONIUM CRUDUM 9 C

- In case of gout that is becoming constant
- Gouty nodes in many joints

BRYONIA ALBA 9 C

- The joint is hot to the touch
- It is always on the same joint that the patient has his attacks
- The skin is red

- The joint is swollen
- The patient is irritable; improved by immobility and strong pressure and aggravated by movement

CINCHONA 9 C

- The joint is very sensitive to touch
- It is always the same joint (*Bryonia*)
- The joint is swollen
- The patient is aggravated by touch
- Improved by strong pressure (*Bryonia*)

COLCHICUM AUTUMNALE 9 C

- The joint is swollen and hot to the touch
- The attacks go from one joint to another (main symptomatic medicine)
- The skin is red
- The pain prevents patient from walking
- Predominantly on the large toe
- Aggravated by movement and by touch
- Aggravated in warm weather but improved by local heat

LEDUM PALUSTRE 9 C

- The joint is cold to the touch
- The skin is white
- The joint is swollen
- Painful tophi (main symptomatic medicine)
- Aggravated by local heat (the patient takes the blankets off the joint)
- Improved by cold baths

NUX VOMICA 9 C

- Gout after indulging in rich food, fat, and alcohol
- The patient is irritable
- The patient is sensitive to cold

SULPHUR 9 C

- Gout after indulging in rich food, fat, and alcohol
- The patient is rather jovial
- The patient is always too hot

High Blood Pressure

In the case of a patient suffering from high blood pressure, it would be unreasonable, and dangerous, to stop all classic medications to give an exclusive homeopathic treatment.

The following medicines could be added, as complementary ones, to the classic treatment in certain specific cases.

PANIC ATTACK ACCOMPANIED BY INCREASE IN BLOOD PRESSURE

Aconitum napellus 9 C

- Major anxiety in a patient who was perfectly healthy until now
- Anxiety felt in the precordial area
- The patient is afraid of dying

HIGH BLOOD PRESSURE AFTER SUNSTROKE

Glonoinum 9 C

- Sudden congestive headache
- You can see the beating of the carotids

HIGH BLOOD PRESSURE OF NERVOUS ORIGIN

Ignatia amara 9 C

- After a contradiction
- The attack can be used as a weapon to frighten the people around him

The medicines mentioned in the arteriosclerosis chapter can also be used as complementary therapy.

Plumbum metallicum 9 C

- To add in case of lesions on the renal arteries

Only a chronic homeopathic treatment would be able, in certain cases, to stabilize a patient's high blood pressure on a long-term basis.

Sexual Disorders

The homeopathic treatment alone is often sufficient. Again, there is no problem associating it with any other sort of treatment. Homeopathy never interferes with other therapies.

ABSTINENCE

Conium maculatum

- Homeopathic medicine classically indicated in abstinent patients
- Desire is increased but sexual "power" is decreased; the patient presents with sexual excitement but weak erections
- This medicine is regularly prescribed to patients who are denied sex

ABSENT OR LOW SEXUAL DESIRES

Graphites

- Sexual weakness with increased desire
- Aversion to intercourse
- Too early or no ejaculation

Sepia officinalis

- Has become indifferent to those around him
- Inferiority complex

PREMATURE EJACULATION

Argentum nitricum

- This symptom belongs to the anticipation anxiety and the precipitation context of the medicine
- He wants to be "finished before starting"

Onosmodium

- Accompanied by psychological impotence
- Weakness of erection
- Major decrease or total loss of libido

Selenium

- With seminal losses coming out drop by drop without erection
- Often linked to prostate hypertrophy

ERECTION DISORDERS

Graphites

- The erection does not last

Cantharis

- In case of priapism

Sports Injuries

Every day sports injuries are at the forefront of homeopathic practice and one of the medicines, *Arnica*, should always be close at hand.

ARNICA MONTANA 9 C

This is to be given systematically after each injury.

Arnica is a capillary protector. In case of trauma it prevents capillary bleeding, and therefore bruising and swelling. It also has a positive action on muscles and cellular tissues. It is used routinely by plastic surgeons to minimize the visible effects of their procedures.

It is to be taken two to three times daily for at least 10 days and may be completed by another medicine according to the trauma's location or its nature:

Black eye: *Ledum palustre* 9 C
Sprain: *Ruta graveolens* 9 C
During physiotherapy: *Rhus toxicodendron* 9 C
Nerve pains, as after fall on the coccyx: *Hypericum* 9 C

Testicular Pathologies

EPIDIDYMITIS

In case of epididymitis three medicines can be very useful:

Berberis vulgaris 9 C

- Epididymitis with pains radiating in the spermatic cords that are inflamed
- Sometimes associated with functional urinary disorder such as tenesmus and red sediment in the urine accompanied by jelly-type mucus

Pulsatilla 9 C

- Acute epididymitis
- Sometimes following gonorrhea
- Associated with orchitis
- The testicles are swollen

Rhododendron chrysanthum

- Epididymitis with sensation as if the testicle were crushed and hot

ORCHITIS

It is the physician's responsibility to choose if he or she wants to treat this condition alone or in association with classic therapy.

Here are a certain number of medicines (in alphabetical order) having the testicle as the target and clinically proven to be effective in orchitis.

Aconitum napellus 9 C

- The testicle is painful and hard
- It is enlarged
- High fever accompanied by agitation and anxiety

Belladonna 9 C

- The testicle is hard and retracted
- Throbbing and burning pain
- Intense fever with prostration
- Aggravated by jolts

Clematis erecta 9 C

- The testicle is painful and retracted
- Aggravated by the heat of the bed
- Often after gonorrhea
- Accompanied by inguinal adenopathies
- Urethral irritation

Hamamelis virginiana 6 C

- The testicle is enlarged and swollen
- The testicle is hot
- Medicine for lingering orchitis with testicle sensitive to the touch
- There is often an important sweating on the scrotum
- Often associated with a varicocele

Pulsatilla 9 C

- One of the most frequently prescribed homeopathic medicines for this condition
- Very specific for orchitis due to mumps
- The testicle is painful with inflammation of the spermatic cord

- There is often an associated epididymitis
- The testicle is retracted

Rhododendron chrysanthum 9 C

- Atrophy of the testicle
- Sensation as if the testicle was crushed
- Indicated in chronic orchitis

Spongia tosta 9 C

- The testicle is hard with a sensation of local heat
- The testicle is enlarged

In conclusion, we have seen that homeopathic medicines can have a real and effective role in everyday medical care for men's health, not only for acute but also for chronic conditions that are difficult to treat with conventional therapies.

10

Men's Integrative Cardiology

CHRISTOPHER J. SUHAR AND CHRISTINA ADAMS

ardiovascular disease (CVD) continues to be the leading cause of death among men (Heron et al., 2009) and is one of the major progressive lifelong diseases of the modern era. 70% to 89% of all sudden cardiac events occur in men, with more than half reporting no previous symptoms (Lloyd-Jones et al., 2010). Although Western allopathic medicine excels in the arena of acute care management such as treating heart attacks and performing lifesaving procedures, it often falls short in prevention and chronic disease management. No field of medicine lends itself better to the integrative approach than cardiology, which uses state-of-the-art technology while mandating the need for aggressive lifestyle change.

Through the broad spectrum of cardiovascular disease, almost all cardiovascular risk factors are associated and dependent on how one lives his or her life. These risk factors are multifactorial and range from hyperlipidemia, inflammation, diabetes mellitus, hypertension, and tobacco use to sedentary lifestyle and social connection. Over 90% of men with heart disease report at least one risk factor, with more than 35% reporting two or more (Centers for Disease Control and Prevention, 2005; Lloyd-Jones et al., 2010). An integrative approach to cardiovascular disease is about treating all cardiac risk factors and getting to the underlying cause, whether it is sedentary lifestyle, hyperlipidemia, or maladaptive responses to stress and tension.

If we hope to decrease the prevalence of CVD, we must shift our emphasis from treatment after disease has developed to a more proactive approach and concentrate on preventative efforts. Holistic integrative medicine offers expertise in nutrition, nutraceuticals, exercise, and mind–body interventions that are pivotal to CVD treatment and prevention. This is a particular challenge in a male population who tends to go without primary care visits during young and middle adulthood and only seeks care when symptomatic. A challenge of integrative men's health is to encourage a relationship with a health care provider who will educate and promote lifestyle change before actual pathology exists.

Assessing Cardiovascular Risk

A fundamental goal of an integrative approach toward cardiovascular disease is aggressive primary prevention, early detection, and risk assessment. If we aim to decrease the prevalence of cardiovascular disease, then there is an urgent need to identify not only those people who are "at higher risk" but also those "at very low risk" in order to prevent the development of disease or arrest its progression. Therefore, *initial* risk assessment, and close follow-up, is particularly important and requires a comprehensive evaluation. This begins with obtaining a thorough history and physical examination, review of systems, and complete, accurate family history. In addition, prior medical conditions not previously associated with cardiovascular risk, such as rheumatoid arthritis, inflammatory bowel disease, lupus, and HIV, cannot be overlooked as contributing to a chronic, proinflammatory state and increased atherosclerotic risk (Forrester and Bick-Oreester, 2005; Libby, 2002). Additional testing that is performed at our early detection center to improve risk stratification includes laboratory evaluation using advanced lipid testing (vertical auto profile or VAP panel), lipoprotein (a), high-sensitivity C-reactive protein (hs-CRP), and HgbA1C, as well as advanced imaging such as computed tomography (CT) and carotid intima-media thickness (IMT) scanning. It is important to emphasize that evaluating risk is a *comprehensive* assessment of an individual as a whole and that there is no one single test that can predict risk.

RISK FACTORS

The Framingham Risk Score is used to calculate the 10-year risk of myocardial infarction or cardiac death based on traditional risk factors of age, gender, total cholesterol, high-density lipoprotein (HDL), tobacco abuse, and systolic blood pressure (Adult Treatment Panel III, 2001). This is commonly used to estimate an individual's risk, but it fails to take into account other contributing factors of coronary disease such as waist-to-hip ratio, lipoprotein subparticle size, obesity, nutritional status, psychological stressors and depression, sedentary lifestyle, and family history. The Reynolds Risk Score (Ridker, Buring, et al., 2007; Ridker, Paynter, et al., 2008) (http://www.reynoldsriskscore.org) adds the components of hs-CRP and parental history of myocardial infarction (MI) to calculate risk. Although these are helpful tools, it is important to remember that atherosclerosis slowly develops over an entire lifetime. Estimating an individual's 10-year risk fails to address the reality that CVD often takes two decades for presentation. In addition, as seen in the Nurses' Health Study, individuals with a healthy lifestyle had an 82% reduced risk of coronary heart disease (CHD), which was *independent* of age, hypertension, lipids, and family history (Stampfer et al., 2000). The findings of the INTERHEART study (Yusuf et al., 2004), which examined modifiable risk factors associated with myocardial infarction in men and women in 52 countries, reflects the importance of lifestyle interventions and the ability to prevent CVD. Nine risk factors emerged as accounting for 90% of the risk of acute myocardial infarction: smoking, diet, exercise, alcohol intake, hypertension, diabetes, abdominal obesity, psychosocial factors, and lipids. These risk factors were consistent across sexes, geographic regions, and ethnic groups. One of the most important points of this trial was the overwhelming effect of the *modifiable* nature of these risk factors in the young. These results again suggest how preventable CVD is and that an early, aggressive approach is warranted.

ADVANCED CARDIAC BIOMARKERS

Vertical auto profile (VAP); Berkley HeartLab

Historically, cholesterol measurement has been simplified into total cholesterol, low-density lipoprotein (LDL) or "bad" cholesterol, HDL or "good" cholesterol, and triglycerides. The standard lipid panel calculates LDL based on the Friedewald equation using independent measurements of total cholesterol, HDL, and triglycerides (Friedewald et al., 1972). Unfortunately, this does not tell the entire story of lipoprotein-associated risk. Although high LDL and low HDL levels are certainly considered primary risk factors, most coronary events occur in patients with "normal" HDL and LDL (Ridker, 2000). The heterogeneity of both LDL and HDL particles has been examined extensively, and it is now recognized that not all particles are equally atherogenic or equally protective, respectively (Austin et al., 1988; Kulkarni, 2006; Tian and Fu, 2010; Von Eckardstein et al., 1994). The vertical auto profile, or VAP panel (http://www.atherotech.com), and the Berkley HeartLab (http://www.bhlinc.com) methods offer a cholesterol profile measurement that simultaneously measures cholesterol concentrations of the lipoprotein classes (Kulkarni, 2006). LDL consists of four density subclasses, LDL_1 through LDL_4, ranging from large, buoyant particles (conferring less risk) to small, dense particles (higher risk). Smaller, more dense particles are more easily oxidized and thus taken up into coronary arterial intima. Individuals vary in their expression of LDL particle size, and this can be significantly modified through lifestyle changes as well as statin/niacin therapy. HDL is also subclassified into more protective and less protective based on size. HDL-2 is a large, buoyant subclass that is associated with reverse cholesterol transport efficiency and is therefore more protective than HDL-3, which is smaller and more dense. This lipoprotein subclass separation offers a direct (rather than calculated) measurement of LDL, improving accuracy, as well as determining lipoprotein subclass that redefines risk (Brook et al., 2005). Both the VAP panel and Berkeley HeartLab also measure apolipoprotein B100. Apo B is considered an aggregate marker of atherogenic particles (LDL, very-low-density lipoprotein [VLDL], intermediate-density lipoprotein [IDL], lipoprotein [a]). Higher levels of apo B positively correlate with cardiovascular risk, similarly to LDL (Brook et al., 2005; Brunzell, 2005; Pischon et al., 2005; Sniderman, 2005).

Particle subclass analysis is an effective tool to more clearly define risk as well as measure response to treatment. We routinely use particle subclass analysis in our patients who are first presenting for risk stratification, but we also use it to follow those patients with established disease to monitor therapeutic interventions. As subclass particle testing becomes more common, we anticipate that national cholesterol treatment guidelines will include atherogenic particle size for diagnostic and treatment purposes.

hs-CRP

hs-CRP is a nonspecific marker of inflammation. CRP may play a direct role in development of atherosclerosis as it binds to oxidized LDL, promoting macrophage uptake of LDL into arterial walls (Ridker, Cushman, et al., 1997; Ridker, Hennekens, et al., 2000). Elevated hs-CRP has been shown to increase the risk of MI, stroke, and sudden cardiac death in the Physicians' Health Study (Ridker, Cushman, et al., 1997; Ridker, Hennekens, et al., 2000; Sniderman, 2005). Exercise and weight loss, as well as statin use, have all been shown to decrease CRP levels (Ridker, Cushman, et al., 1997; Ridker, Hennekens, et al., 2000). Individuals who have an elevated hs-CRP, despite normal lipids, benefit from statin initiation (AFCAPS/TexCAPS). The JUPITER trial (Pearson et al., 2003) revealed a 44% reduction in cardiovascular events in patients with an LDL less than 130 mg/dl and hs-CRP greater than 2.0 mg/L treated with rosuvastatin. American Heart Association (AHA)/Centers for Disease Control and Prevention (CDC) guidelines have established levels of risk based on hs-CRP.

Lp(a)

Lipoprotein (a) is a lipoprotein similar in structure to LDL but with the addition of apolipoprotein A, which is a highly glycosylated protein. It has been found to be a highly atherogenic particle as well as a marker for thrombosis (Erquo et al., 2009; Ridker, Danielson, et al., 2008). It is now considered to be a strong, independent, inheritable marker for coronary disease (Clarke et al., 2009). Individual levels are highly heritable and there are currently no therapies known to lower levels of Lp(a). In addition, it is not known if decreasing levels of Lp(a) result in improved cardiovascular outcomes. It can be used to further stratify an individual's risk; however, therapy guidelines in patients with elevated Lp(a) are not generally recognized. In our early detection clinic, we routinely screen for Lp(a). Patients in whom an elevated Lp(a) level (despite a normal LDL level) is found are considered at higher risk. Initiation with L-carnitine or niacin is considered, although there are currently no randomized, controlled trials examining the effectiveness of L-carnitine nor niacin in lowering Lp(a) levels.

HgbA1c

The cardiovascular risk associated with the development of diabetes is well known. Diabetes accelerates the atherosclerosis process and is linked with worsening hypertension, hyperlipidemia, and obesity (Kannel, 1985). Furthermore, diabetic patients often present with atypical chest pain and/ or an absence of chest pain, which can delay the diagnosis. Large angiographic studies have revealed that diabetics consistently demonstrate more extensive coronary artery disease (CAD), increased plaque burden, and decreased collateral vessels (Burchfiel et al., 1993). In addition, patients with a borderline normal HgbA1c of 6% have been shown to have an increased risk of microvascular complications (Khaw et al., 2004). Therefore, screening for diabetes becomes an important part of early preventative efforts. A prospective cohort study over 3 years following approximately1,250 patients in the Veterans Administration (VA) system found that HgbA1c testing in nondiabetic outpatients helped to predict the likelihood that patients would develop diabetes in the future (Edelman et al., 2004). Baseline HgbA1c and body mass index (BMI) were both significant predictors of new-onset diabetes; however, HgbA1c was more strongly correlated with diabetes development than obesity. High "normal" HgbA1c levels of 5.6% to 6% resulted in an increased incidence of diabetes over a 1-year period. Identifying these patients *early* by screening and instituting lifestyle changes or pharmacotherapy may prevent or delay the development of diabetes. Our early detection center measures HgbA1c at all initial visits, regardless of a previous diagnosis of diabetes. Patients with no known history of diabetes who have a borderline high-normal level are treated with aggressive nutritional intervention by recommending a low-glycemic-index diet and exercise prescription with follow-up of HgbA1c within 3 to 6 months to assess changes.

ADVANCED IMAGING

As atherosclerosis can be a dormant disease for a considerable amount of time, questions remain as to how to stratify asymptomatic patients' long-term risk and what role stress testing and imaging can play for primary prevention. In addition, the use of risk models such as the Framingham Risk Score to improve prediction is not 100% accurate (D'Agostino et al., 2001). Therefore, the ability to visualize coronary anatomy for atherosclerotic burden or to stress a patient's heart to unveil electrocardiographic (ECG) changes or symptoms is an attractive means to diagnose disease *before* significant symptoms occur. However, stress tests have their own limitations, and appropriate screening of individuals who will most benefit continues to be debated.

Exercise Stress Testing

Several studies have shown that exercise-induced ischemia in healthy men with coronary risk factors is associated with an increased risk of future myocardial infarction and sudden death compared with the same population with normal findings on stress testing (Bruce et al., 1983; Gordon et al., 1986). Even among men with a *single* coronary risk factor, an abnormal result on electrocardiographic exercise testing was associated with a relative risk of death from coronary cause ranging from 8 to 10, compared with similar men with normal stress tests (Gibbons et al., 2000). Often overlooked but critically valuable information that should be obtained from stress testing includes exercise capacity, heart rate recovery, blood pressure response, presence of arrhythmia, and hemodynamic response (Greenland and Gaziano, 2003). Using all of this information can be a critical tool in speaking to patients about the importance of fitness, setting an exercise prescription, and discussing symptoms of chest pain and dyspnea, in addition to the evaluation for chest pain.

Critics of stress testing note the low specificity and sensitivity in asymptomatic patients who are at low risk (Gibbons et al., 2002). The ideal patient for stress testing is a patient at intermediate risk. The addition of imaging to exercise stress by using perfusion scintigraphy or stress echo improves diagnostic capabilities and predictive capability compared to use of exercise stress alone.

Carotid IMT/Duplex Ultrasound

Carotid IMT has long been used as a surrogate marker for cardiovascular disease, the prevalence of atherosclerosis in other arterial beds, and an endpoint for determining the success of interventions that lower levels of LDL cholesterol. Approximately 50% to 60% of patients with carotid disease have severe CAD; however, only 10% of patients with CAD have severe carotid disease (O'Holleran et al., 1987). Carotid duplex ultrasound is the most widely used method for detection and quantification of carotid artery disease and reports a sensitivity and specificity of greater than 80% (Nederkoorn et al., 2002). It should be noted that accuracy of carotid IMT is lower among patients with only mild to moderate disease. Elevated carotid IMT is associated with prevalence and incidence of CHD and stroke (O'Leary et al., 1999). Asymptomatic patients with 60% stenosis or more have an annual stroke risk of approximately 2% per year (Wolf et al., 1981). The recent ARIC study argues that adding plaque and carotid IMT to traditional risk factors can improve the early detection and diagnosis of silent CVD (Nambi et al., 2010).

Critics of carotid IMT argue that regression of carotid IMT is poorly predictive of cardiovascular risk reduction and that the addition of carotid IMT does not reclassify a patient's CVD risk. This may be in part due to the pathophysiology of intimal thickening, which is due not only to atherosclerosis but also to hemodynamics, such as blood pressure and shear stress associated with the vessel. Currently, the American Heart Association validates the use of IMT in individuals who are at intermediate risk for CVD.

Coronary Artery Calcium (CAC) Score

A CAC score aims to identify *subclinical* atherosclerosis by the observation that coronary calcium is a surrogate marker for coronary atherosclerotic plaque (Agatston et al., 1990; Arad et al., 2000; Detrano et al., 2008; Wong et al., 2000). Detection and quantification of coronary calcium is achieved by ECG-gated electron-beam CT, generating a coronary calcium score. The most commonly used scoring system is the Agatston coronary artery calcium volume score (Agatston et al., 1990; Arad et al., 2000). It is derived by measuring the area of each calcified coronary lesion and multiplying it by a coefficient of 1 to 4, depending on the maximum CT attenuation within that lesion. Scores are classified into five groups: 0: no coronary calcium; 100: mild coronary calcium; 101 to 399: moderate calcification; 400 to 999: severe calcification; greater than 1,000: extensive coronary calcium. Higher calcium scores correlate with older age, higher levels of risk factors, and extent of coronary atherosclerosis. Men and individuals with renal insufficiency and diabetes tend to have higher scores and therefore scores are age and gender specific. Numerous investigations of CAC reveal that the majority of coronary events occur in individuals in whom the CAC score is greater than 100 (Achenbach et al., 2004; Nasir et al., 2012; O'Rourke et al., 2000; Pletcher et al., Wong et al., 2000). The MESA (Multi-Ethnic Study of Atherosclerosis) and HNR (Heinz Nixdorf Recall) prospective registries both support previous research of the strong prognostic value of CAC in predicting CVD events (Budoff et al., 2009; Erbel et al., 2010). Individuals with severe CAC had a nine- to 16-fold increased hazard ratio in predicting CVD events compared to individuals with a CAC score of zero. A high Agatston score greater than 300 has been shown to be associated with an elevated risk beyond measured Framingham Risk Score (Pletcher et al., 2004), and therefore may reclassify an individual's risk of CVD from patients who were previously intermediate risk into a high-risk category. Finally, emerging evidence suggests that individuals with higher CAC scores are more likely to engage in lifestyle changes and medication adherence. Critics of CAC as a primary prevention tool note that the absolute event rate, despite an elevated level, remains modest. It is important to acknowledge that not all atherosclerotic plaque is calcified and that the presence of a large amount of calcium does not imply the presence of significant stenoses. Published literature suggests an unacceptably high false-positive rate when the test is applied to low-risk patients. In addition, there is a small, although real radiation exposure risk (Hunold et al., 2003). The mean effective dose is ~1 mSv compared to the average annual exposure in the United States of ~3 mSv. This dose is comparable to a mammogram screen. Finally, CAC may result in increased downstream testing and costs. Our recommendation is that coronary calcium scoring is best utilized in patients with intermediate-risk classification whose scores may reclassify them to a higher or lower risk group.

Coronary CT Angiography (CCTA)

The ability to visualize coronary arteries noninvasively is an attractive alternative to an invasive procedure and explains the recent rapid evolution of cardiac CT as a screening and diagnostic tool. Multidetector computed tomography allows for spatial resolution of 0.4 mm, compared to 0.2 mm for invasive angiography, the gold standard. The indications are vast and include the evaluation of chest pain (MI, pulmonary embolism [PE], dissection), suspicion of coronary anomalies, evaluation of cardiac masses, pericardial disease, aortic disease, pulmonary vein evaluation, congenital heart disease, and assessing graft patency from prior bypass. From a perspective of visualizing coronaries, CCTA has been shown to be an accurate noninvasive modality with high sensitivity (85% to 95%) and specificity (95% to 98%) when compared to invasive angiography (Leber et al., 2007). It is most useful in low-/intermediate-risk patients with chest pain. Proponents for CCTA argue that there is a uniformly high negative predictive value of coronary CT, reported as 93% to 100%. The appropriate use of CCTA includes patients with an intermediate pretest probability of CAD whose ECG may be uninterpretable, who are unable to exercise, or who have had an equivocal stress test (O'Rourke et al., 2000).

There are few absolute contraindications to CT; however, these include renal insufficiency, iodine allergy, atrial fibrillation (due to necessity for ECG gating), or an inability to hold one's breath for 10 seconds.

Lifestyle Change Intervention

As medicine is becoming more dependent on the pharmaceutical industry, a focus has shifted from treating every aspect of a patient's health to a disease-driven model of treatment focused on the presenting disease and not necessarily the root cause of disease. Furthermore, medicine has also focused heavily on treating the disease at hand in lieu of preventing the disease to come. Affecting one's lifestyle continues to be the single most effective prevention and treatment of most cardiovascular diseases. Unfortunately, in a recent survey of primary care physicians and cardiologists, discussing and affecting lifestyle including nutrition, exercise, and psychosocial stressors continues to be poorly addressed (Integrative Cardiology textbook; Mosca et al., 2005).

Almost all CVD is closely related to and affected by inflammation, which is a direct result of obesity, poor nutrition, sedentary lifestyle, and maladaptive responses to stress and tension. In fact, poor nutrition and physical inactivity are identified as probably the true leading "actual" causes of death in the United States (Mokdad et al., 2004). Increasing BMI has been shown to worsen diabetes, cholesterol, and blood pressure in a linear fashion. Inversely, as the BMI is lowered, there is improvement in all risk factors in the same linear fashion. Multiple avenues of research have shown lifestyle intervention alone can alter the course of disease. For example, in the Diabetes Prevention Study, type 2 diabetes was prevented in high-risk individuals who underwent individualized counseling on weight loss and physical activity alone when compared to appropriately matched controls (Tuomilehto et al., 2001).

An integrative approach to cardiovascular care broadens the traditional diagnosis and treatment of disease utilizing both the Western-based diagnostic tests and pharmaceuticals and an aggressive focus on all aspects of health including nutrition, exercise, and psychosocial stress. In almost all cases, a comprehensive lifestyle change approach is necessary.

NUTRITION

What a patient puts into his or her mouth can directly affect his or her cardiovascular health. In fact, a single high-fat meal transiently impairs arterial endothelial function and blood flow (Vogel et al., 1997). Although multiple studies have shown benefit from various different diets, nutrition continues to be underemphasized in the primary care setting. A very large epidemiological study evaluated the effect of nutrition in the United States versus rural China. In this study of over 10,000 individuals, the U.S. fat intake was twice as high, fiber intake was three times lower, and animal protein intake was 90% higher. The heart disease death rate was 16.7-fold greater for men. Other diseases were also higher in the United States, including cancers, osteoporosis, diabetes, and hypertension (Junshi et al., 1990). Importantly, when the study evaluated Asian people immigrating to the United States, it showed that they reached the U.S. level of heart disease and cancer deaths within two generations.

An initial approach to one's nutrition should simply start with total caloric consumption, which is the most important variable affecting obesity. From 1990 to 2000, the Department of Agriculture reported an 8% increase in food consumption. Concordantly, the CDC reported a doubling in the prevalence of obesity between 1971 and 2000, which correlated with a 22% increase in calorie consumption for women and a 9% increase for men (CDC, 2004). Interestingly, despite indications that the percentage of calories consumed as fat is decreasing, surveys indicate that we are consuming more calories overall (Eckle and Krauss, 1998). Reduction in total caloric intake should be emphasized as a first-line approach to weight loss.

Fats and carbohydrates are the major macronutrients affecting cardiovascular health. Fats are broken down into saturated, monounsaturated, and polyunsaturated fatty acids. Saturated fatty acids contain no double bonds in their fatty acid chains and they are typically solid at room temperature. They are the predominant fats in dairy products, red meat, and tropical oils, such as coconut oil. Saturated fats increase both total and LDL cholesterol and overall, the intake of saturated fat is associated with an increase in the incidence of cardiovascular disease (Ascherio, 2002). However, the Nurses' Health Study showed that when you simply replace saturated fat intake with carbohydrate intake, there is a very small reduction in cardiovascular risk. In contrast, replacement with monounsaturated or polyunsaturated fats was associated with an almost 10-fold greater decrease in risk (Hu et al., 1997).

Monounsaturated fatty acids contain only one double bond in their fatty acid side chains. These are typically liquid at room temperature but become cloudy and thicken when cooled. Foods rich in monounsaturated fat include olive oil, canola oil, many types of nuts, and avocados. Monounsaturated fats have been associated with lower CVD risk. This is best shown through the Mediterranean diet, which is high in monounsaturated fats. One of the main characteristics of this diet is the use of olive oil as the main source of fat in the form of monounsaturated fat. The largest prospective study to look at the benefits of monounsaturated fats and the Mediterranean diet is the Lyons Diet Heart study (De Lorgeril et al., 1999). This study randomized patients with known CVD to receive either the Mediterranean diet or the AHA step 1 diet and showed a very impressive protective effect with the Mediterranean diet. One must remember, though, that this diet has several other distinguishing characteristics, including a high consumption of fresh fruits and vegetables; the use of whole-grain rather than refined carbohydrates; low to moderate amounts of dairy, fish, and poultry; low amounts of red meat; minimal amounts of processed foods; and a low to moderate consumption of wine. Although many people have focused on the use of the monounsaturated olive oil as a primary fat source, there are many other dietary and social components to this diet that likely provide significant cardiovascular benefit.

Polyunsaturated fats contain multiple double bonds in their fatty acid chains. These are typically liquid at room temperature and in the refrigerator. Foods rich in polyunsaturated fats include most seeds and their oils, such as corn, sunflower, and safflower oil, and meats from animals fed on seeds. Omega-6 fatty acids and omega-3 fatty acids are in the family of polyunsaturated fats and are becoming increasingly important to the diet and CVD risk prevention. The Nurses' Health Study evaluated the effect of substituting dietary fat for an equivalent energy from carbohydrates (Junshi et al., 1990). While substituting with monounsaturated fats showed a 19% reduction in cardiovascular risk, a more significant reduction of 38% was seen when substituting with polyunsaturated fats. This finding demonstrates a more cardioprotective effect from polyunsaturated fats.

Carbohydrates represent the other major macronutrient affecting cardiovascular health. They are composed of isomers and polymers of monosaccharides and there are several forms, including mono-, di-, oligo-, and polysaccharides. The digestible forms of carbohydrates are starches and simple sugars; nondigestible forms make up the various types of fibers. Importantly, monosaccharides represent simple sugars such as glucose and fructose and polysaccharides represent dietary fibers. Most research related to carbohydrates and their effect on cardiovascular health has been on the glycemic index/load and dietary fiber.

The glycemic index (GI) represents the type and quality of the carbohydrate. This was developed by studying the effects of various carbohydrates on blood glucose levels (Jenkins et al., 1981). The glycemic load is the product of the glycemic index value and the carbohydrate content and represents a better idea of the functional impact on cardiovascular risk. Liu et al. studied 75,000 women and found that a high dietary glycemic load from refined carbohydrates increases the risk of CVD, independent of known coronary disease risk factors (Liu et al., 2000). They also demonstrated that high-carbohydrate, low-fat diets increased triglyceride levels and decreased HDL cholesterol levels in postmenopausal women. Several controlled clinical trials have found that subjects consuming low-glycemic-index meals have improved glycemic control and improved lipid profiles primarily affecting HDL and triglycerides (Eckle and Krauss, 1998; Gordon and Rifkind, 1989; Wolever, 1992).

Dietary fibers are polysaccharides that have been linked to cardiovascular risk reduction as well as multiple other diseases. They can be divided into two groups, soluble and insoluble fiber. High-fiber diets have been shown to aid in minimizing constipation, increasing satiety, slowing glucose absorption from the small bowel, and inhibiting cholesterol absorption from the small intestine, thereby reducing serum cholesterol levels. Numerous studies have shown that daily dietary fiber can reduce total cholesterol and LDL cholesterol levels (Brown et al., 1999; CDC, 2004). Furthermore, the Nurses' Health Study and the Health Professionals' Study showed reduced risk for fatal and nonfatal myocardial infarction in both men and women in the highest quartile of fiber intake when compared to the lowest quartile of fiber intake (Rimm et al., 1996; Wolk et al., 1999).

Hu and Willett (2002) reviewed 147 epidemiologic and dietary intervention studies and developed these nutrition principles for prevention of CVD:

1. Increase consumption of omega-3 fatty acids from fish, fish oil supplementation, and plant sources.
2. Substitute nonhydrogenated unsaturated fats for saturated and trans fats.
3. Consume a diet high in fruits, vegetables, nuts, and whole grain and low in sugar and refined grain products.

EXERCISE

A sedentary life is detrimental to general health. Almost all cardiovascular diseases and diabetes have been shown to worsen in patients with sedentary lives. The Health Professionals' Follow-Up Study evaluated 44,452 men and demonstrated that the adjusted 12-year relative risk for fatal and nonfatal MI across increasing quintiles of total physical activity progressively fell (Tanasescu et al., 2002). Looking at patients after MI, percutaneous coronary intervention (PCI), or coronary artery bypass grafting (CABG), the study determined that those who participate in a comprehensive exercise rehab program have a sixfold decrease in cardiac death as compared to those patients not undergoing rehab (Taylor et al., 2004). Despite these and many other findings showing the benefits of exercise, physicians reported spending an average of 8 minutes counseling their patients on lifestyle change at routine annual visits. Furthermore, less than 5% of physicians advise patients to engage in physical activity at least 6 days per week as recommended by national guidelines.

A provocative study looking at exercise versus PCI in patients with CAD determined by greater than 75% stenosis by angiography showed that daily exercise over a 12-month period had a lower cardiovascular event–free survival and equal angina symptom improvement (Rainer, 2004). This and other studies such as the recently published Courage trial suggests that aggressive medical management including comprehensive exercise can alter the course and management of CAD.

Time and effort must be made to counsel all patients about the benefits of exercise, especially those with cardiovascular risk factors. Patients should be instructed to perform aerobic exercise in some form every day and try to reach at least 40 minutes. The aerobic exercise should be combined with muscle-building activity at least three times per week (Thompson et al., 2003). However, even mild to moderate levels of exercise have a significant impact on cardiovascular mortality, so efforts should be made to encourage the most "exercise-resistant" patients to simply be more active (Wen et al., 2011). A novel new approach for exercise-resistant patients is listed in Table 10.1. When possible, patients should be referred to exercise physiologists to learn how to

Table 10.1: 5 "Minutes to Exercise". This exercise program is meant for people who are "exercise resistant." The goal is to first focus on creating an exercise routine, then work on increasing the effort. This program is meant to be very simple and basic and therefore easy to accomplish.

5 Minutes to Exercise
• Exercise for only 5 minutes *every* day (cannot skip)
• Exercise for no more than the allotted time
• Exercise at any pace
• If bored, then increase the pace—not the time
• If sick or tired, slow down—do not skip the exercise
• After the first month, increase the duration by 5 minutes
• Increase the duration by 5 minutes each month

Table 10.2: Top 10 Dietary Supplements in Cardiovascular Disease

Supplement	CV Condition	Dose	Level of Evidence	Comments
Red yeast rice	Hyperlipidemia	1,200 mg bid	Effective	Chemical constituents similar to lovastatin Lowers LDL ~20% Significant product variability
Nicotinic acid (niacin)	Dyslipidemia	1,000 mg bid	Effective	Raises HDL ~20% Lowers TG ~27% Lowers LDL ~8%–10% May not add add'l clinical benefit if LDL already at goal <70
Omega-3 oils	All-cause/cardiac mortality Arrhythmia prevention Hypertriglyceridemia	1,800 mg EPA/DHA (combined)	Effective for all conditions	Decreased all-cause mortality 16% in secondary CAD prevention May decrease TG ~20%–50%
Coenzyme Q10	CHF Statin-induced myopathy	50–20 mg daily	Effective for CHF; possibly effective for statin-induced myopathy	Deficiency recognized as independent predictor of morbidity and mortality in CHF Statins deplete CoQ10 levels No large trials to determine clinical endpoints
Magnesium	ArrhythmiaHTN	250–1,000 mg depending on formulation (chelated and slo-mag are best absorbed)	Effective for arrhythmia; possibly effective for HTN	Arrhythmia, torsades de Pointes, VPCs, and APCs Dose-dependent lowering of 4.3 mm Hg systolic to 2.3 mm Hg diastolic for each 10-mmol/day increase

Supplement	Condition	Dose	Effectiveness	Comments
Hawthorn	CHF	160–1,800 mg of standardized extract	Possibly effective	May improve EF and exercise tolerance and reduce subjective symptoms associated with NYHA stage II heart failure
β-Sitosterol (sterol/stanol)	Dyslipidemia CAD	800mg to 2 g daily	Effective	Lowers LDL by 10% Lowers LDL by 20% when added to a low-fat/low-cholesterol diet
D-Ribose	Myopathy CHF	15g	Possibly effective	More studies are needed
Glucomannan (soluble fiber)	Dyslipidemia Weight loss	1.2–15 g/day	Possibly effective	Beneficial in decreasing total cholesterol, LDL cholesterol, TG, and fasting glucose Increased satiety may decrease body weight
Artichoke extract	Dyslipidemia	500–1,500 mg daily	Possibly effective	Up to 23% decrease in LDL cholesterol; however, larger studies are needed to confirm effectiveness

APCs = atrial premature contractions; CAD = coronary artery disease; CHF = congestive heart failure; HDL = high-density lipoprotein; HTN = hypertension; LDL = low-density lipoprotein; NYHA = New York Heart Association; TG = triglycerides; VPCs = ventricular premature contractions.

Adapted from Vogel JHK, Krocoff MW, eds. *Integrative Cardiology: Complementary and Alternative Medicine for the Heart.* New York: McGraw Hill; 2007.

appropriately exercise based on their medical conditions and to learn various forms of exercise in hopes of finding one that they will enjoy.

NUTRACEUTICALS

A number of vitamins and supplements have been shown to be of benefit in CVD. A recent survey of cardiac patients found that 40% use supplements and 35% use megadose vitamins, many of whom reported using the supplements specifically for heart health (Bin and Kiat, 2010). Furthermore, most physicians surveyed were unaware of patients' supplement use. Table 10.2 outlines a number of vitamins and supplements that have a role in the prevention and treatment of CVD. It is important that the physician tailor the supplement profile to a patient's specific need with recommendations geared toward avoiding potential adverse events and supplement–drug interactions.

PSYCHOLOGICAL RISK FACTORS IN THE DEVELOPMENT OF CARDIOVASCULAR DISEASE

The INTERHEART study defined the relative risks for acute myocardial infarction of the various cardiovascular risk factors in a population of 29,972 individuals from 52 different countries. Nine risk factors were found to account for 90% of the populations' attributable risk in men. Of these risk factors, psychosocial factors including depression, stress, and anxiety were independently found to lead to a higher relative risk of developing CVD than most other traditional risk factors including hypertension, diabetes, and obesity (Yusuf et al., 2004). Furthermore, these psychosocial factors were found to dependently increase the incidence or worsen the severity of the traditional cardiac risk factors.

Although stress may at times be an adaptive response to ensure survival, stress hormones—most notably epinephrine, cortisol, and aldosterone—are associated with impaired glucose metabolism, weight gain, arrhythmia, hypertension, hyperlipidemia, inflammation, and coronary spasm. In addition, stress can adversely affect autonomic and vascular tone, immune function, coagulation, and the perception of pain.

A growing body of evidence suggests that depression may predispose people to cardiovascular events (Frasure-Smith et al., 1995). Depression is common after an acute MI and is associated with an increased risk of mortality for at least 18 months. Ziegelstein and colleagues (2000) found that patients who were identified with at least mild to moderate depression or major depression reported lower adherence to a low-fat diet, regular exercise, and stress management. Individuals with major depression or dysthymia reported taking their medications less often than prescribed.

Individuals with mental stress during daily life have twice the risk of myocardial ischemia. Anger was found to increase the risk of an acute myocardial infarction by 230% (Mittleman et al., 1995). In a recent study evaluating the psychological stress associated with the death of a significant person in one's life, the incidence rate of an MI increased 21-fold within the first 24 hours (Mostofsky et al., 2010). Yet this aspect of mental health is often ignored, underdiagnosed, and inadequately treated in the cardiovascular patient.

Evidence-Based Mind–Body Therapies

Multiple studies have demonstrated the impact of stress reduction using various nonpharmacological modalities in cardiovascular mortality. Blumenthal et al. (2005) demonstrated a 50% reduction in 5-year cardiovascular events with the use of biofeedback and progressive muscle relaxation when compared to patients receiving usual care. Dusseldorp et al. (1999) in a meta-analysis of psychoeducational programs for CVD, demonstrated a 29% reduction in MI recurrence and a 34% reduction in overall cardiovascular mortality.

Traditional Western medicine offers few therapeutic options for a patient who is identified with a significant stressor affecting his or her health. Fortunately, there are various nonpharmacological, mind–body therapies for coping with and preventing stress. Everyone reacts to stress differently, and therefore treatment should be tailored to the individual. These therapies can be as simple as addressing diet and exercise coupled with meditation to a multidisciplinary lifestyle change program utilizing multiple modalities such as group support, music therapy, specialized meditation, guided imagery, and/ or healing touch. These mind–body interventions can be implemented in both the inpatient and outpatient care settings, and many of these techniques can be taught to patients for self-administration.

BIOFEEDBACK

Biofeedback is a mind–body technique that incorporates physiological markers such as heart rate, blood pressure, skin temperature, and muscle tension to train people to change habitual reactions to stress. It usually displays visual or auditory feedback to raise a patient's awareness and conscious control of various relaxation techniques such as deep breathing and muscle relaxation.

In CVD patients, biofeedback has been used to reduce stress, lower blood pressure, and increase heart rate variability (HRV). Lehrer et al. (2000) demonstrated that training individuals to maximize peak heart rate differences using biofeedback could increase homeostatic reflexes, lower blood pressure, and improve lung function. Nakao et al. (1997; 2000) demonstrated that biofeedback can effectively lower both systolic and diastolic blood pressure in patients with essential hypertension. Where low HRV is an independent risk factor for sudden cardiac death, all-cause death, and cardiac event recurrence, studies support the use of biofeedback to increase heart rate variability (Bigger et al., 1993; Kleiger et al., 1987). Del Pozo et al. (2004) examined the use of biofeedback in patients with coronary artery disease and found that this technique increases heart rate variability in this patient population, supporting biofeedback as a potential tool for improving cardiac morbidity and mortality rates.

MEDITATION

Meditation has been part of various spiritual traditions for thousands of years. Interest in meditation was rekindled in the United States with the introduction of transcendental meditation (TM) in the late 1960s and with mindfulness-based stress reduction (MBSR) the following decade.

TM offers a unique technique for meditation and relaxation. It is one of the most studied integrative medicine mind–body therapies, with research dating back to the 1970s. TM is practiced for 20 minutes twice daily. Schneider et al. (2005) have demonstrated improvement in hypertension and cardiovascular morbidity and mortality in patients who practice TM daily. Furthermore, TM has been shown to improve not only blood pressure but also the insulin resistance components of the metabolic syndrome as well as cardiac autonomic nervous system tone (Paul-Labrador et al., 2006). This form of meditation can be quickly learned and performed in almost all clinical situations.

MBSR is a structured group program that teaches meditation focused on moment-to-moment awareness. MBSR employs the techniques of mindfulness meditation, gentle yoga, and coordinated deep breathing to decrease pain and anxiety. MBSR has been used not only for stress reduction but also for other conditions such as CAD, chronic pain, hypertension, and anxiety.

In a meta-analysis looking at MBSR for a wide spectrum of clinical populations, it was shown that MBSR may help individuals alleviate stress and suffering associated with various diseases (Grossman et al., 2004). Numerous studies have shown perceived improvement in quality of life, mood, symptoms of stress, and quality of sleep (Carlson et al., 2004; Robert et al., 2004; Tacon et al., 2003).

TAI CHI

Tai chi is a form of traditional Chinese medicine that applies very natural postures and body motions while using relaxation and breathing to generate health, longevity, and internal strength and power.

In a trial sponsored by the National Institutes of Health (NIH) (Yeh et al., 2011), 100 outpatients with stable chronic heart failure (ejection fraction <40% and New York Heart Association class I–III) were randomized to receive either 12 weeks of tai chi training or usual care. The patients receiving tai chi had a statistically significant increase in quality-of-life scores, mood, and exercise self-efficacy. More aggressive tai chi techniques have been shown to not only improve life scores but also improve 6-minute walk distances in a similar group of patients (Yeh et al., 2004). These benefits of tai chi in heart failure should not be underscored in this population of patients who often live with a debilitating illness.

PET OWNERSHIP

Pet ownership not only provides the medical benefits associated with stress reduction but also can convey a sense of companionship and purpose. Social science research studies via surveys have shown a self-reported benefit of both physical and psychological health, leading to fewer physician visits (Headey, 1999; Siegel, 1990). In an effort to have a more direct medical correlation, studies were performed linking pet ownership to lower blood pressure, ultimately resulting in lower cardiovascular risk (Anderson et al., 1992). Also, pet ownership was shown to be associated with increased HRV in patients with CVD (Friedman et al., 2003).

GUIDED IMAGERY

Guided imagery uses the power of thought to influence psychologic and physiologic states. Guided imagery is a therapeutic technique that allows an individual to use his or her own imagination to achieve desirable outcomes such as decreased pain perception and reduced anxiety. Imagery has been successfully used as an intervention in patients with pain, cancer, insomnia, posttraumatic stress disorder, and surgery.

Guided imagery has been studied as a pre- and postsurgical intervention for cardiothoracic surgery patients. A study from the Cleveland Clinic demonstrated that both pain and anxiety decreased significantly with guided imagery (Kshettry et al., 2006). When combined with healing touch, guided imagery resulted in significant decreases in posttraumatic stress disorder, depression, and cynicism while increasing mental quality of life for active marines returning from combat in an ongoing trial from Scripps Clinic. Hypnosis-like guided imagery is also successful in decreasing anxiety and reducing blood pressure (Gay, 2007). Hypnosis has been shown to affect heart rate variability by reducing the sympathetic and enhancing the parasympathetic tone (Hippel et al., 2001).

Our Integrative Approach to Cardiovascular Disease

An integrative approach to cardiovascular disease requires a redefinition of disease state and a recalibration of what is defined as "health." Our early detection and prevention clinic recommends that a comprehensive, individual approach be undertaken. First, in addition to usual "vital signs" obtained at the beginning of a clinic visit, additional measurements including waist circumference and body mass index should be recorded and followed longitudinally for trends. This brings awareness to both physician and patient of potential increasing risk as well as measuring ongoing efforts of lifestyle change and optimal health. A thorough history, physical examination, and accurate family history are then undertaken. The history obtained not only seeks evidence of chest pain or shortness of breath but also includes specific questions about daily exercise, dietary intake, alcohol consumption, and life stressors and coping skills. We recommend obtaining screening laboratory data including VAP panel, hs-CRP, HgbA1c, Lp(a), comprehensive metabolic panel, and complete blood count prior to an initial visit in order to educate our patients and develop a thorough plan at the initial visit.

An important component of an integrative approach relies on forming a trusting relationship between physician and patient. Routine follow-up can serve as a means to check on the success of lifestyle and therapeutic interventions, providing guidance and accountability. This also allows for the identification of trends and listening for subtle cues of a change in health, which can perhaps improve outcomes. Instructing our patients to redefine health not based on a lack of chest pain or shortness of breath but rather with an emphasis on achieving excellent exercise tolerance, stress management, and healthy proper nutrition will undoubtedly help decrease index cardiac events and improve overall quality of life.

REFERENCES

Achenbach S, Moseleweski F, Ropers D, et al. Detection of calcified and noncalcified coronary atherosclerotic plaque by contrast-enhanced, submillimeter multidetector spiral coputed tomography: a segment based comparison with intravascular ultracound. Circulation. 2004;109:14–17.

Agatston AS, Janowitz WR, Hildner FJ, Zusmer NR, Viamonte M Jr, Detrano R. Quantification of coronary artery calcium using ultrafast computed tomography. J Am Coll Cardiol. 1990;15:827–832.

Anderson WP, Reid CM, Jennings GL. Pet ownership and risk factors for cardiovascular disease. Med J Aust. 1992;157:298–301.

Arad Y, Spadaro LA, Goodman K, Newstein D, Guerci AD. Prediction of coronary events with electron beam computed tomography. J Am Coll Cardiol. 2000;36:1253–1260.

Ascherio A. Epidemiologic studies on dietary fats and coronary heart disease. Am J Med. 2002;113(Suppl 9B):9S–12S.

Austin M, Breslow J, Hennekens C, et al. Low-density lipoproteins subclass patterns and risk of myocardial infarction. JAMA. 1988;260:1917–1921.

Bigger JT, Fleiss JL, Rolnitzky LM, et al. The ability of several short-term measures of RR variability to predict mortality after myocardial infarction. Circulation. 1993;88:927–934.

Bin YS, Kiat H. Prevalence of dietary supplement use in patients with proven or suspected cardiovascular disease. Evidence-Based Complement Altern Med. 2010. doi:10.1155/2011/632829

Blumenthal JA, Sherwood A, Babyak MA, et al. Effects of exercise and stress management training on markers of cardiovascular risk in patients with ischemic heart disease: a randomized controlled trial. JAMA. 2005;293:1626–1634.

Brook RD, Kansal M, Bard RL, Eagle K, et al. Usefulness of low-density lipoprotein particle size measurement in cardiovascular disease prevention. Clin Cardio. 2005;28:534–537.

Brown L, et al. Cholesterol-lowering effects of dietary fiber: a meta-analysis. Am J Clin Nutr. 1999;69(1):30–42.

Bruce RA, Hossack KF, DeRouen TA, Hofer V. Enhanced risk assessment for primary coronary heart disease events by maximal exercise testing: 10 years' experience of Seattle Heart Watch. J Am Coll Cardiol. 1983;2:565–573.

Brunzell J. Increased apoB in small dense LDL particles predicts premature coronary artery disease. Arterioscler Thromb Vasc Biol. 2005;25:553–559.

Budoff MJ, McClelland RL, Nasir K, et al. Cardiovascular events with absent or minimal coronary calcification: the Multi-Ethnic Study of Atherosclerosis (MESA). Am Heart J. 2009;158:554–561.

Burchfiel CM, Reed DM, Marcus EB, et al. Association of diabetes mellitus with coronary atherosclerosis and myocardial lesions: an autopsy report fomr the Honollu Heart Program. Am J Epidemiol. 1993;137:1328–1340.

Carlson LE, Speca M, Patel KD, Goodey E. Mindfulness-based stress reduction in relation to quality of life, mood, symptoms of stress and levels of cortisol, dehydroepiandrosterone sulfate (DHEAS) and melatonin in breast and prostate cancer outpatients. Psychoneuroendocrinology. 2004;29(4):448–474.

CDC. Trends in intake of energy and macronutrients—United States, 1971–2000. MMWR. 2004;53:80–82.

Centers for Disease Control and Prevention. Racial/ethnic and socioeconomic disparities in multiple risk factors for heart disease and stroke—United States, 2003. MMWR. 2005;54(5):113–117.

Clarke R, Peden JF, Hopewell JC, Kyroakou T et al. Genetic variants associated with Lp(a) lipoprotein level and coronary disease. N Engl J Med. 2009;361:2518–2528.

D'Agostino RB Sr, Grundy S, Sullivan LM, Wilson P. Validation of the Framingham coronary heart disease prediction scores: results of a multiple ethinic groups investigation. JAMA. 2001;286:180–187.

De Lorgeril M, Salen P, Martin JL, Monjaud I, Delaye J, Mamelle N. Mediterranean diet, traditional risk factors, and the rate of cardiovascular complications after myocardial infarction: final report of the Lyon Diet Heart Study. Circulation. 1999;99:779–785.

Del Pozo JM, Gevertz RN, Scher B, Guarneri E. Biofeedback treatment increases heart rate variability in patients with known coronary artery disease. Am Heart J. 2004;147:e11.

Detrano R, Guerci AD, Carr JJ, et al. Coronary calcium as a predictor of coronary events in four racial or ethnic groups. N Engl J Med. 2008;358:1336–1345.

Dusseldorp E, van Elderen T, Maes S, Meulman J, Kraaij V. A meta-analysis of psychoeducational programs for coronary heart disease patients. Health Psychol. 1999;18:506–519.

Eckle RH, Krauss RM. American Heart Association call to action: obesity as a major risk factor for coronary heart disease. Circulation. 1998;97:2099–2100.

Edelman D, Olsen MK, Dudley TK, Harris AC, Oddone E. Utility of hemoglobin A1c in predicting diabetes risk. J Gen Intern Med. 2004;19:1175–1180.

Erbel R, Mohlenkamp S, Moebus S, et al. Heinz Nixdorf Recall Study Investifative Group. Coronary risk stratification, discrimination, and reclassification improvement based on quantification of subclinical coronary atherosclerosis. The Heize Nixdorf Recall Study. J Am Coll Cardiolo. 2010;56:1397–1406.

Erquo S, Kaptoge S, Perry PL, Di Angelantonio E, et al. Lipoprotein(a) concentration and the risk of coronary heart disease, stroke, and nonvascular mortality. JAMA. 2009;302(4):412–423.

Forrester JS, Bick-Oreester J. Persistence of inflammation is a cause of chronigc progressive diseases. Med Hypotheses. 2005;65:227–231.

Frasure-Smith N, Lesperance F, Talajic M. Depression and 18-month prognosis after myocardial infarction. Circulation. 1995;91:999–1005.

Friedewald W, Levy R, Fredrickson D. Estimation of concentration of low-density lipoprotein cholesterol in plasma, without the use of preparative ultracentrifuge. *Clin Chem.* 1972;18:499–502.

Friedman E, Thomas SA, Stein P, Kleiger R. Relation between pet ownership and heart rate variability in patients with healed myocardial infarcts. JACC. 2003;91:718–721.

Gay MC. Effectiveness of hypnosis in reducing mild essential hypertension: a one-year follow-up. Int J Clin Exp Hypn. 2007;55:67–83.

Gibbons LW, Mitchell TL, Wei M, Blair SN, Cooper KH. Maximal exercise test as a predictor of risk for mortality from coronary heart disease in asymptomatic men. Am J Cardiol. 2000;86:53–58.

Gibbons RJ, Balady GJ, Bricker JT, et al. ACC/AHA 2002 guideline update for exercise testing: summary article: a report pf the American College of Cardiology/American Heart Association Task Force on Practice Guidelines (Committee to Update 1997 Exercise Testing Guidelines). Circulation. 2002;106:1883–1892.

Gordon DJ, Ekelund LG, Karon JM, et al. Predictive value of the exercise tolerance test for mortality in North American men: the Lipid Research Clinics Mortality Follow-up Study. Circulation. 1986;74:252–261.

Gordon DJ, Rifkind BM. High-density lipoprotein—the clinical implications of recent studies. NEJM. 1989;321(19):1311–1316.

Greenland P, Gaziano JM. Selecting asymptomatic patients for coronary computed tomography or electrocardiographic exercise testing. N Engl J Med. 2003;349:465–473.

Grossman P, Neimann L, Schmidt S, Walach H. Mindfulness-based stress reduction and health benefits. A meta-analysis. J Psychosom Res. 2004;57(1):35–43.

Headey B. Health benefits and health cost savings due to pets: preliminary results from an Australian national survey. Soc Indicators Res. 1999;47:233–243.

Heron MP, Hoyert DL, Murphy SL, Xu JQ, Kochanek KD, Tejada-Vera B. *Deaths: Final data for 2006 National Vital Statistics Reports*; Vol. 57, No. 14. Hyattsville, MD: National Center for Health Statistics, 2009.

Hippel CV, Hole G, Kaschka WP. Autonomic profile under hypnosis as assessed by heart rate variability and spectral analysis. Pharmacopsychiatry. 2001;34:111–113.

Hu FB, Stampfer MJ, Manson JE, et al. Dietary fat intake and the risk of coronary heart disease in women. NEJM. 1997;337:1491.

Hu FB, Willett WC. Optimal diets for prevention of coronary heart disease. JAMA. 2002;288:2569–2578.

Hunold P, Vogt FM, Schmermund A, et al. Radiation exposure during cardiac CT: effetive doses at multi-detector row CT and electron-beam CT. Radiology. 2003;226:145–152.

Jenkins DJ, et al. Glycemic index of foods: a physiological basis for carbohydrate exchange. Am J Clin Nutr. 1981;34(3):362–366.

Junshi, Chen; T. Colin; Junyao, Li et al., eds. (1990). *Diet, lifestyle, and mortality in China: a study of the characteristics of 65 Chinese counties*. Oxford University Press.

Kannel WB. Lipids, diabetes, and coronary heart disease: insights from the Framingham Study. Am Heart J. 1985;110:1100–1107.

Khaw K, Waremah N, Bingham S, Lubon R. Association of hemoglobin A1c with cardiovascular disease and mortality in adults: the European prospective invetigation into cancer in Norfolk. Ann Int Med. 2004;114:413–420.

Kleiger RE, Miller JP, Bigger JT, et al., and the Multicenter Post-Infarction Research Group. Decreased heart rate variability and its association with increased mortality after acute myocardial infarction. Am J Cardiol. 1987;59:256–262.

Kshettry VR, Carole LF, Henly SJ, Sendelbach S, Kummer B. Complementary alternative medical therapies for heart surgery patients: feasibility, safety, and impact. Ann Thorac Surg. 2006;81(1):201–205.

Kulkarni K. Cholesterol profile measurement by vertical auto profile method. Clin Lab Med. 2006;26:787–802.

Leber AW, Knez A, Becker A, et al. Accuracy of multidetector spiral computed tomography in indentifying and differentiating the composition of coronary atherosclerotic plaques: a comparative study with intracoronary ultrasound. J Am Coll Cardiol. 2007;49:946–950.

Lehrer PM, Vaschillo E, Vaschillo B. Resonant frequency biofeedback training to increase cardiac variability: rationale and manual for training. Appl Psychophysiol Biofeedback. 2000;25:177–191.

Libby P. Inflammation in atherosclerosis. Nature. 2002;420:868–874.

Liu S, et al. A prospective study of dietary glycemic load, carbohydrate intake, and risk of coronary heart disease in US women. Am J Clin Nutr. 2000;71(6):1455–1461.

Lloyd-Jones D, Adams RJ, Brown TM, et al. Heart disease and stroke statistics—2010 update. A report from the American Heart Association Statistics Committee and Stroke Statistics Subcommitee. Circulation. 2010;121:e1–e170.

Mittleman MA, Maclure M, Sherwood JB, et al. Triggering of acute myocardial infarction onset by episodes of anger. Circulation. 1995;92:1720–1725.

Mokdad AH, Marks JS, Stroup DF, Gerberding JL. Actual causes of death in the United States, 2000. JAMA. 2004;291:1238–1245.

Mosca L, Linfante AH, Benjamin EJ, Berra K, Hayes SN, Walsh BW, Fabunmi RP, Kwan J, Mills T, Simpson SL. National study of physician awareness and adherence to cardiovascular disease prevention guidelines. Circulation. 2005;111:499–510.

Mostofsky E, Malcolm M, Sherwood JB, Tofler GH, Muller JE, Mittleman MA. Risk of acute myocardial infarction after the death of a significant person in one's life. Circulation. 2010;125:491–496.

Nakao M, Nomura S, Shimosawa T, Yoshiuchi K, Kumano H, Kuboki T, et al. Blood pressure biofeedback treatment of white-coat hypertension. J Psychosom Res. 2000;48(2):161–169.

Nakao M, Nomura S, Shimosawa T, Yoshiuchi K, Kumano H, Kuboki T, et al. Clinical effects of blood pressure biofeedback treatment on hypertension by auto-shaping. Psychosom Med. 1997;59(3):331–338.

Nambi V, Chambless L, Folsom AR, He M, et al. Carotid intima-mediat thichness and presence or absence of plaque improves prediction of coronary heart disease risk, The ARIC (atherosclerosis risk in communities) study. J Am Coll Cardiol. 2010;55:1600–1607.

Nasir K, Shaw LJ, Budoff MJ, Ridker PM, Pena JM. Coronary artery calcium scanning should be used for primary prevention. Pros and cons. J Am Coll Cardiol: Cardiovascular Imaging. 2012;5(1):111–118.

Nederkoorn PJ, Mali WP, Eikelboom BC, et al. Preoperative diagnosis of carotid plaque: accuracy of noninvasive testing. Stroke. 2002;33:2003–2008.

O'Holleran LW, Kennelly NM, McClurken M, et al. Natural history of asymptomatic carotid plaque. Five year follow-up study. Am J Surg. 1987;154:659–662.

O'Leary D, Polak JF, Kronmal RA, Manolio TA, et al. Carotid-artery intima and media thickness as a risk factor for myocardial infarction and stroke in older patients. N Engl J Med. 1999;340:14–22.

O'Rourke RA, Brundage BH, Froelicher VF, GreenlandP, et al. American College of Cardiology/Amrican Heart Association expert consensus document on electron-beam computed tomography for the diagnosis and prognosis of coronary artery disease. J Am Coll Cardiol. 2000;36:326–340.

Paul-Labrador M, Polk D, Dwyer JH, Velasquez I, Nidich S, Rainforth M, et al. Effects of a randomized controlled trial of transcendental meditation on components of the metabolic syndrome in subjects with coronary heart disease. Arch Intern Med. 2006;166:1218–1224.

Pearson TA, Mensah GA, Alexander RW, et al. Markers of inflammation and cardiovascular disease: application to clinical and public health practice; a statement for healthcare professionals from the Centers for Disease Control and Prevention and the American Heart Association. Circulation. 2003;107:499–511.

Pischon T, Girman CJ, Sacks FM, Rifai N, Stampfer MJ, Rimm EB. Non–high-density lipoprotein cholesterol and apolipoprotein B in the pre- diction of coronary heart disease in men. Circulation. 2005;112:3375–3383.

Pletcher MJ, Tice JA, Pignone M, McCulloch C, et al. What does my patient's coronary artery calcium score mean? Combining information from the coronary artery calcium score with information from convenstional risk factors to estimate coronary heart disease risk. BMC Medicine. 2004;2:31–42.

Rainer H. Percutaneous coronary angioplasty compared with exercise training in patients with stable coronary artery disease: a randomized trial. Circulation. 2004;109:1371–1378.

Ridker P. Beyond cholesterol: C-reactive protein and homocysteine as predictors of cardiovascular risk. In Rifai N, Warnick GR, Dominiczak MH, Eds. *Handbook of lipoprotein testing.* 2nd Edition. Washington (DC): AACC Press; 2000. pp61–75.

Ridker PM, Buring JE, Rifai N, Cook NR. Development and validation of improved algorithms for the assessment of global cardiovascular risk in women: The Reynolds Risk Score. JAMA. 2007;297:611–619.

Ridker PM, Cushman M, Stampfer MJ, et al. Inflammatio, aspirin, and the risk of coronary heart disease in apparently health men. N Engl J Med. 1997;336:973–979.

Ridker PM, Danielson E, Fonseca, FAH, et al., Sc.D. for the JUPITER Study Group. Rosuvastatin to prevent vascular events in men and women with elevated C-reactive protein. N Engl J Med. 2008; 359:2195–2207.

Ridker PM, Hennekens CH, Buring JE, et al. C-reactive protein and other markers of inflammation in the prediction of cardiovascular disease in women. N Engl J Med. 2000;342:836–843.

Ridker PM, Paynter NP, Rifai N, Gaziano JM, Cook NR. C-reactive protein and parental history improve global cardiovascular risk prediction: The Reynolds Risk Score for men. Circulation. 2008;118(25):2243–2251.

Rimm EB, et al. Vegetable, fruit, and cereal fiber intake and risk of coronary heart disease among men. JAMA. 1996;275(6):447–451.

Robert McComb JJ, Tacon A, Randolph P, Caldera Y. A pilot study to examine the effects of a mindfulness-based stress-reduction and relaxation program on levels of stress hormones, physical functioning, and submaximal exercise responses. J Altern Complement Med. 2004;10(5):819–827.

Schneider RH, Alexander CN, Staggers F, Rainforth M, Salerno J, Hartz A, et al. Long-term effects of stress reduction on mortality in persons >55 years of age with systemic hypertension. Am J Cardiol. 2005;95:1060–1064.

Siegel JM. Stressful life events and use of physician services among the elderly: the moderating effects of pet ownership. J Pers Soc Psychol. 1990;58:1081–1086.

Sniderman AD. Editorial: Apolipoprotein B versus non-high-density lipoprotein cholesterol. And the winner is.... Circulation. 2005;112:3366–3367.

Stampfer MJ, Hu FB, Manson JE, Rimm EB, Willett WC. Primary Prevention of cornary heart disease in women through diet and lifestyle. N Engl J Med. 2000;343(1):16–22.

Tacon AM, McComb J, Caldera Y, Randolph P. Mindfulness meditation, anxiety reduction, and heart disease: a pilot study. Fam Community Health. 2003;26(1):25–33.

Tanasescu M, et al. Exercise type and intensity in relation to coronary heart disease in men. JAMA. 2002;288(16):1994–2000.

Taylor R, Brown A, Ebrahm S, et al. Exercise-based rehabilitation for patients with coronary heart disease: systematic review and meta-analysis of randomized controlled trials. Am J Med. 2004;116(10):682–692.

Third report of the expert panel on detection, evaluation, and treatment of high blood cholesterol in adults (Adult Treatment Panel III): 10-year risk calculator. Bethesda, MdL National Heart, Lung, and Blood Institute, May 2001. http://www/nhlbi.nih.gov/guidelines/cholesterol/index.htm.

Thompson PD, et al. Exercise and physical activity in the prevention and treatment of atherosclerotic cardiovascular disease: a statement from the council on clinical cardiology. Circulation. 2003;107:3109–3116.

Tian L, Fu M. The relationship between high density lipoprotein subclass profile and plasma lipids concentrations. Lipids in Health and Disease. 2010;9:118.

Tuomilehto J, et al. Prevention of type 2 diabetes mellitus by changes in lifestyle among subjects with impaired glucose tolerance. NEJM. 2001;344(18):1343–1350.

Vogel JHK, Krocoff MW, eds. Integrative Cardiology: Complementary and Alternative Medicine for the Heart. New York: McGraw Hill; 2007.

Vogel RA, Corretti MC, Plotnick GD. Effect of a single high-fat meal on endothelial function in healthy subjects. Am J Cardiology. 1997;79:350–354.

Von Eckardstein A, Huang Y, Assmann G. Physiologic role and clinical relevance of high-density lipoprotein subclasses. Curr Opin Lipidol. 1994;5:404–416.

Wen CP, et al. Minimum amount of physical activity for reduced mortality and extended life expectancy: a prospective cohort study. Lancet. 2011;378:1244–1253.

Wolever TM. Beneficial effect of a low glycemic index diet in type 2 diabetes. Diabet Med. 1992;9(5):451–458.

Wolf PA, Kannel WB, Sorlie P, et al. Asymptomatic carotid bruit and risk of stroke. The Framingham Study. JAMA. 1981;245:1442–1445.

Wolk A, et al. Long-term intake of dietary fiber and decreased risk of coronary heart disease among women. JAMA. 1999;281(21):1998–2004.

Wong ND, Hsu JC, Detrano RC, Diamond G, Eisenberg H, Gardin JM. Coronary artery calcium evaluation by electron beam computed tomography and its relation to new cardiovascular events. Am J Cardiol. 2000;86:495–498.

Yeh GY, McCarthy EP, Phillips RS, et al. Tai chi exercise in patients with chronic heart failure. Arch Intern Med. 2011;171(8):750–757.

Yeh GY, Wood MJ, Lorell BH, et al. Effects of tai chi mind-body movement therapy on functional status and exercise capacity in patients with chronic heart failure: a randomized controlled trial. Am J Med. 2004;117:541–548.

Yusuf S, Hawken S, Ounpuu S, Dans T, et al. Effect of potentially modifiable risk factors associated with myocardial infarction in 52 countries (the INTERHEART study): case-control study. Lancet. 2004;364:937–952.

Yusuf S, Hawken S, Ounpuu S, on behalf of the INTERHEART Study Investigators. Effect of potentially modifiable risk factors associated with myocardial infarction in 52 countries (the INTERHEART study): case-control study. Lancet. 2004;364:937–952.

Ziegelstein RC, Fauerbach JA, Stevens SS, Romanelli J, Richter DP, Bush DE. Patients with depression are less likely to follow recommendations to reduce cardiac risk during recovery from a myocardial infarction. Arch Intern Med. 2000;160:1818–1823.

11

Urology

ERIC YARNELL

Conditions affecting the male reproductive tract are common and often overlooked, undertreated, or misunderstood. Though these conditions are rarely life threatening, they can have substantial morbidity. One reason men are less likely to seek professional medical help is that far too often they do not receive the help, support, and unbiased information they are seeking. This chapter will seek to improve understanding of these conditions and provide a wider array of options than are available in conventional medicine, along with an approach to individualizing treatments.

Benign Prostatic Hyperplasia and Lower Urinary Tract Symptoms

Benign prostatic hyperplasia (BPH) plagues many men as they grow older. Hyperplastic overgrowth of the transitional zone and periurethral stromal smooth muscle and fibroblasts, hyperplastic overgrowth of the secretory epithelium, or both result in a set of symptoms called lower urinary tract symptoms (LUTSs), though other conditions can also cause these symptoms (Kirby et al., 2005). Microscopic BPH is a universal condition of male aging, though only a fraction of men develop clinical symptoms (Campbell, 2004; Gu et al., 1994). Far more men in the developed world develop clinical BPH, and as areas of the developing world adopt a Western lifestyle, clinical BPH rates are skyrocketing there (Gu, 1997; Terai et al., 2000).

It has been estimated that in the year 2000, 25% of white men ages 50 to 79 years had symptomatic BPH in the United States alone, or at least 6.5 million men (Wei et al., 2005). There were millions of medical visits to treat BPH, with 87,400 prostatectomies for this condition done in that year, contributing to a total of nondrug costs of $1.1 billion spent to treat it.

The etiology of BPH is unknown, though it is likely multifactorial. Androgens are known to be a permissive factor in allowing hyperplasia to occur, though they do not necessarily cause the condition (Ho and Habib, 2011). High serum androgens and testosterone therapy do not clearly correlate to causing or aggravating clinical BPH (Page et al., 2011; Shigehara et al., 2011). It is possible that androgen levels in the prostatic venous plexus are elevated far beyond what is present in the general circulation due to back-pressure from compromised spermatic veins, a common condition associated with aging (Gat et al., 2008). Alternatively, an excess of estrogens, possibly due to increased adiposity that develops with age, aromatizing androgens, or environmental xenoestrogenic chemicals, has also been reasonably posited to contribute to BPH (Griffiths et al., 2002). Excess oxidation has also been linked to BPH, though only weakly (Aydin et al., 2006). Insulin resistance and obesity have been repeatedly linked to BPH, which may explain the increased incidence in developed countries (Nandeesha et al., 2006).

LUTSs are generally divided into two groups: irritative symptoms (frequency, urgency, nocturia) and storage/obstructive symptoms (slow stream, hesitancy, dribbling, incomplete emptying). The diagnosis of BPH is usually a clinical one based on the presence of LUTSs and palpable enlargement of the prostate on digital exam. The International Prostate Symptom Score, a 7-item questionnaire, is commonly used to assess severity and to semiquantitatively monitor therapeutic progress. Digital prostate exam, peak flow rate (Qmax), and postvoid residual (PVR) urine levels assessed by ultrasound are also frequently employed to help determine if a man has BPH causing his LUTSs.

Lifestyle and nutritional approaches are recommended to prevent BPH, including avoiding excessive animal product intake, increasing vegetable intake, maintaining healthy weight, exercising regularly, and not smoking (Barnard et al., 2008; Cimino et al., 2012; De Nunzio et al., 2012). Garlic and onions have shown the most protective effect among vegetables (Galeone et al., 2007). Intake of more than 5 mg of isoflavones from food such as whole soy products also significantly reduces the risk of developing severe BPH (Wong et al., 2007).

The two types of medications currently used to treat symptoms of BPH are α blockers, specific or nonspecific, and 5-α-reductase inhibitors (5aRi) (see Table 11.1). Nonspecific α₁-adrenergic receptor antagonists such as terazosin and doxazosin act to relax blood vessels, as well as being spasmolytic in the prostate and bladder, but can cause dizziness, hypotension (particularly at drug initiation), fatigue, and edema and are associated with increased cardiovascular mortality (ALLHAT, 2003). Selective α blockers such as tamsulosin

Table 11.1: Dosing Treatments for Benign Prostatic Hypertrophy

Agent	Action	Usual Oral Starting Dose*	Contraindications	Adverse Effects
Ammi visnaga fruit FPT	Spasmolytic	1 ml tid	None established	Mild sedation
Piscidia piscipula bark DPT	Spasmolytic	1 ml tid	None established	Sedation
Lobelia inflata aerial parts FPT	Spasmolytic	10 gtt tid	None established	Nausea, vomiting
Valeriana spp root FPT	Spasmolytic	2–3 ml tid	None established	Mild sedation
Gelsemium sempervirens root FPT	Spasmolytic	10 gtt tid	Operation of heavy machinery	Sedation
Niu Che Sen Qi Wan granules	Spasmolytic, anticholinergic	2.5 g tid	Arrhythmias	Arrhythmias (rare but potentially fatal)
Finasteride	5aRI	5 mg qd	Prostate <40 g	ED, low libido, gynecomastia, increased prostate cancer severity (?)
Dutasteride	5aRI	0.5 mg qd	Prostate <40 g	as finasteride
Tamsulosin	α_1 Blocker	0.2–0.8 mg qd	Cataract surgery	EjD, hypotension
Alfuzosin	α_1 Blocker	5 mg bid (10 mg qd SR)	Cataract surgery	as tamsulosin
Serenoa repens standardized extract	Phytoestrogen, 5aRI, α_1 blocker	320 mg qd	None established	Minimal

(continued)

Table 11.1: (continued)

Agent	Action	Usual Oral Starting Dose*	Contraindications	Adverse Effects
Urtica dioica root extract	Aromatase inhibitor, SHBG inhibitor	1–2 g bid	None established	Minimal
Polygonum multiflorum decocted root	Hormone modulator	2.5 g tid (granules); 2–3 ml tid (DPT)	None established	Minimal
Epimedium grandiflorum herb	Hormone modulator	2.5 g tid (granules); 2–3 ml tid (DPT)	None established	Minimal

* Always modify to suit the individual patient's situation as warranted.

5aRI = 5-α-reductase inhibitor; DPT = dry plant tincture; ED = erectile dysfunction; EjD = ejaculatory dysfunction; FPT = fresh plant tincture; SHBG = sex hormone–binding globulin; SR = sustained release.

and alfuzosin have fewer adverse effects and largely do not act on blood vessels, and thus are likely to be safer. Tamsulosin is slightly more effective than terazosin in comparative clinical trials and has fewer adverse effects (Dong et al., 2009). α Blockers do not prevent progression of BPH. 5aRi drugs such as finasteride and dutasteride reduce prostate volume, albeit very slowly (often taking >6 months to do so), and only work in men with a larger baseline prostate volume (generally 40 g or higher, though some studies show it is helpful even at 30 g) (Kaplan and colleagues, 2011; Neal, 1997).

To effectively treat patients with clinical BPH requires assessing their clinical phenotype. The most common type is spasmodic BPH, with a predominance of irritative symptoms, prostate volume less than 40 ml, PVR less than 50 ml, Qmax greater than 10 ml/sec, and relief of symptoms by use of α blockers. These patients' symptoms respond most when they are given spasmolytics to relax the excessive stromal tissue in their prostates. Unfortunately, there has been no published clinical research on natural Western botanical spasmolytics, but their use has a long tradition, with a beneficial effect on symptoms and minimal side effects being commonplace. Moderately potent herbal spasmolytics such as *Ammi visnaga* (khella) fruit, *Piscidia piscipula* (Jamaica dogwood) bark, *Lobelia inflata* (lobelia) aerial parts, *Valeriana officinalis* (valerian) or *V. sitchensis* (Pacific valerian) root, and even *Gelsemium sempervirens* (gelsemium) root are recommended for initial therapy. The Chinese herbal formula Niu Che Sen Qi Wan, known in Japanese as Gosha-jinki-gan, contains *Aconitum* spp. (aconite, *fu zi*) processed lateral roots and other herbs that have been shown to have anticholinergic and spasmolytic effects on the prostate and is effective in trials for BPH patients at a dose of 2.5 g tid (Fujiuchi et al., 2008; Gotoh et al., 2004; Nishijima et al., 2007; Ogushi and Takahashi, 2007). This provides at least some research-based support for the idea of using herbal spasmolytics in patients with spasmodic BPH.

Hormonally active herbs such as *Serenoa repens* (saw palmetto) fruit, *Prunus africanum* (pygeum) bark, and *Urtica dioica* (nettle) root are commonly thought of when considering natural therapies for men with BPH. These herbs are more appropriate for men with obstructive BPH, though often their prostates are greater than 50 ml in volume, which is too large for herbs alone to correct. Other signs of obstructive BPH are predominance of obstructive symptoms, PVR greater than 50 ml, Qmax less than 10 ml/sec, and minimal improvement by α blockers. Natural therapies may have a role in supporting conventional therapy in such patients (primarily 5aRi) or for long-term prevention of progression. Empirically, a combination of saw palmetto, nettle root, and *Polygonum multiflorum* (he shou wu) decocted root or *Epimedium grandiflorum* (yin yang huo) herb, the latter two of which are Kidney Yang tonics (basically, hormone modulators) in Chinese medicine, has been helpful clinically to augment 5aRi therapy and to maintain patients' prostate volumes after they stop a pharmaceutical agent (Bensky et al., 2004).

The two largest and most rigorous clinical trials of saw palmetto standardized extract failed to show it was superior to placebo for symptoms of uncharacterized clinical phenotype BPH (Barry et al., 2011; Bent et al., 2006). However, these trials did not include an active control arm, and prior clinical trials have shown that saw palmetto extract is as effective as finasteride and only slightly inferior to tamsulosin (Hizli and Uygur, 2007; Tacklind et al., 2009). Longer term (2-year) open trials still suggest that saw palmetto extract can reduce risk in men with BPH ultimately requiring surgery (Djavan et al., 2005). One meta-analysis of studies on purified β-sitosterol (at a dose of 15 to 65 mg tid), a key component of saw palmetto and pygeum, has shown that it can relieve symptoms due to BPH, but few long-term studies have been published (Wilt et al., 1999). One open 18-month follow-up of a 6-month double-blind β-sitosterol study found the benefits durable for at least that length of time (Berges et al., 2000). Pygeum has very similar chemistry to saw palmetto and is effective, but it is overharvested in the wild in Africa (primarily the country of Cameroon), which has led to this slow-growing, uncommon tree becoming an endangered species (Stewart, 2003). It is therefore not recommended for use under any circumstance.

Nettle root appears to act completely differently from saw palmetto. It is a mild sex hormone–binding globulin receptor antagonist and mild aromatase inhibitor, and effectively alleviates BPH symptoms clinically (Chrubasik et al., 2007). It is very safe. The usual dose is 1 to 3 g bid to tid of crude root.

Other treatments that have been reported helpful in patients with BPH (subtype unclear) include pumpkin seeds and pumpkin seed oil, lycopene, and *Linum usitatissimum* (flax) seed. A typical daily dose of pumpkin seeds is one handful; long-term randomized clinical trials have used concentrated extracts at a dose of 500 mg bid (Bach, 2000). This is likely related to the essential fatty acids in pumpkin seeds and not zinc. There is really no credible evidence that oral supplementation of zinc is helpful for BPH patients (Moyad, 2004). Lycopene at a dose of 15 mg qd has been shown to inhibit prostate growth in one 6-month clinical trial (Schwarz et al., 2008). Lycopene can be found in red fruits and vegetables. For example, tomato paste contains 20 to 30 mg lycopene/100 g, about 4 mg/100 g of canned tomatoes. The lycopene from tomatoes is made more bioavailable with heating and combining the tomatoes with some form of fat, such as olive oil. Flax seed extracts at doses of lignans 300 to 600 mg/day have helped reduce symptoms in clinical trials (Zhang et al., 2008).

In most patients, improvement in symptoms can be achieved with careful clinical assessment and matching therapy to the particulars of the case. Unfortunately, medical therapy is not always effective, and some patients present with such advanced and severe disease that there is little chance of natural therapies or medications helping. It has been particularly difficult clinically to nonsurgically help patients who develop a median bar (prostate tissue that pushes into the bladder). Patients who develop acute urinary retention, sustained PVR greater than 200 ml, infectious cystitis, signs of renal failure, or other serious consequences, or in whom natural and conventional therapies do not bring relief, should be referred to a urologist for a surgical consult.

Chronic Prostatitis and Chronic Pelvic Pain

Chronic prostatitis is a misleadingly named condition affecting a large number of men, which has only really come to be widely appreciated in the past decade. Most men present with symptoms of intermittent pelvic/ urethral discomfort or pain of varying severity that may radiate, but other symptoms including fatigue, depression, sexual dysfunction, and irritative voiding are also common. Chronic prostatitis and chronic pelvic pain syndrome (CPPS) are very common, with an estimated prevalence of 9% in U.S. men (Krieger et al., 2002). Though chronic prostatitis is not thought to reduce lifespan, it can significantly degrade quality of life (McNaughton Collins et al., 2001).

Originally believed to be a chronic infection of the prostate, a causative bacterium has since been determined to only occur in a minority of patients with chronic prostatitis. Some do have demonstrable prostatic inflammation without any clear infection, but most men (90%+) who suffer symptoms have no inflammation or infection (Krieger et al., 1999). Thus, the term *chronic pelvic pain syndrome* is now used more often to characterize this condition. The National Institute of Diabetes and Digestive and Kidney Diseases (NIDDK) recognizes five prostatitis syndromes (see list), with type III being by far the most common. To truly distinguish these syndromes clinically requires a digital rectal exam (DRE) followed by culturing of and looking for leukocytes in expressed prostatic secretions (EPSs), or the same analysis of post-DRE urine specimens (Ludwig et al., 2000). It should also be noted that chronic prostatitis and interstitial cystitis are clinically identical, and modern studies show that men affected by this syndrome are frequently diagnosed with prostatitis but never undergo cystoscopy (Forrest and Schmit, 2004).

NIDDK-Recognized Prostatitis Syndromes
Type I: Acute bacterial prostatitis
Type II: Chronic bacterial prostatitis (bacteria can be cultured from semen or post-DRE urine)

Type III: Chronic abacterial prostatitis, CPPS
  Type IIIA: Inflammatory CPPS (leukocytes >10/hpf in EPSs/post-DRE urine)
  Type IIIB: Noninflammatory CPPS (leukocytes <10/hpf in EPSs/post-DRE urine)
Type IV: Asymptomatic inflammatory prostatitis

A more recent approach has been to categorize patients into one of six clinical phenotypes in order to individualize therapy (Shoskes et al., 2009). These are urinary, psychosocial, organ specific, infection, neurologic, and pelvic floor dysfunction (trigger points in pelvic floor). The National Institutes of Health Chronic Prostatitis Symptom Index (CPSI) has three subdomains that can be used to help distinguish these phenotypes. The treatments mentioned later for each phenotype are primarily focused on alleviating symptoms, though in some cases they may treat and eliminate causes. In many cases, the underlying problem has actually turned out to be in the gut (discussed more later). It is critical in all cases to try to find and treat the causes and not to be content with symptom relief. The classic waxing–waning pattern of symptoms in these patients means that it is difficult to determine if treatments are actually the cause of symptom improvement or if time has simply passed and symptoms improved on their own. Only durable relief from recurrent symptoms for years should be considered consistent with efficacy or cure.

Patients with the urinary phenotype appear initially to primarily have BPH, with symptoms of urinary frequency, urgency, nocturia, weak stream, dribbling, and hesitancy. The CPSI urinary score will be greater than 4, and these patients may have PVR greater than 100 ml and Qmax less than 5 ml/min. The initial natural treatment is essentially the same as that for spasmodic BPH as outlined previously. If this fails, then α blockers are used, which clinical trials show can be helpful (Yang et al., 2006).

In the psychosocial phenotype, signs and symptoms of depression, anxiety, stress, and/or abuse predominate. The CPSI scores will all be low, but questionnaires like the Patient Health Questionnaire 9 (PHQ-9) will often show depression or anxiety. There are no localizing findings (e.g., pelvic floor and prostate nontender on palpation, urine and EPSs normal). Such patients usually respond best to therapy with adaptogen and nervine herbs, counseling, and help developing stress coping and understanding the mind–body connection in illness. Validation that the patient's symptoms represent a real clinical condition that is known to be exacerbated by stress is important. Although Western pharmaceutical treatment may be indicated, the sexual side effects of many antidepressants make herbal therapies an attractive option. *Withania somnifera* (ashwagandha) root is a calming adaptogen traditionally used for men and is a good option in many of these cases. A typical dose is 1 to 2 g tid in capsules or 3 to 5 ml tincture tid. Kava should be added in men with significant anxiety. For men with predominant depression, consider *Hypericum perforatum* (St. John's wort) flowering tops, *Turnera aphrodisiaca* (damiana) flowering tops, and/or *Oplopanax horridum* (devil's club) root bark. Typical doses of tincture of all of these are 3 to 5 ml tid. Note that St. John's wort can interact with many medications. If those do not help, then *Gelsemium sempervirens* (yellow Jessamine) root tincture, 5 to 10 gtt tid, can be attempted. If this doesn't work, then tricyclic antidepressants and/or anxiolytic medications may be helpful.

In the inflammatory or organ-specific phenotype, patients have predominant pelvic pain and a CPSI pain score greater than 5. There are usually leukocytes in the post-DRE urine or EPSs, and such patients may have inflammatory epididymitis, seminal vesiculitis, prostatitis, and/or interstitial cystitis. These patients respond well to cold sitz baths. The approach here focuses on reducing inflammation with inflammation modulators and demulcents such as *Curcuma longa* (turmeric) rhizome (2 to 5 g powder tid) or purified curcumin (1 to 2 g tid), bromelain (3200 mcu or 2,400 gdu potency, 1 to 2 g tid away from food), and quercetin (1 g tid). These three natural therapies are available in combinations from many manufacturers. Other botanical options include *Zea mays* (corn) silk (1 tbsp/cup of water cold infused over 12 hours, 1 cup tid or more) and *Eryngium yuccafolium* (rattlesnake master) root (1 to 2 ml tincture tid) (Shoskes et al., 1999). Yellow Jessamine or *Pulsatilla occidentalis* (Western pasque flower) flowering top, 3 to 5 gtt tid, may help relieve pain. If natural therapies are insufficient, then nonsteroidal anti-inflammatory (NSAIDs) drugs or cyclooxygenase-2 inhibitors may be tried, though these can increase gastrointestinal permeability, which may be the underlying cause of many cases of CPPS, as well as having other significant chronic adverse effects (Higuchi et al., 2009; Nickel et al., 2003).

Patients with the infection subtype have both bacteria and white blood cells (WBCs) in their post-DRE urine and EPSs, and would be said to have type II bacterial prostatitis. Their CPSI pain score is generally greater than 5. Antibiotics are the primary treatment for chronic prostatitis and CPPS in conventional medicine, often without regard to whether or not a significant number of organisms can be cultured from post-DRE or EPSs. Unfortunately, even such positive cultures do not correlate to who will respond to antibiotic therapy (Nickel et al., 2001). One study in the Veterans Administration found that, "Despite evidence that antibiotics are not effective in the majority of men with chronic pelvic pain syndrome, they were prescribed in 69% of men with this diagnosis." (Taylor et al., 2008). One of the largest clinical trials to date on ciprofloxacin, which along with levofloxacin is among the most common antibiotics prescribed to men with

CPPS, found it and tamsulosin were ineffective for men with chronic disease and moderate symptomatic severity (Alexander et al., 2004). Though little studied, there is evidence that chronic antibiotic therapy in CPPS patients can result in colonization with new Gram-negative bacteria in the prostate not present at baseline (Bergen et al., 1989). Fluoroquinolones are also now known to cause specific changes to the connective tissue, which can result in spontaneous rupture of tendons and ligaments, sometimes delayed after treatment is discontinued. Preliminary animal research suggests magnesium and vitamin E together may decrease chondrotoxicity of fluoroquinolones (Pfister et al., 2007). Magnesium should be taken at least 2 hours apart from these drugs, as it can decrease its absorption. Response to an antibiotic does not prove a patient had or has a meaningful bacterial infection, as fluoroquinolones and other antibiotics have anti-inflammatory and other actions that could affect symptoms of CPPS (Takahashi et al., 2005). Antibiotics should be reserved for patients who absolutely do not respond to natural therapies, for those with heavy (>10^5 CFU) bacterial colonization of the urine and/or EPSs, and for those with systemic signs of infection (particularly fever). Probiotics (at least 50 billion organisms/day) should always be given with antibiotics.

Patients with the neurological phenotype typically present with irritable bowel syndrome, chronic fatigue syndrome, fibromyalgia, migraines, and/or low back pain. Their quality of life CPSI score is typically greater than 5. There are often no localizing findings to the prostate. Contrast sitz baths can be helpful. Adaptogens such as *Centella asiatica* (gotu kola) whole plant (glycerite or tincture 3 to 5 ml tid) is a calming choice (ashwagandha would also be appropriate here), and devil's club is a more stimulating agent depending on the patient's energy level. Digestive bitters (for constipation/hypoactive-predominant symptoms) such as *Achillea millefolium* (yarrow) flowering top (tincture 2 to 3 ml sipped before meals in water) or carminatives (for diarrhea/hyperactivity-predominant symptoms) such as *Foeniculum vulgare* (fennel) fruit (same dose as yarrow) are indicated. These patients should always be assessed and treated with an elimination/challenge diet and gut support work as discussed later.

The trigger point phenotype (pelvic floor dysfunction) is associated with pain on perineal or anal palpation, has a CPSI pain score greater than 5, and frequently has symptoms exacerbated by prolonged sitting (particularly driving, bicycle riding, rowing, or horse riding). No leukocytes or bacteria are present. Manual therapy including osteopathic manipulation as well as an anti-inflammatory approach as discussed previously may be helpful for men presenting with this scenario. In addition, acupuncture and the use of magnesium orally and in baths (as Epsom salts) can be helpful.

Case Presentation: CPPS

M. was a 31-year-old White heterosexual man who developed irritation after voiding 14 months prior to presenting to see me. The onset was associated with a time of great stress. His symptoms persisted for 2 weeks, at which point he saw a local naturopathic doctor who found nothing on DRE, urinalysis (UA), or a screen for sexually transmitted diseases. Rye pollen, saw palmetto, bilberry extracts, zinc picolinate, and avoiding alcohol and coffee did not help, so after a month of trying them he took a course of ciprofloxacin prescribed by a urologist. He had only minor relief at best. Avoiding citrus and chocolate did not help. Tamsulosin made him extremely dizzy and tired. He had a cystoscopy, which he found very painful and nearly caused him to vomit, and which showed only slight bladder inflammation. He also experienced a prickling sensation at the base of his penis and occasional pain on ejaculation. Riding a stationary exercise bicycle worsened his symptoms. His medical history was also notable for mental fog accompanied by a modestly elevated thyroid-stimulating hormone (TSH) level, which improved upon taking levothyroxine, and chronic insomnia long predating his prostate symptoms. His mother and all six siblings (two brothers and four sisters) also have thyroid problems and all take thyroid hormones. His mother also has depression, and his father was a chronic alcoholic who died during surgery after a stroke.

At this point no phenotype was clear, so a broad approach to likely exacerbating factors was initiated. This included recommendations to address likely mind–body contributing factors through the use of journaling, minimizing possible dietary contributing factors through a strict elimination/challenge diet, and the use of a program of supplements to rebuild the urothelium, reduce inflammation, and improve intestinal permeability with N-acetylglucosamine 750 mg bid, glutamine 2 g bid, bromelain 2 cap tid, probiotics 12.5 billion organisms bid, fish oil 6 g qd, and curcumin 1 g bid. However, the patient decided instead to take doxycycline and have craniosacral therapy. He returned to clinic exactly 4 years later having tried several other therapies including a gluten-free diet for 6 weeks and seeing a physical therapist, but he felt he was no better off. This time a more thorough pelvic exam revealed quite a bit of tenderness in the pelvic floor, which activated his urethral irritation, and an otherwise normal prostate. Based on this, he was felt to have pelvic floor dysfunction (despite lack of improvement with physical therapy). He was recommended to take hot Epsom salts sitz baths twice daily for 4 days and then daily for 2 weeks, oral magnesium citrate providing 400 mg elemental magnesium per day, and a combination of kava and Jamaica dogwood tincture (75%/25%) 1 tsp four times per day; to set an alarm so he would stand up and stretch every 30 minutes at work; and to receive acupuncture and more craniosacral work. Within 1 month of doing most of this (he didn't get acupuncture or craniosacral work and took 1 dropperful of tinctures tid in reality), he was dramatically improved. He continued on a reduced program for another 2 to 3 months and felt he was nearly 100% better at that point. He has not had a relapse for 1 year as of April 2012. As noted previously, many patients with CPPS have been observed to have increased intestinal permeability, or leaky gut (as assessed by lactulose/mannitol testing), regardless of phenotype. If this is not addressed, then symptoms will often recur. An extensive and often difficult elimination/challenge diet has been effective clinically in a substantial number of these cases, sometimes leading to durable cure. Two weeks of eating very few foods (generally only those rarely consumed and not known to be common allergens such as sweet potato, white rice, quinoa, lamb, ostrich, and pears) is followed by introducing one new food every 48 hours, any of which provoke symptoms are then avoided for at least 1 year. Glutamine 1 to 3 g tid, probiotics (50 billion organisms qd), and *Aloe vera* juice (1 to 2 oz bid) are typically instituted to help repair intestinal leakiness once reaction-inducing foods are removed (so that they will not keep constantly triggering new damage and symptoms). There are several commercially available combinations of herbs and supplements that are helpful with leaky gut, especially when used in combination with the identification of symptom-causing foods. Because the majority of our immune system surrounds the gut via gut-associated lymphoid tissue, any inflammatory condition such as CPPS may be traced back to gastrointestinal causes. The chapter on gastroenterology has a more extensive description on gut repair and the 4R approach often used.

Intestinal leakiness can lead to food sensitivities and chronic systemic inflammation, which in some patients appear to present as urothelial damage and leakiness, with CPPS as the clinical expression (Kirby et al., 1982). Urothelial leakiness is now sometimes confirmed by potassium sensitivity testing, though this is painful and not recommended for most patients (Parsons, 2009). N-Acetyl glycosamine 750 mg bid for at least 6 months is recommended to help resolve urothelial damage (so far only validated in cats with interstitial cystitis) (Panchaphanpong et al., 2011); pentosan sulfate may also be used for this purpose.

Epididymitis and Seminal Vesiculitis

Inflammation of the epididymis or seminal vesicles is difficult to detect or diagnose. The symptoms typically mirror those of chronic prostatitis or CPPS but with more pronounced scrotal discomfort. There is no readily available test to diagnose these conditions, so the diagnosis is usually made clinically based on presence of scrotal discomfort with no clear identifiable cause. Biopsy or ultrasound may be necessary to rule out anatomic or pathologic causes. When those are negative, treatment is essentially the same as for chronic prostatitis and CPPS.

Chronic low-grade traumatic epididymitis is a separate case where treatment may differ. This is typically seen in patients who wear either no underwear or only boxer-type loose underwear. They typically are very physically active, either in athletics or with exercise, particularly running or jogging. Simply ensuring these patients wear tight underwear or an athletic supporter during activity will often resolve symptoms and certainly should be advocated for prevention. In some cases, topical icing or cold sitz baths along with analgesic and inflammation-modulating herbs (similar to organ-specific CPPS phenotype) may be necessary orally to help relieve pain.

Case Presentation: Epididymitis

J.is a 40-year-old White heterosexual male with onset of persistent hematuria and hematospermia as well as persistent scrotal pain after vasectomy. Prolonged sitting, particularly while driving, exacerbated the pain. No intratesticular pathology has been detected so far (including after ultrasound), but the left epididymis (side where incision for vasectomy occurred) was slightly enlarged. Naproxen and more frequent ejaculation did not resolve symptoms. His urologist prescribed ciprofloxacin and his naturopathic doctor prescribed hydrotherapy and homeopathic arnica, but he still did not improve. After 8 weeks on ciprofloxacin, he was switched to meloxicam and cefuroxime, which helped minimally. Ibuprofen and naproxen were not helpful, whereas acetaminophen and topical ice did temporarily relieve pain. He also tried having acupuncture with minimal relief. Finally, he was given a gentamicin injection intramuscularly, which did temporarily relieve his symptoms. He began giving himself such an injection once every 5 days but felt this was not a sustainable approach.

A combination of elimination/challenge diet, glutamine 10 g qd, probiotics 25 billion organisms per day, curcumin 1 g tid, topical ice as needed, and an herbal formula (containing gotu kola glycerite 30%, kava tincture 30%, *Glycyrrhiza glabra* [licorice] root 20%, *Mahonia aquifolium* [Oregon grape] root tincture 10%, *Anemone pulsatilla* [pasque flower] herb tincture 5%, and *Fouquieria splendens* [ocotillo] bark tincture 5%; 1 tsp tid) enabled him to discontinue all conventional medications with a durable 50% reduction in his symptoms all the time. He also was having prolonged periods with no symptoms for the first time since this started 14 months prior. Excessive exercise involving the legs would still trigger a flare-up. Treatment is continuing, and he is avoiding eggs, cow milk, and nuts on an ongoing basis.

Varicocele

Varicocele is a common condition in which the pampiniform venous plexus dilates due to incompetent venous valves. This is particularly common in the left scrotum because the left testicular vein typically drains into the left renal vein while the right drains directly into the inferior vena cava. This means there is significantly more back-pressure on the left. Surprisingly though, close examination reveals bilateral lesions in half the cases; the remaining half have left-sided lesions (Kupeli et al., 1991). Chronic gravitational strain is the leading theory for the cause of varicocele (Biase and Nagler, 1992). Though occasionally varicoceles can cause significant discomfort or pain, the major problem with them is heat-induced infertility. Varicocele in such situations is usually treated surgically.

Herbs that are traditionally used to treat varicosities in other parts of the body may have application in men with varicoceles. In support of this was a randomized trial in Chinese men with chronic varicocele-related infertility who were randomized to varicocelectomy or oral treatment with escin (a saponin complex from *Aesculus hippocastanum*, horse chestnut, a common treatment for varicosities) 30 mg bid or vitamin E 20 mg, pentoxifylline 400 mg qd, and clomiphene 50 mg qd for 2 months (Fang et al., 2010). The men in the surgery and escin groups had significantly higher sperm density than the other group; sperm motility only improved in the surgical group. Other herbs that may be beneficial, particularly in mild disease, are *Collinsonia canadensis* (stoneroot), *Fagopyrum esculentum* (buckwheat), *Hamamelis virginiana* (witch hazel), *Ruscus aculeatus* (butcher's broom), and *Vitis vinifera* (grape seed). Oral and topical application should both be considered.

Seminal coenzyme Q10 levels are reduced in patients with varicocele compared to those without (Mancini et al., 2005). This suggests either that there is increased oxidative stress caused by varicocele or that there is decreased intake or production somehow related to varicocele.

Spermatocele

Spermatocele, or cystic accumulation of sperm, is most often an adverse effect of vasectomy, though they sometimes occur spontaneously as men get older (generally after age 40). A sometimes tender, mobile, soft mass develops that appears to be adherent to the testicle or epididymis. Ultrasound is indicated to confirm the diagnosis. No treatment is required in most cases beyond reassurance, as it is benign. If there is persistent pain or discomfort, then contrast sitz baths, topical ice, and treatments similar to inflammatory CPPS can be helpful. In extreme cases not responding to other treatment, referral to a urologist for a surgical consult is warranted.

Hydrocele

Hydrocele is an accumulation of fluid in the tunica vaginalis or along the spermatic cord. The least common form (congenital or communicating) occurs when the tunica vaginalis does not normally separate from the abdominal cavity, and fluid drains into it due to gravity. This generally occurs in infants and is easily remedied surgically. The much more common form is acquired (noncommunicating), in which some imbalance between fluid creation and absorption causes fluid to build up. The usual causes are some inflammatory processes in the scrotum such as epididymitis, orchitis, or testicular cancer. Some cases are idiopathic and may be due to tunica vaginalis inflammation or dysfunction. The author has particularly noticed a surprisingly high rate of idiopathic hydroceles in men over the age of 60 who have been sexually active for many years. However, increased rates of ejaculation have not consistently helped.

If epididymitis is suspected as the cause, particularly in men who wear no or only loose underwear, then the treatments mentioned previously for that condition should be implemented. In sexually active men with risk factors, chlamydia and gonorrhea should be ruled out as a cause of the epididymitis. Obviously if testicular cancer is suspected, referral for confirmation of the diagnosis is mandatory. In idiopathic cases, oral inflammation modulators such as curcumin and bromelain or oral NSAIDs may be helpful along with topical ice and tight underwear. Internal use of the traditional pelvic lymphagogue *Fouquieria splendens* (ocotillo) bark (tincture dose 1 to 2 ml tid) may also help resolve the lesion.

Peyronie's Disease

Peyronie's disease is a common condition believed to be an autoimmune fibrotic condition that affects the tunica albuginea of the penis. The definitive etiology and pathophysiology are still not known. Insulin resistance syndromes, Paget's disease of bone, and Dupuytren's contracture are associated with increased risk of Peyronie's disease. Though plaques develop in the tunica albuginea, these are not clearly and directly related to trauma or to symptoms except in extreme cases, which variably consist of excessive curvature of the erect penis (usually dorsal, but can be at any angle), pain on erection, penile shortening, indentations of the penis, and erectile dysfunction. Some percentage of patients with Peyronie's disease spontaneously remit, though this may be as low as 12% according to large modern patient cohorts (Mulhall et al., 2006). A rare condition that can look like Peyronie's disease is superficial thrombophlebitis of the dorsal vein of the penis, or Mondor's disease, which should be suspected when there is no penile curvature and prominent tenderness of the dorsal vein; ultrasound is the best way to rule out this condition.

Any risk factors that can be eliminated should be, including treating metabolic syndrome/insulin resistance if present. Most patients should decrease or eliminate sexual activity to reduce the risk of penile reinjury given the weight of evidence suggesting sexual trauma plays a role in the condition (Casabé et al., 2011). It is otherwise difficult to individualize therapy due to overall lack of understanding of the etiology and pathophysiology of the disease.

I generally start by having the patient apply a combination of *Centella asiatica* (gotu kola) whole herb glycerite and vitamin E mixed into any available cream base. Generally this is done twice daily, and patients are advised that this will disrupt efficacy of condoms when this is relevant (but should not harm any sexual partner if it gets in or on them). Though there is scant evidence for these treatments in the published literature, I have found it empirically helpful.

Other oral treatments may be helpful in some patients, though certainly not all. Mixed natural tocotrienols 400 to 1,200 IU qd, acetyl-L-carnitine 500 mg bid to tid, bromelain (3,200 mcu or 2,400 gdu potency) 1 to 2 g tid to qid, para-aminobenzoic acid 3 g tid (increased by 1 g per dose per week until the patient starts to have pruritus, at which point decrease to prior safe dose, or patient reaches 7 g tid), propolis 300 to 1,000 mg tid, and pentoxifylline 400 mg bid all have some research support or have shown benefit clinically (Hauck et al., 2006).

If some combination of the gotu kola and vitamin E cream with safer oral treatments is not effective, then one can try topical potassium iodide 5 gtt qd to bid in patients not sensitive to iodine (this will stain the skin) and/or topical dimethylsulfoxide 70% at nighttime (has offensive sulfurous odor), sometimes along with the gotu kola and vitamin E combination. I have had patients purchase small iontophoresis machines so they can drive in topical verapamil 15% cream at least once a day (Montorsi et al., 1995). Superoxide dismutase, lidocaine, and corticosteroids have also been used topically with iontophoresis. Oral tamoxifen 20 mg bid is also sometimes helpful but can have significant adverse effects. Oral *Colchicum autumnale* (autumn crocus) corm tincture 5 gtt bid or purified colchicine 0.5 mg qd 5 days per week is sometimes helpful. Both forms are contraindicated in patients with significant liver or kidney disease or with bone marrow problems; complete blood count and serum transaminases need to be monitored monthly in patients taking any colchicine-containing medicine. If none of these are effective, then patients should be referred for intralesional injection treatments or surgery.

Case Presentation: Peyronie's

M. is a 48-year-old White man with a 10-year history of difficulty achieving and maintaining erections without phosphodiesterase-5 inhibitor drugs. The erectile dysfunction was not related to any psychoemotional problems he could identify and occurred with three different female sexual partners (a former wife and his current wife included). He had urethral surgery, apparently for urethral stricture, 20 years prior. He has long had an hourglass deformity of the penis with prominent inability to fully engorge the distal tip of the glans. He has no penile curvature but has a band of palpable plaque encircling the glans, and no pain associated with this. He was 10 pounds overweight and working a sedentary job with some exposure to industrial solvents and heavy metals. On the theory that he had a combination of early metabolic syndrome with postsurgical Peyronie's disease, I recommended a pescovegan diet with ample quantities of garlic, intensification of his minimal exercise program, and stress reduction. After 3 months of following these directions closely, he had dramatic improvement in his erectile function but became overly sexually active and severely aggravated his Peyronie's disease. Incidentally, his blood pressure improved dramatically and his weight and muscle mass improved with this lifestyle approach. He had opposite reactions than are usual to arginine and *Pausinystalia yohimbe* bark tincture—both caused erectile dysfunction. This seemed to further signal that the Peyronie's disease was impairing function quite significantly. If he took gotu kola he got pruritus unless he took very tiny doses (5 drops), which he felt helped reduce anxiety and did (after discontinuation and restarting it) lead to noticeable improvement in his Peyronie's disease symptoms. Topical gotu kola cream had a mild positive effect. Oral PABA and bromelain helped alleviated the hour glassing and penile dip detumescence problems and he continues to take them daily. After trying many other treatments, iontophoretic verapamil also seemed somewhat helpful. The patient is able to have sex without pain with his wife on a regular basis without aggravating his condition. He continues to eat well and exercise regularly and has maintained his overall health. Although the Peyronie's disease has not completely resolved, he feels he has control over it.

Phimosis

Phimosis is a state of adhesion between the foreskin and glans and is normal in infancy. In most boys it spontaneously clears and the foreskin becomes freely and fully retractable by age 3 to 4 years. In one British series pathological phimosis was present at a rate of 0.4/1,000 boys by age 15 years (Shankar and Rickwood, 1999). Of the 51 foreskins that were removed and examined histologically in this series, 43 (84%) had balanitis xerotica obliterans (male genital lichen sclerosus). In a large Danish series, only 1% of boys still had phimosis by age 17 years (Øster, 1968). Therefore, it is critical to note that most phimosis is normal and is not an indication for circumcision. Only phimosis that is causing pain on erection, obstructing urinary outflow, or causing recurrent infections should be treated, and all but the most advanced cases can be rectified with medical therapy short of circumcision. It is important that parents and caregivers be instructed to avoid forcing retraction of the foreskin in infants as this may actually cause increased scarring. It has also been proposed that masturbation by rubbing the genitals forcefully against a pillow or bed may cause some causes of pathological phimosis and so this practice should be avoided (Sank, 1998).

Gentle daily stretching, preferably in a hot shower or bath, is the basis of treatment of problem phimosis. This has not been studied as sole treatment but generally only combined with topical corticosteroids such as fluticasone 0.05% or betamethasone 0.05% applied twice daily (Ghysel et al., 2009; Zavras et al., 2009). This approach is highly effective and avoids the need for circumcision in most cases. In mild, early cases, topical application of *Calendula officinalis* (calendula) flower cream saturated with *Centella asiatica* (gotu kola) herb glycerite and compounded 5% vitamin E applied twice daily has also been effective combined with gentle stretching in my experience.

Paraphimosis

Paraphimosis occurs when the foreskin is pulled back off the head of the penis and is inflamed (usually secondary to bacterial infection) and cannot be retracted. Fluid and pressure begin to build up. The patient usually presents with a hardened, painful ring of foreskin tissue trapped around the glans. The initial treatment is to attempt to reduce this by applying firm, steady pressure with both thumbs (wearing gloves of course) to the head of the penis for a full 5 minutes. Meanwhile, the patient very gently attempts to retract the foreskin over the nearly bloodless glans. If this fails, then the patient should be referred for an emergency dorsal slit or circumcision. If it does work, then treatments for the presumed infection should be commenced. Usually this occurs in the setting of patients who are immunosuppressed, particularly patients with poorly controlled diabetes mellitus.

Some topical natural antimicrobials to consider include *Hydrastis canadensis* (goldenseal) cultivated root powder, *Mahonia aquifolium* (Oregon grape) root powder, *Thymus vulgaris* (thyme) leaf volatile oil (diluted with 75% jojoba oil), and propolis. These should be applied at least twice a day. Thyme oil 2 to 3 gtt tid and propolis 1 g tid should also be taken internally along with the macrophage stimulator, inflammation modulator, and antimicrobial *Echinacea angustifolia* root (tincture 3 to 5 ml tid, capsules 1 to 2 g tid). *E. purpurea* does not have these same effects (it is primarily an immunomodulator) and is not particularly indicated here except possibly for prevention of recurrence. If there is not significant improvement within 48 hours or if there is deterioration of the infection, then oral antibiotics should be commenced.

Urethritis

Acute urethritis remains a fairly common occurrence in sexually active men. Any patient with acute urethritis should of course be tested for gonorrhea and chlamydia, usually by urine polymerase chain reaction (PCR). Both of these infections should be treated with antibiotics if detected based on local health department guidelines regarding community susceptibility patterns. Probiotics should be combined with this, as well as *Camellia sinensis* (green tea) leaf as an antimicrobial resistance inhibitor. Urine culture is indicated if symptoms persist or are severe despite negative gonorrhea/chlamydia testing. However, many patients with acute urethritis have no identifiable pathogen (Wetmore et al., 2009). Any obvious cause of urethral irritation such as known food allergies, unusual sexual practices, and the like should also be ruled out in all cases.

The oral antimicrobial herbs mentioned under paraphimosis earlier coupled with the inflammation-modulating treatments for the inflammatory phenotype of chronic prostatitis are recommended as initial treatment in patients with idiopathic acute urethritis. Cranberry and blueberry juices (8 oz per day diluted with water) or capsules (1 to 2 g tid) are also recommended to reduce adhesion of any bacteria that might be involved. If this fails then a course of empiric antibiotics may be warranted.

Patients with chronic urethritis will generally also have no identifiable organism, and it is recommended that they be assessed and treated essentially as if they had chronic prostatitis (see earlier for details).

Male Infertility

Male factor infertility is more and more recognized to be common and much more of an issue in cases of infertility (defined as failure to become pregnant after 1 year of trying with good technique). Therefore, it is reasonable to assess both the male and female partner in any infertility case. Assuming physical examination and history reveal no obvious causes of male infertility, the next step would be semen analysis. It is unclear whether computer-assisted or entirely human semen analysis is superior. If semen analysis is abnormal, it should be repeated before any further testing is considered. Note that if varicocele is present, the section on that condition should be referenced as this can contribute to sperm abnormalities.

In patients with azoospermia (no production of sperm), a full hormonal assessment should be ordered including free and total testosterone, luteinizing hormone (LH) and follicle-stimulating hormone (FSH), total estrogens, sex hormone–binding globulin, and prolactin. In patients with only moderate oligospermia or normal sperm counts and the absence of any other symptoms, it is highly unlikely that there is a severe hormonal imbalance to explain their problem, and so a hormonal workup would be unnecessary (Frey and Patel, 2004). In patients with low testosterone, high estrogens, and lack of virilization, Klinefelter syndrome should be suspected and a karyotype ordered. Screening for hereditary hemochromatosis is also warranted in men with otherwise idiopathic infertility and oligospermia or azoospermia.

Natural medicine is less likely to be helpful in oligospermic and azoospermic men. However, shilajit, a mineral-rich pitch containing various organic acids and triterpenoids, 100 mg bid has been shown helpful in raising sperm counts and testosterone levels in one trial of oligospermic men (Biswas et al., 2010). Acupuncture combined with clomiphene was significantly more effective than clomiphene alone at raising pregnancy rates in nonhypogonadal, oligospermic men (He, 1998).

If hyperprolactinemia is the problem with no obvious cause, then a magnetic resonance image of the brain is ordered to rule out pituitary adenoma. If there is no visible adenoma, then pyridoxine 500 mg bid, *Vitex agnus-castus* (chaste tree) fruit tincture 1 to 2 ml tid, *Glycyrrhiza glabra* (licorice) root glycerite 1 to 2 ml tid, and *Paeonia lactiflora* (bai shao) root without bark tincture 2 to 3 ml tid can be tried. If these fail, then bromocriptine or similar drugs are used. Visible adenomas or prolactin levels greater than 100 ng/ml are generally indications for surgical treatment.

Asthenospermia, or impaired sperm motility with a normal sperm count, is an area in which natural medicine can be very helpful. Redox modulator supplementation is often helpful (after ensuring the patient's diet is already replete with micronutrient-dense vegetables and fruits); the ideal supplement to choose in such cases is uncertain. Vitamin C 1 g tid is simple and cheap, and though it results in pregnancy in only ~15% of patients taking it in clinical trials, this rate is similar to the efficacy of clomiphene and mesterolone (Martin-Du Pan and Sakkas, 1998). Selenium 100 to 200 mcg (an amount that can also be attained by eating four to five Brazil nuts per day) has also been shown to improve sperm motility in patients with marginal selenium nutriture (a common occurrence).

Carnitine 1 g tid is also often effective at improving sperm motility and raising pregnancy rates with minimal adverse effects (Zhou et al., 2007). Adaptogens such as *Panax ginseng* (Asian red ginseng, ren shen) steamed root 1 to 2 g tid, *Astragalus membranaceus* (huang qi) root 1 to 3 g tid, and *Withania somnifera* (ashwagandha) root 1 to 2 g tid can also have a positive effect in such cases.

Patients can generally benefit from a review of ideal timing of sexual intercourse to maximize conception (in and around the time of ovulation, and every 48 hours to allow time to recover sperm count). Avoidance of any pelvic excess heat may help, though switching to looser underwear is controversial.

If simple measures fail, then referral to an infertility specialist or endocrinologist is recommended.

Conclusion

There is a great deal of potential for natural approaches to the miscellaneous men's health conditions discussed here. Improved knowledge of diagnosis and management of these conditions is one important factor for men to feel comfortable seeking medical help. Integration of natural treatments with conventional treatments is practical in many cases, though natural methods alone are often sufficient.

REFERENCES

Alexander RB, Propert KJ, Schaeffer AJ, et al. Ciprofloxacin or tamsulosin in men with chronic prostatitis/chronic pelvic pain syndrome: a randomized, double-blind trial. Ann Intern Med. 2004;141:581–589.

Antihypertensive and Lipid-Lowering Treatment to Prevent Heart Attack Trial Collaborative Research Group. Diuretic versus alpha-blocker as first-step antihypertensive therapy: final results from the Antihypertensive and Lipid-Lowering Treatment to Prevent Heart Attack Trial (ALLHAT). Hypertension. 2003;42(3):239–246.

Aydin A, Arsova-Sarafinovska Z, Sayal A, et al. Oxidative stress and antioxidant status in non-metastatic prostate cancer and benign prostatic hyperplasia. Clin Biochem. 2006;39(2):176–179.

Bach D. Placebo-controlled, long-term therapeutic study of a pumpkin seed extract product in patients with micturitions complaints from benign prostatic hyperplasia. Urologe B. 2000;40(5):437–443 [in German].

Barnard RJ, Koabayashi N, Aronson WJ. Effect of diet and exercise intervention on growth of prostate epithelial cells. Prostate Cancer Prostatic Dis. 2008;11:362–366.

Barry MJ, Meleth S, Lee JY, et al. Effect of increasing doses of saw palmetto extract on lower urinary tract symptoms: a randomized trial. JAMA. 2011;306:1344–1351.

Bensky D, Clavey S, Stöger E, Gamble A. *Chinese Herbal Medicine Materia Medica* 3rd ed. (Seattle: Eastland Press, 2004).

Bent S, Kane C, Shinohara K, et al. Saw palmetto for benign prostatic hyperplasia. N Engl J Med. 2006;354(6):557–566.

Bergen B, Wedren H, Holm SE. Long-term antibiotic treatment of chronic bacterial prostatitis. Effect on bacterial flora. Br J Urol. 1989;63:503–507.

Berges RR, Kassen A, Senge T. Treatment of symptomatic benign prostatic hyperplasia with beta-sitosterol: an 18-month follow-up. BJU Int. 2000;85(7):842–846.

Biase JN, Nagler HM. The varicocele: current concepts and controversies. Curr Opin Urol. 1992;2:463–466.

Biswas KK, Pandit S, Mondal S, et al. Clinical evaluation of spermatogenic activity of processed shilajit in oligospermia. Andrologia. 2010;42(1):48–56.

Campbell B. High rate of prostate symptoms among Ariaal men from Northern Kenya. Prostate. 2004;62:83–90.

Casabé A, Bechara A, Cheliz G, et al. Risk factors of Peyronie's disease. What does our clinical experience show? J Sex Med. 2011;8(2):518–523.

Chrubasik JE, Roufogalis BD, Wagner H, Chrubasik S. A comprehensive review on the stinging nettle effect and efficacy profiles. Part II: urticae radix. Phytomedicine. 2007;14:568–579.

Cimino S, Favilla V, Castelli T, et al. Dietary patterns and prostatic diseases. Front Biosci (Elite Ed). 2012;4:195–204.

De Nunzio C, Aronson W, Freedland SJ, et al. The correlation between metabolic syndrome and prostatic diseases. Eur Urol. 2012;61(3):560–570.

Djavan B, Fong YK, Chaudry A, et al. Progression delay in men with mild symptoms of bladder outlet obstruction: a comparative study of phytotherapy and watchful waiting. World J Urol. 2005;23:253–256.

Dong Z, Wang Z, Yang K, et al. Tamsulosin versus terazosin for benign prostatic hyperplasia: a systematic review. Syst Biol Reprod Med. 2009;55(4):129–136.

Fang YJ, Zhao L, Yan F, et al. Escin improves sperm quality in male patients with varicocele-associated infertility. Phytomedicine. 2010;17(3–4):192–196.

Forrest JB, Schmit S. Interstitial cystitis, chronic nonbacterial prostatitis and chronic pelvic pain syndrome in men: a common and frequently identical clinical entity. J Urol. 2004;172:2561–2562.

Frey KA, Patel KS. Initial evaluation and management of infertility by the primary care physician. Mayo Clin Proc. 2004;79(11):1439–1443.

Fujiuchi Y, Watanabe A, Fuse H. Effect of Goshajinkigan on storage symptoms in prostatic disease—fundamental researches of Chinese herbal medicine for voiding dysfunction and its future aspects. Hinyokika Kiyo. 2008;54(6):463–466 [in Japanese].

Galeone C, Pelucchi C, Talamini R, et al. Onion and garlic intake and the odds of benign protatic hyperplasia. Urology. 2007;70:672–676.

Gat Y, Gornish M, Heiblum M, Joshua S. Reversal of benign prostate hyperplasia by selective occlusion of impaired venous drainage in the male reproductive system: novel mechanism, new treatment. Andrologia. 2008;40(5):273–281.

Ghysel C, Vander Eeckt K, Bogaert GA. Long-term efficiency of skin stretching and a topical corticoid cream application for unretractable foreskin and phimosis in prepubertal boys. Urol Int. 2009;82:81–88.

Gotoh A, Goto K, Sengoku A, et al. Inhibition mechanism of Gosha-jinki-gan on the micturition reflex in rats. J Pharmacol Sci. 2004;96(2):115–123.

Griffiths K, Denis LI, Turkes A. *Oestrogens, Phyto-oestrogens and the Pathogenesis of Prostatic Disease* (London: Martin Dunitz, 2002).

Gu F. Changes in the prevalence of benign prostatic hyperplasia in China. Chin Med J (Engl). 1997;110(3):163–166.

Gu FL, Xia TL, Kong XT. Preliminary study of the frequency of benign prostatic hyperplasia and prostatic cancer in China. Urology. 1994;44(5):688–691.

Hauck EW, Diemer T, Schmelz HU, Weidner W. A critical analysis of nonsurgical treatment of Peyronie's disease. Eur Urol. 2006;49:987–997.

He XY. Acupuncture plus medication for male idiopathic oligospermatic sterility. Shanghai J Acupunct Moxibustion. 1998;2:35–37.

Higuchi K, Umegaki E, Watanabe T, et al. Present status and strategy of NSAIDs-induced small bowel injury. J Gastroenterol. 2009;44(9):879–888.

Hizli F, Uygur MC. A prospective study of the efficacy of *Serenoa repens*, tamsulosin, and *Serenoa repens* plus tamsulosin treatment for patients with benign prostate hyperplasia. Int Urol Nephrol. 2007;39:879–886.

Ho CKM, Habib FK. Estrogen and androgen signaling in the pathogenesis of BPH. Nat Rev Urol. 2011;8:29–41.

Kaplan SA, Lee JY, Meehan AG, Kusek JW; MTOPS Research Group. Long-term treatment with finasteride improves clinical progression of benign prostatic hyperplasia in men with an enlarged versus a smaller prostate: data from the MTOPS trial. J Urol. 2011;185(4):1369–1373.

Kirby RS, Lowe D, Bultitude MI, Shuttleworth KED. Intra-prostatic urinary reflux: an aetiological factor in abacterial prostatitis. Br J Urol. 1982;54:729–731.

Kirby RS, McConnell JD, Fitzpatrick JM, et al. (eds.). *Textbook of Benign Prostatic Hyperplasia*, 2nd ed. (London: Taylor and Francis, 2005).

Krieger JN, Nyberg L Jr, Nickel JC. NIH consensus definition and classification of prostatitis. JAMA. 1999;282(3):236–237.

Krieger JN, Ross SO, Riley DE. Chronic prostatitis: epidemiology and role of infection. Urology. 2002;60(6 Suppl):8–12.

Kupeli S, Arikan N, Aydos K, Aytac S. Multiparametric evaluation of testicular atrophy due to varicocele. Urol Int. 1991;46:189–192.

Ludwig M, Schroeder-Printzen I, Lüdecke G, Weidner W. Comparison of expressed prostatic secretions with urine after prostatic massage—a means to diagnose chronic prostatitis/inflammatory chronic pelvic pain syndrome. Urology. 2000;55:175–175.

Mancini A, Milardi D, Conte G, et al. Seminal antioxidants in humans: pre-operative and postoperative evaluation of coenzyme Q10 in varicocele patients. Horm Metab Res. 2005;37(7):428–432.

Martin-Du Pan RC, Sakkas D. Is antioxidant therapy a promising strategy to improve human reproduction? Are anti-oxidants useful in the treatment of male infertility? Human Reproduction. 1998;13:2984–2985.

McNaughton Collins M, Pontari MA, O'Leary MP, et al. Chronic Prostatitis Collaborative Research Network. Quality of life is impaired in men with chronic prostatitis. J Gen Intern Med. 2001;16(10):656–662.

Montorsi F, Guazzoni G, Bocciardi A, et al. Transdermal electromotive multi-drug administration for Peyronie's disease: a randomized, double-blind, placebo-controlled, partial crossover study. J Urol. 1995;153(suppl):472 [abstract 973].

Moyad MA. Zinc for prostate disease and other conditions: a little evidence, a lot of hype, and a significant potential problem. Urol Nurs. 2004;24(1):49–52.

Mulhall JP, Schiff J, Guhring P. An analysis of the natural history of Peyronie's disease. J Urol. 2006;175:2115–2118.

Nandeesha H, Koner BC, Dorairajan LN, Sen SK. Hyperinsulinemia and dyslipidemia in non-diabetic benign prostatic hyperplasia. Clin Chim Acta. 2006;370(1–2):89–93.

Neal DE. Watchful waiting or drug therapy for benign prostatic hyperplasia? Lancet. 1997;350:305–306.

Nickel JC, Downey J, Johnston B, et al. Predictors of patient response to antibiotic therapy for the chronic prostatitis/chronic pelvic pain syndrome: a prospective multicenter clinical trial. J Urol. 2001;165:1539–1544.

Nickel JC, Pontari M, Moon T, et al. Rofecoxib Prostatitis Investigator Team. A randomized, placebo controlled, multicenter study to evaluate the safety and efficacy of rofecoxib in the treatment of chronic nonbacterial prostatitis. J Urol. 2003;169(4):1401–1405.

Nishijima S, Sugaya K, Miyazato M, Ogawa Y. Effect of Gosha-jinki-gan, a blended herbal medicine, on bladder activity in rats. J Urol. 2007;177(2):762–765.

Ogushi T, Takahashi S. Effect of Chinese herbal medicine on overactive bladder. Hinyokika Kiyo. 2007;53(12):857–862.

Øster J. Further fate of the foreskin. Arch Dis Child. 1968;43:200–203.

Page ST, Hirano L, Gilchriest J, et al. Dutasteride reduces prostate size and prostate specific antigen in older hypogonadal men with benign prostatic hyperplasia undergoing testosterone replacement therapy. J Urol. 2011;186(1):191–197.

Panchaphanpong J, Asawakarn T, Pusoonthornthum R. Effects of oral administration of N-acetyl-d-glucosamine on plasma and urine concentrations of glycosaminoglycans in cats with idiopathic cystitis. Am J Vet Res. 2011;72(6):843–850.

Parsons CL. The potassium sensitivity test: a new gold standard for diagnosing and understanding the pathophysiology of interstitial cystitis. J Urol. 2009;182(2):432–434.

Pfister K, Mazur D, Vormann J, Stahlmann R. Diminished ciprofloxacin-induced chondrotoxicity by supplementation with magnesium and vitamin E in immature rats. Antimicrob Agents Chemother. 2007;51(3):1022–1027.

Sank LI. Traumatic masturbatory syndrome. J Sex Marital Therapy. 1998;24:37–42.

Schwarz S, Obermüller-Jevic UC, Hellmis E, et al. Lycopene inhibits disease progression in patients with benign prostate hyperplasia. J Nutr. 2008;138(1):49–53.

Shankar KR, Rickwood AM. The incidence of phimosis in boys. BJU Int. 1999;84(1):101–102.

Shigehara K, Sugimoto K, Konaka H, et al. Androgen replacement therapy contributes to improving lower urinary tract symptoms in patients with hypogonadism and benign prostate hypertrophy: a randomised controlled study. Aging Male. 2011;14(1):53–58.

Shoskes DA, Nickel JC, Rackley RR, Pontari MA. Clinical phenotyping in chronic prostatitis/chronic pelvic pain syndrome and interstitial cystitis: a management strategy for urologic chronic pelvic pain syndromes. Prost Cancer Prost Dis. 2009;12:177–183.

Shoskes DA, Zeitlin SI, Shahed A, Rajfer J. Quercetin in men with category III chronic prostatitis: a preliminary prospective, double-blind, placebo-controlled trial. Urology. 1999;54:960–963.

Stewart KM. The African cherry (*Prunus africana*): can lessons be learned from an over-exploited medicinal tree? J Ethnopharmacol. 2003;89:3–13.

Tacklind J, MacDonald R, Rutks I, Wilt TJ. *Serenoa repens* for benign prostatic hyperplasia. Cochrane Database Syst Rev. 2009;(2):CD001423.

Takahashi HK, Iwagaki H, Xue D, et al. Effect of ciprofloxacin-induced prostaglandin E2 on interleukin-18-treated monocytes. Antimicrob Agents Chemother. 2005;49(8):3228–3233.

Taylor BC, Noorbaloochi S, McNaughtn-Collins M, et al. Excessive antibiotic use in men with prostatitis. Am J Med. 2008;121(5):444–449.

Terai A, Kakehi Y, Terachi T, Ogawa O. National trend of management of benign prostatic hyperplasia in Japan during 1990s: analysis of national health statistics. Hinyokika Kiyo. 2000;46(8):537–544 [in Japanese].

Wei JT, Calhoun E, Jacobsen SJ. Urologic diseases in America project: benign prostatic hyperplasia. J Urol. 2005;173(4):1256–1261.

Wetmore CM, Manhart LE, Golden MR. Idiopathic urethritis in young men in the United States: prevalence and comparison to infections with known sexually transmitted pathogens. J Adolescent Health. 2009;45:463–472.

Wilt TJ, MacDonald R, Ishani A. Beta-Sitosterol for the treatment of benign prostatic hyperplasia: a systematic review. BJU Int. 1999;83:976–983.

Wong SYS, Lau WWY, Leung PC, et al. The association between isoflavone and lower urinary tract symptoms in elderly men. Br J Nutr. 2007;98(6):1237–1242.

Yang G, Hei Q, Li H, et al. The effect of alpha-adrenergic antagonists in chronic prostatitis/chronic pelvic pain syndrome: a meta-analysis of randomized controlled trials. J Androl. 2006;27:847–852.

Zavras N, Christianakis E, Mpourikas D, Ereikat K. Conservative treatment of phimosis with fluticasone proprionate 0.05%: a clinical study in 1185 boys. J Pediatr Urol. 2009;5:181–185.

Zhang W, Wang X, Liu Y, et al. Effects of dietary flaxseed lignan extract on symptoms of benign prostatic hyperplasia. J Med Food. 2008;11(2):207–214.

Zhou X, Liu F, Zhai S. Effect of L-carnitine and/or L-acetyl-carnitine in nutrition treatment for male infertility: a systematic review. Asia Pac J Clin Nutr. 2007;16(Suppl 1):383–390.

12

Integrative Men's Sexual Health

JOEL J. HEIDELBAUGH

Key Concepts

- Worldwide, men are increasingly embracing alternative therapies for treatment of sexual dysfunction.
- Currently, there is a lack of rigorous, randomized, controlled trials comparing the efficacy of standard pharmacotherapy with complementary and alternative treatments for sexual dysfunction.

Sexual Health and Complementary and Alternative Medicine

Although the focus of sexual health in men commonly centers on the use of phosphodiesterase type 5 (PDE5) inhibitors for improvement of symptoms of erectile dysfunction, men are increasingly embracing alternative therapies for treatment of various forms of sexual dysfunction, including both erectile dysfunction and premature ejaculation. Most studies to date on therapies for these conditions lack substantial rigor and large sample sizes, and there are no definitive head-to-head trials comparing effects of standard pharmacotherapy to complementary and alternative medicine (CAM) therapies. Moreover, most CAM options for treatment of sexual dysfunction have not defined specific mechanisms of action for proposed treatments (Park et al., 2008). Nonetheless, current literature on these conditions posits a favorable benefit over potential harm.

Erectile Dysfunction

PATHOPHYSIOLOGY

Erectile dysfunction (ED) is defined by the National Institutes of Health (NIH) as "the inability to achieve or maintain an erection sufficient for satisfactory sexual performance" (NIH, 1992, p 1). ED often causes serious psychological distress to men, as it often has a profound effect on their intimate relationships, quality of life, and overall self-esteem. A large cross-sectional, community-based study in men ages 40 to 49 years found a prevalence of complete or severe ED to be 5% and the prevalence of moderate erectile dysfunction to be 17%; in men ages 70 to 79 years, estimated prevalences were 15% and 34%, respectively (Feldman et al., 1994). The economic impact of ED is multifactorial and is most heavily weighted by direct costs including physician evaluation, pharmacotherapy, and diagnostic testing (Heidelbaugh, 2010).

Normal male sexual function is a complex biologic and psychological interaction (McVary et al., 2007). Erections result from a combination of the interaction between neurotransmitters and vascular smooth muscle responses that results in increased arterial flow and signaling between endothelial-lined cavernosal sinusoids and the underlying smooth muscle cells. Nitric oxide produced by the parasympathetic nonadrenergic, noncholinergic neurons and endothelial cells triggers a molecular cascade that results in the relaxation of smooth muscle cells, then occludes venous return through passive compression of the subtunical venules, resulting in an erection.

DIAGNOSIS AND EVALUATION

A man's medical history may reveal comorbid conditions and risk factors that predispose him to develop ED, including advanced age, cardiovascular disease, cigarette smoking, diabetes mellitus, hormonal disorders (e.g., hypogonadism, hypothyroidism, hyperprolactinemia), hypercholesterolemia, hypertension, obesity, psychological conditions (e.g., anxiety, depression, guilt, history of sexual abuse, marital or relationship problems, stress), and a sedentary lifestyle. Illicit drug use and various medications (e.g., antihistamines, benzodiazepines, β blockers, serotonin-specific reuptake inhibitors) may also play a role in the development of ED (American Urological Association Erectile Dysfunction Clinical Guidelines Panel, 1996). The International Index of Erectile Function Questionnaire (IIEF-5) can be used to assess the severity of symptoms of erectile dysfunction (Table 12.1).

Table 12.1: International Index of Erectile Function (IIEF-5) Questionnaire

Scores	1	2	3	4	5
1. How do you rate your confidence that you could get and keep an erection?	very low	low	moderate	high	very high
2. When you had erections with sexual stimulation, how often were your erections hard enough for penetration?	never or almost never	a few times	sometimes	most times	almost alwaysor always
3. During sexual intercourse, how often were you able to maintain your erection after you had penetrated (entered) your partner?	never or almost never	a few times	sometimes	most times	almost always or always
4. During sexual intercourse, how difficult was it to maintain your erection	extremely difficult	very difficult	difficult	slightly difficult	not difficult

(continued)

Table 12.1: (continued)

Scores	1	2	3	4	5
to completion of intercourse?					
5. When you attempted sexual intercourse, how often was it satisfactory for you?	never or almost never	a few times	sometimes	most times	almost always or always

The IIEF-5 score is the sum of the above five question responses.

ED is classified based on these scores as:

Mild	17–21
Mild to moderate	12–16
Moderate	8–11
Severe	5–7

Adapted from Rosen, R.C., Cappelleri, J.C., Smith, M.D., Lipsky, J., Pena, B.M. (1999). Development and evaluation of an abridged, 5-item version of the International Index of Erectile Function (IIEF-5) as a diagnostic tool for erectile dysfunction. Int J Impot Res. 11,319–326.

CONVENTIONAL THERAPY

First-line therapy for treatment of male sexual dysfunction should center on modification of lifestyle and chronic health parameters in the primary and secondary prevention of cardiovascular diseases. Significant attention should be paid to the appropriate treatment of hypertension, hyperlipidemia, obesity, metabolic syndrome, and testosterone deficiency, when applicable. Caution should be taken when prescribing α, β, and calcium channel blockers, as these medications may worsen erectile function. Cessation of cigarette smoking and illicit drug use, as well as minimization of alcohol, is paramount.

The mainstay of pharmacotherapy for treatment of ED is the PDE5 inhibitors (sildenafil, vardenafil, tadalafil), as they have proven to be the most effective drugs (Carson & Lue, 2005). A meta-analysis using an intention-to-treat analysis determined that sildenafil, compared to placebo, improved erectile function by 74% with a number needed to treat of two patients, as sildenafil improved such function in a dose-dependent fashion (Burls et al., 2001). If a man exhibits signs and symptoms of testicular hypogonadism and has decreased levels of bioavailable serum testosterone, then supplementation is advised, as this may increase normal erectile function (Shabsigh & Anastasiadis, 2003).

Randomized double-blind controlled trials have determined that sildenafil is safe and effective for treatment of ED in men with diabetes (Rendell et al., 1999; Vardi & Nini, 2007). Many antidepressants, including the selective serotonin reuptake inhibitors (SSRIs), have been implicated in decreasing libido and erectile function in men. PDE5 inhibitors have been found to be safe and effective in men with depression treated with SSRIs (Nurnberg et al., 2003).

Patients taking PDE5 inhibitors should not take nitrates concomitantly. Although no safe dosing interval has been determined between these classes, it is suggested that a 24-hour "washout" interval be used for sildenafil and vardenafil, and a 48-hour "washout" interval be used for tadalafil (Shabsigh & Anastasiadis, 2003). Common side effects of PDE5 inhibitors include headache, facial flushing, indigestion, and nasal congestion. Drugs that are metabolized via the CYP3A4 pathway should be dosed appropriately when used in conjunction with PDE5 inhibitors.

YOHIMBINE

Yohimbine is derived from the bark extract of the *Pausinystalia yohimbe* tree in Western Africa. It is an α_2-adrenergic receptor antagonist that has been used in the treatment of ED for many decades. There is no standard accepted dose or preparation that is recommended for treatment of ED. A meta-analysis found that oral yohimbine was superior to placebo for the effective treatment of ED, defined as satisfactory improvement in erectile function, and side effects were both limited and manageable (Ernst & Pittler, 1998). A three-arm randomized trial comparing placebo, yohimbine, and a combination of yohimbine and L-arginine yielded a statistically significant improvement in erectile function in both treatment groups (Lebret et al., 2002). Yohimbine may increase blood pressure and heart rate and cause harmful drug interactions with monoamine oxidase inhibitors or tricyclic antidepressants. Other adverse effects include headache, insomnia, sweating, and agitation.

Countless medications marketed to men to treat ED are available on the Internet and in vitamin and supplement stores for sale, many of which contain yohimbine or similar related compounds. In patients with cardiovascular disease, use of these compounds can result in an unpredictable decrease in blood pressure, as several cases of fatal syncope have been reported. As with all medications used to treat all disorders, a detailed discussion between provider and patient should review nonprescription formulations to minimize unintended side effects and interactions with standard pharmaceutical preparations.

L-ARGININE

L-arginine is a biologic precursor to nitric oxide, which plays a key role in endothelial function for normal erectile function (Wu & Meininger, 2000). An impaired relationship between L-arginine and nitrous oxide in endothelial function has been demonstrated to have a negative effect on erectile function.

Most studies have positive results, with some trials revealing modest improvement in male sexual function, whereas others suggest no significant improvement over placebo. One trial involved treating men with 5 g of L-arginine daily compared to placebo over a period of 6 weeks, with 31% of men in the treatment group reporting an improvement in erectile function (Chen et al., 1999).

Pycnogenols, phytochemicals isolated from pine bark, have also been found to play a role in improvement of erectile function when combined with L-arginine, likely due to enhanced stimulation of nitric oxide pathways. A 3-month trial in 40 men aged 25 to 45 treated men with 1.7 g of L-arginine daily for the first month, adding 40 mg Pycnogenol twice daily to the first regimen in the second month, then increasing to 40 mg Pycnogenol three times daily with the L-arginine in the third month. With addition of Pycnogenol, by the second month of the study, 80% of men reported normal erectile function, and 92% reported normal function at the end of 3 months (Stanislavov & Nikolova, 2003).

KOREAN RED GINSENG (PANAX GINSENG)

Panax ginseng was initially investigated for the treatment of ED in a double-blind, placebo-controlled, cross-over study over a decade ago (Hong et al., 2002).

Men who took Korean red ginseng dosed three times daily for 8 weeks exhibited higher mean International Index of Erectile Function scores, particularly in terms of penetration and maintenance, as well as higher penile tip rigidity on RigiScan testing, but overall sexual experience was not improved. The mechanism of action of red ginseng is not well understood, yet possible theories include a relationship in mechanism of action to testosterone and relaxation of smooth muscle via the nitrous oxide pathway.

A meta-analysis of seven randomized controlled trials found that panax ginseng is effective and safe in the treatment of ED, yet optimal dosing has not been established (Jang et al., 2008). Most trials used unstandardized doses of 1,800 to 3,000 mg, whereas some used as little as 900 to 1,000 mg. Rarely reported adverse effects included headache, insomnia, and gastric upset. Overall, it is considered that Korean red ginseng can be recommended as a cost-effective alternative to PDE5 inhibitors (Price & Gazewood, 2003).

MACA

Lepidium meyenii (maca) is a root related to the mustard family that is largely found in the Andes mountains in Peru. Historically, it is considered to have aphrodisiac properties and may improve fertility, but it has not been found to have a demonstrable effect on testosterone levels. It has been used for millennia safely without report of significant adverse effects. More significantly, a recent trial showed improvement in sexual side effects from SSRI antidepressant medications when maca was added to the patients regimen (Shin et al., 2010).

MIND–BODY THERAPY AND ACUPUNCTURE

Men with sexual dysfunction, especially those with psychosocial stressors related to both their relationship(s) and their goals of sexual performance, may benefit from behavioral therapy. In many men without prominent underlying cardiovascular diseases, targeted education, physician support, and reassurance may be sufficient to restore acceptable sexual function in some men with ED. One intervention randomized men to sex-group therapy plus sildenafil and found significant improvement in successful intercourse, defined as improved erectile function among the psychotherapy group, and they were less likely than those receiving only sildenafil to drop out of therapy (Melnik et al.,

2007). Group psychotherapy has also been shown to significantly improve ED compared to therapy with sildenafil alone.

Acupuncture has proven to have promising benefits of therapy in a variety of medical conditions in recent years. With or without moxibustion, some trials utilizing acupuncture have proven some benefit without significant harm in the treatment of nonorganic or psychogenic ED. In a randomized, controlled pilot trial in patients with psychogenic ED, a satisfactory response was achieved in 68.4% of the treatment group and 9% of the placebo group (Englehardt et al., 2003).

Premature Ejaculation

Premature ejaculation is reported by 20% to 30% of men. The condition is a source of significant stress not only for the man but also for the relationship he may be in. Men with premature ejaculation have a higher incidence of anxiety and depression related to the disorder. Defining a precise and consistent characterization continues to be a challenge. Common tenets include short intravaginal ejaculatory latency time, lack of control, and dissatisfaction with sexual performance (Lue & Broderick, 2007). Clinical research on treatment of premature ejaculation is continually presented with the challenge of subjectivity of the complaint itself, as well as a bona fide lack of true understanding of pathophysiology of the disorder.

CONVENTIONAL THERAPY

The first pharmacotherapeutic agents used in the treatment of premature ejaculation were α blockers (e.g., terazosin, alfuzosin), monoamine oxidase inhibitors, and phenelzine. Adverse side effects proved to be more common than desired benefits. SSRIs are currently the recommended therapy, as their ability to delay ejaculation was discovered unintentionally as a side effect noted in the treatment of men with major depressive disorder.

Subsequently, several studies have shown benefit in increasing latency, while proving to have a favorable side effect profile. A double-blind, placebo-controlled trial with either 20 or 40 mg of paroxetine demonstrated significantly improved ejaculation times (Waldinger et al., 1997). Since this trial, dozens of other placebo-controlled trials have examined the efficacy of SSRIs in the treatment of premature ejaculation, nearly all of which have shown some improvement across the spectrum of SSRIs.

Although PDE5 inhibitors are nearly exclusively considered to be therapy for ED, there is some proven benefit in the treatment of premature ejaculation. Patients with lifelong premature ejaculation are reported to have nearly a 50% rate of concomitant ED. A review found that three of five studies determined that PDE5 inhibitors were superior to placebo in improving ejaculatory time, whereas two placebo-controlled studies found no significant improvement (Chen et al., 2007).

YOGA

Yoga has also been compared to SSRIs as a potential therapeutic option for the treatment of premature ejaculation. A trial of 68 men with premature ejaculation randomized the men to either yoga (38 men) or fluoxetine (30 men). All men randomized to the yoga group reported improved intravaginal latencies defined as "good" to "fair" improvement, whereas 25 of 30 men reported symptomatic improvement in the fluoxetine group (Dhikav et al., 2007). Yoga is considered to be a safe and effective treatment in premature ejaculation, but more rigorous trials are needed to claim definitive efficacy.

ACUPUNCTURE

A randomized trial of acupuncture compared to paroxetine proved superiority of paroxetine in improving overall symptomatology, but acupuncture had a significant stronger ejaculation-delaying effect compared to placebo (Sunay et al., 2011). Acupuncture pressure points utilized in this study included the second metacarpal bone, calcaneal tendon, tibialis anterior muscle, metatarsal bone, and prominence of the medial malleolus. Additional studies using larger numbers of patients across various populations are needed to further elucidate efficacy.

CONCLUSION

Offering our male patients CAM therapies for the treatment of sexual dysfunction is a reasonable approach to therapy, without significant demonstrated harm. Patients should be advised that CAM options composed of medicinal extracts may interact with other medications and may have adverse effects. Future studies are needed to determine long-term efficacy, safety, and comparability to conventional pharmacotherapeutic options.

REFERENCES

American Urological Association Erectile Dysfunction Clinical Guidelines Panel. Report on the Treatment of Organic Erectile Dysfunction. The American Urological Association, Baltimore, Maryland, 1996. Updated guideline at: http://www.ngc.gov/summary/summary.aspx?doc_id=10018& nbr=005332&string=erectile+AND+dysfunction. Accessed January 14, 2012.

Burls, A., Gold, L., Clark, W. (2001). Systematic review of randomized controlled trials of sildenafil (Viagra) in the treatment of male erectile dysfunction. Br J Gen Pract. 51,1004–1012.

Carson, C.C., Lue, T.F. (2005). Phosphodiesterase type 5 inhibitors for erectile dysfunction. BJU Int. 96(3),257–280.

Chen, J., Keren-Paz, G., Bar-Josef, Y., Matzkin, H. (2007). The role of phosphodiesterase type 5 inhibitors in the management of premature ejaculation: a critical analysis of basic science and clinical data. Eur Urol. 52,1331–1339.

Chen, J., Wollman, Y., Chernichovsky, T. (1999). Effect of oral administration of high-dose nitric-oxide donor L-arginine in men with organic erectile dysfunction: results of a double-blind, randomized, placebo-controlled study. BJU Int. 83,269–273.

Dhikav, V., Karmarkar, G., Gupta, M., Anand, K.S. (2007). Yoga in premature ejaculation: a comparative trial with fluoxetine. J Sex Med. 4,1726–1732.

Engelhardt, P.F., Daha, L.K., Zils, T., Simak, R., Konig, K., Pfluger, H. (2003). Acupuncture in the treatment of psychogenic erectile dysfunction: first results of a prospective randomized placebo-controlled study. Int J Impot. 15,343–346.

Ernst, E., Pittler, M.H. (1998). Yohimbine for erectile dysfunction: a systematic review and meta-analysis of randomized clinical trials. J Urol. 159,433–436.

Feldman, H.A., Goldstein, I., Hatzichristou, D.G., Krane, R.J., McKinlay, J.B. (1994). Impotence and its medical and psychosocial correlates: results of the Massachusetts Male Aging Study. J Urol. 151,54–61.

Heidelbaugh, J. (2010). Management of erectile dysfunction. Am Fam Physician. 81(3):305–312.

Hong, B., Ji, Y.H., Hong, J.H., Nam, K.Y., Ahn, T.Y. (2002). A double-blind crossover study evaluating the efficacy of Korean red ginseng in patients with erectile dysfunction: a preliminary report. J Urol. 168,2070–2073.

Jang, D.J., Lee, M.S., Shin, B.C., Lee, Y.C., Ernst, E. (2008). Red ginseng for treating erectile dysfunction: a systematic review. Br J Clin Pharmacol. 66(4),444–450.

Lebret, T., Herve, J.M., Gorny, P., Worcel, M., Botto, H. (2002). Efficacy and safety of a novel combination of L-arginine glutamate and yohimbine hydrochloride: a new oral therapy for erectile dysfunction. Eur Urol. 41,608–613.

Lue, T., Broderick, G. (2007). Evaluation and nonsurgical management of erectile dysfunction and premature ejaculation. In: Walsh, P.C., Retik, A.B., Vaughn, E.D., Wein, A.J., Kavoussi, L.R., Novick, A.C., Partin, A.W., Peters, C.A., eds. Campbell-Walsh Urology. 9th edition, Vol. 1. Philadelphia, PA: Saunders-Elsevier; 750–787.

McVary, K.T. (2007). Erectile dysfunction. NEJM. 357(24),2472–2481.

Melnik, T., Soares, B.G., Nasselo, A.G. (2007). Psychosocial interventions for erectile dysfunction. Cochrane Database Syst Rev. CD004825.

National Institutes of Health. (1992). NIH Consensus Statement, Impotence. 10(4),1–31.

Nurnberg, H.G., Hensley, P.L., Gelenberg, A.J., Fava, M., Lauriello, J., Paine, S. (2003). Treatment of antidepressant-associated sexual dysfunction with sildenafil. A randomized controlled trial. JAMA. 289,56–64.

Park, J., Shin, D.W., Ahn, T.Y. (2008). Complimentary and alternative medicine in men's health. JMH. 5(4),305–313.

Price, A., Gazewood, J. (2003). Korean red ginseng effective for treatment of erectile dysfunction. J Fam Pract. 52,20–1.

Rendell, M.S., Raifer, J., Wicker, P.A., Smith, M.D. (1999). Sildenafil for treatment of erectile dysfunction in men with diabetes: a randomized controlled trial. JAMA. 281,421–426.

Shabsigh, R., Anastasiadis, A.G. (2003). Erectile dysfunction. Annu Rev Med. 54,153–168.

Shin, B.C., Lee, M.S., Yang, E.J., Lim, H.S., Ernst, E. (2010). Maca (L. meyenii) for improving sexual function: a systematic review. BMC Complement Altern Med. 10,44.

Stanislavov, R., Nikolova, V. (2003). Treatment of erectile dysfunction with pycnogenol and L-arginine. J Sex Marital Ther. 29,207–213.

Sunay, D., Sunay, M., Aydogmus, Y., Bagbanci, S., Arslan, H., Karabulut, A., Emir, L. (2011). Acupuncture versus paroxetine for the treatment of premature ejaculation: a randomized, placebo-controlled clinical trial. Eur Urol. 59,765–771.

Vardi, M., Nini, A. (2007). Phosphodiesterase inhibitors for erectile dysfunction in patients with diabetes mellitus (Cochrane Review). In: *The Cochrane Library 2007 Issue 1*. Chichester, UK: John Wiley and Sons, Ltd.

Waldinger, M.D., Hengeveld, M.W., Zwinderman, A.H. (1997). Ejaculation-retarding properties of paroxetine in patients with primary premature ejaculation: a double-blind, randomized, dose-response study. Br J Urol. 79,592–595.

Wu, G., Meininger, C.J. (2000). Arginine nutrition and cardiovascular function. J Nutr. 130,2626–2629.

13

Testosterone Deficiency and Complementary and Alternative Medicine (CAM)

MARTIN M. MINER

The Clinical Problem

Hypogonadism, henceforth referred to as testosterone deficiency (TD), afflicts approximately 30% of men ages 40 to 79, and its prevalence is associated with aging (Allan and McLachan, 2004). The prevalence values differ among the different studies (Mulligan et al., 2006; Tajar et al., 2010; Wu et al., 2008; Zitzmann, 2009) due to assessment based on population surveys or clinical settings. Clinical symptoms of TD include fatigue, decreased libido, erectile dysfunction (ED), and negative mood states (Araujo et al., 2007; Dandona and Rosenberg, 2010; Kaufman and Vermeulen, 2005; Zitzmann et al., 2006). TD is also associated with changes in body composition, including decreased lean body mass, increased fat mass, and decreased bone mineral density (Araujo et al., 2007; Dandona and Rosenberg, 2010; Kaufman and Vermeulen, 2005; Zitzmann et al., 2006). A significant increased risk of TD is noted in association with common medical conditions, such as obesity, type 2 diabetes mellitus (T2DM), and hypertension (Araujo et al., 2007; Dandona and Rosenberg, 2010; Kaufman and Vermeulen, 2005; Zitzmann et al., 2006). In addition, a strong relationship was observed between TD and the metabolic syndrome (MetS) (Kupelian et al., 2006; Laaksonen et al., 2003; Laaksonen et al., 2004; Muller et al., 2005; Wang et al., 2000). Whereas treatment of TD has been initiated primarily for relief of sexual symptoms, there is now increasing interest among clinicians in addressing the potential adverse metabolic and general health issues associated with TD. However, there are limited sources to guide decision-making in commonly seen cases where testosterone replacement therapy (TRT) may be considered.

TESTOSTERONE DEFICIENCY: SIGNS, SYMPTOMS, AND PREVALENCE

Table 13.1 lists the signs and symptoms of TD, and the most common symptoms are sexual dysfunction (low libido and/or ED) and chronic fatigue (Bhasin et al., 2006). The prevalence of TD increases with age, ranging from 9% in men in their 50s to 91% of those in their 80s (Bhasin et al., 2006). Mulligan et al. found that the rate of TD was ~38.7% in men 45 years old or older (N = 2,165) who visited a primary care provider's office (Mulligan et al., 2006). Although TD is more common among men with certain comorbidities (Harman et al., 2001), the decline in testosterone (T) levels observed with age appears unrelated to illness. Free T fell by about 1.4% per year in men ages 39 to 70 (N = 1,709) (Gray et al., 1991). Data from the Massachusetts Male Aging Study of approximately 1,700 community-dwelling men showed that T levels among men with one or more comorbid conditions (e.g., obesity, cancer, coronary heart disease, hypertension, diabetes, prostate problems) remained 10% to 15% lower than those of the control group of subjects, but the rate of decline in free T was similar (Travison et al., 2007). The clinical question is whether there is a role for testosterone replacement therapy (TRT) as treatment for the patient's sexual symptoms and MetS.

Table 13.1: Clinical Manifestations of Testosterone Deficiency

Physical	Psychological	Sexual
Decreased BMD	Depressed mood	Diminished libido
Decreased muscle mass and strength	Diminished energy, sense of vitality, or well-being	Erectile dysfunction
Increased body fat or BMI	Impaired cognition and memory	Difficulty achieving orgasm
Gynecomastia		Decreased morning erections
Anemia		Decreased performance
Frailty		
Fatigue		

BMD = bone mineral density; BMI = body mass index.

Adapted from Petak SM, Nankin HR, Spark RF, et al., for the AACE Hypogonadism Task Force. American Association of Clinical Endocrinologists medical guidelines for clinical practice for the evaluation and treatment of hypogonadism in adult male patients—2002 update. Endocr Pract. 2002;8:440-456.

Bhasin S, Cunningham GR, Hayes FJ, et al., for the Androgen Deficiency Syndromes in Men Guideline Task Force. Testosterone therapy in adult men with androgen deficiency syndromes: An Endocrine Society Clinical Practice Guideline. J Clin Endocrinol Metab. 2006;91:1995-2010.

The Evidence of Testosterone Replacement Therapy and Broader Health Implications

RELATIONSHIP BETWEEN TESTOSTERONE DEFICIENCY AND METABOLIC SYNDROME AND DIABETES

The relationship between TD and MetS is bidirectional and complex and involves multiple pathophysiological pathways (Figure 13.1) (Traish, Guay, et al., 2009; Traish, Saad and Guay, 2009; Traish, Saad, et al., 2009; Zitzmann, 2009). Evidence derived from epidemiological and clinical studies (Akishita et al., 2007; Akishita et al., 2009; Allan et al., 2008; Basaria et al., 2006; Fukui et al., 2007; Haidar et al., 2007; Hak et al., 2002; Kapoor et al., 2006; Makinen et al., 2005; Makinen, et al., 2008; Oh et al., 2002; Phillips et al., 1994; Pitteloud, Hardin, et al., 2005; Pitteloud, Mootha, et al., 2005; Selvin et al., 2007; Simon et al., 1997; Srinivas-Shankar et al., 2010; Stellato et al., 2000; van Pottelbergh et al., 2003; Yeap et al., 2009; Yialamas et al., 2007; Traish et al., 2009) with TRT in hypogonadal men, as well as androgen deprivation therapy (ADT) in prostate cancer (PCa) patients, suggests that the link between TD and MetS encompasses multiple pathways including increased insulin resistance (IR), hyperglycemia, visceral fat accumulation, dyslipidemia, increased inflammatory cytokines, and endothelial dysfunction, leading to vascular disease (Akishita et al., 2007; Akishita et al., 2009; Caminiti et al., 2009; Fukui et al., 2007; Malkin et al., 2004; Nettleship et al., 2007; Oh et al., 2002; Phillips et al., 1994; Pitteloud, Hardin, et al., 2005; Pitteloud, Mootha, et al., 2005; Selvin et al., 2007; Stellato et al., 2000; Traish, Abdou, et al., 2009; Traish, Feeley, et al., 2009; Yeap et al., 2009).

Emerging evidence links TD to multiple cardiovascular risk factors including obesity, diabetes, hypertension, and altered lipid profiles, suggesting that T plays an important role in the regulation of metabolic homeostasis. TD is an independent determinant of endothelial dysfunction (Akishita et al., 2009; Malkin et al., 2004; Nettleship et al., 2007), thus contributing to vascular pathology. TRT in men with TD produced significant improvement in lipid profiles, reduced body fat and increased lean muscle mass, and decreased fasting glucose levels (Basaria et al., 2010; Caminiti et al., 2009; Heufelder et al., 2009; Shores et al., 2006; Tajar et al., 2010; Wang et al., 2000).

TESTOSTERONE DEFICIENCY AND ALL-CAUSE MORTALITY AND CARDIOVASCULAR DISEASE RISK

Epidemiologic studies have identified significant associations between T levels and all-cause and cardiovascular (CV) death in general populations of men 40 years old or older (Figure 13.2) (Bhasin et al., 2010; Khaw et al., 2007;

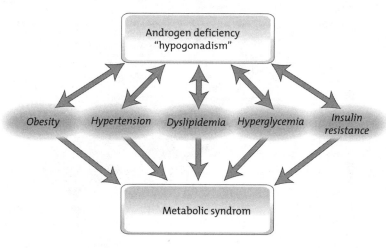

FIGURE 13.1. Relationship between testosterone deficiency (TD) and metabolic syndrome (MetS) is bidirectional.

Laughlin et al., 2008). Mortality rate over a mean of 4.3 years for 858 veterans with normal, equivocal (one normal, one low measurement), and low T levels was 20.1%, 24.6%, and 34.9%, respectively (Shores et al., 2006). A larger (2,314 men, aged 40 to 79 years), longer (average 7-year follow-up) nested case-control study found that every 173 ng/dl (6.0 nmol/L) increase in serum T was associated with a 21% lower risk of all-cause death after excluding deaths within the first 2 years and controlling for multiple variables (age, body mass index [BMI], systolic blood pressure, cholesterol, cigarette smoking, diabetes, alcohol intake, physical activity, social class, education, and sex hormone–binding globulin [SHBG]) (Laughlin et al., 2008). The Rancho Bernardo study (N = 794 men, aged 50 to 91 years; average follow-up, 11.8 years, but up to 20 years) also found that total and bioavailable T were inversely related to risk of death (Khaw et al., 2007). Low total T also predicted increased risk of death due to CV and respiratory disease (Bhasin et al., 2010).

Data from recent randomized placebo-controlled trials of TRT in elderly frail men with limited mobility suggested potential improvements in physical function (Srinivas-Shankar et al., 2010) when T levels were maintained in the physiological range. Caminiti et al. (2009) showed, in a double-blind, placebo-controlled, randomized trial of 70 elderly patients with chronic heart failure, that long-acting intramuscular T supplementation on top of optimal therapy improves functional exercise capacity, muscle strength, insulin levels, and baroreflex sensitivity (Caminiti et al., 2009).

However, negative cardiovascular risks in an older, sicker group of men with subclinical vascular disease were noted when T levels were maintained in the higher range (Basaria et al., 2010). It should be noted that in the latter

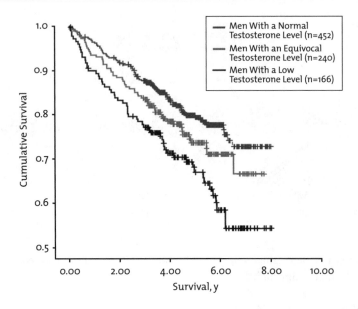

FIGURE 13.2. Low testosterone associated with shorter survival. Unadjusted Kaplan-Meier survival curves for 3 T level groups. Men with low and equivocal (one normal and one low measurement) had a significantly shorter survival than men with normal T levels (log-rank test; p = .001). N Low testosterone = total T <250 ng/dL (8.7 nmol/L) or free T <0.75 ng/dL (0.03 nmol/L).

Adopted from Shores MM, Matsumoto AM, Sloan KL, Kivlahan DR. Low serum testosterone and mortality in male veterans. *Arch Intern Med.* 2006;166:1660–1665.

study, the small sample size, older and sicker population, and mobility limitations preclude the generalizability of these findings. This study, known as the TOM (Testosterone on Mobility) study, raised questions regarding use of rather large doses of T in older frail men with subclinical vascular disease.

In contrast to the study by Srinivas-Shankar et al. (2010) which showed no serious cardiac adverse events, the TOM study (Basaria et al., 2010) suffers from serious limitations: (a) patients with subclinical cardiovascular diseases and high prevalence of hypertension, diabetes, hyperlipidemia, and obesity; (b) selection of subjects based on T levels only instead of combination with clinical symptoms; (c) inadequate randomization; and (d) a dose-seeking study with T doses administered that exceeded those cited in the Endocrine Society recommendations (Bhasin et al., 2010).

It should be pointed out that monitoring of the adverse events was not the primary endpoints and reporting of these events was carried out by telephone interviews of subjects or reviewing external medical records. Thus, subjective feelings of tachycardia, syncope of unknown origin, arterial hypertension, and myocardial infarctions were all used as cardiovascular adverse events. In fact, in a recent meta-analysis it was concluded that "the adverse effects of testosterone therapy include an increase in hemoglobin and hematocrit and a small decrease in high-density lipoprotein cholesterol but pointed to no cardiovascular events." (Haddad RM et al., 2007). However, the authors drew broad conclusions on the adverse effect of TRT on cardiovascular health in these frail and immobile men. Indeed, the authors stated that "the lack of a consistent pattern in these events and the small number of overall events suggest the possibility that the differences detected between the two trial groups may have been due to chance alone." (Basaria et al., 2010).

Can Testosterone Replacement Therapy Reverse or Ameliorate Metabolic Syndrome or Early Type 2 Diabetes?

MetS is associated with the risk of developing insulin resistance, T2DM, and cardiovascular disease (CVD) and a higher risk of incident CVD and mortality (Lorenzo et al., 2007). MetS is associated with a twofold increase of 5- to 10-year risk of CVD (Esposito et al., 2005). Furthermore, the syndrome confers a fivefold increase in risk for T2DM (Osuna et al., 2006). Despite this evidence, the clinical use of this category, and in particular its utility as a predictor of CVD, has been the subject of vigorous criticism (Guembe et al., 2010; Hobbs et al., 1993; Kalinchenko et al., 2010; Osuna et al., 2006; Singh et al., 2006). Accordingly, recent data from a survey involving 880 community-dwelling men supported the construct that MetS is not better than the sum of its components in addressing cardiovascular risk (Aversa, Bruzziches, Francomano, et al., 2010).

The level of evidence supporting TRT in the treatment of MetS, T2DM, and CVD varies because TRT administered in various formulations has differing outcomes on different aspects of clinical endpoints investigated. Specifically, reduction of body fat, especially intra-abdominal fat, is a key component in treating most individuals with MetS or T2DM, as well as many patients with atherosclerotic cardiovascular disease and dyslipidemia. We consider the evidence supporting TRT in reducing fat mass to be quite rigorous (Hobbs et al., 1993; Singh et al., 2006). Several randomized clinical trials (Aversa et al., 2010a, b; Heufelder et al., 2009; La Vignera et al., 2008; Saad, 2010) that enrolled 306 patients with MetS with had a mean follow-up of 58 weeks have been reported. In addition, TRT was associated with a significant reduction of fasting plasma glucose, Homeostasis Model Assessment (HOMA) index, triglycerides, and waist circumference. It should be noted that in the aforementioned studies some, but not all, of the patients recruited were receiving statins to reduce cholesterol. The levels of T may be affected by the use of statins because it has been reported that statin use may reduce total but not bioavailable T (Kapoor et al., 2008; Stanworth et al., 2009).

VALUE OF TESTOSTERONE REPLACEMENT THERAPY IN TESTOSTERONE DEFICIENCY PATIENTS WITH ERECTILE DYSFUNCTION AND LOW LIBIDO

Studies of TRT on sexual function and performance vary in quality, though findings are generally consistent. Most studies show that TRT increased sexual awareness and arousal, erectile function, and the frequency of spontaneous erections but is less consistent in enhancing sexual behavior and performance (Anderson et al., 1992; Aversa et al., 2003; Benkert et al., 1979; Cavallini et al., 2004; Corona et al., 2010; Kunelius et al., 2002; Park et al., 2003; Schiavi et al., 1997; Shabsigh et al., 2004; Shabsigh, 2005; Svartberg et al., 2004). Overall, the evidence demonstrates that TRT benefits some aspects of sexual desire, erectile function, and performance. This assessment is consistent with a recently published review (Bolona et al., 2007) and meta-analyses of randomized, placebo-controlled trials of TRT in men with sexual dysfunction and varying endogenous T levels (Isidori et al., 2005). It is also worth noting that, because vasculopathy is the most common cause of ED, it can also serve as an early marker for CVD (Miner and Kuritzky, 2007). It is reasonable to obtain T results in men with ED, especially if associated with diminished libido or fatigue, and in men with an inadequate response to phosphodiesterase type 5 (PDE5) inhibitors. T action in these vascular beds may be mediated by several pathways including vasodilation of blood vessels via activation of K^+ channels or inhibition of Ca^{++} channels (Yildiz and Seyrek, 2007).

Treatment of Testosterone Deficiency

A number of TRT preparations are currently available in the U.S. market (Table 13.2). Intramuscular injections of short-acting T derivatives achieve good serum concentrations within 2 to 3 days, with levels returning to baseline in most men by 2 weeks, resulting in an injection schedule of 1 to 2 weeks. Men or their partners may be taught to perform the injection at home. Topical gels or patches provide a more stable serum T concentration over time than injections. Currently available patches in the United States are associated with a high rate of skin reaction, and their use has been largely supplanted by T gels. The main disadvantage of T gels is cost and a black box warning concerning transfer potential to women and children (Zitzmann, 2010). An

Table 13.2: Testosterone Replacement Therapy Preparations

Generic Name (Sample Brands)	Route	Dosing Regimen	Advantages	Disadvantages
T cypionate (Depo-Testosterone), T enanthate (aka ethanate) (Delatestryl), T mixed esters (Sutanon)	IM	200 mg/2 weeks300mg/3 weeks 400 mg/4 weeks	Long acting, relatively inexpensive if self-administered, flexibility of dosing	Requires IM injection, does not mimic physiologic levels, creates peaks and troughs
Injectable long-acting T undecanoate in oil (Nebido)	IM	1000 mg, followed by 1000 mg at 6 weeks, and 1000 mg every 12 weeks	Infrequent administration	Not approved in the United States, IM injection of large volume (4 ml)
Transdermal hydroalcoholic gel (AndroGel, Testim) or compounded testosterone creams and gels	Topical	5–10 g, delivers 50–100-mg dose daily	Flexible dosing, ease of application, good skin tolerability	Risk of transfer to a female partner or child by skin-to-skin contact if gel not completely dry, moderately high DHT levels
Transdermal T patch (Androderm, Testoderm TTS)	Topical	5mg/day, applied to skin at bedtime	Mimics physiologic levels and diurnal pattern, ease of application, lesser increase in hemoglobin than injectable esters	Mimics physiologic dosing, contact dermatitis

(continued)

Table 13.2: (continued)

Generic Name (Sample Brands)	Route	Dosing Regimen	Advantages	Disadvantages
Scrotal T patch (Testoderm)	Topical	One patch delivers 6 mg over 24 hr, applied daily	Mimics physiologic levels	To promote adherence, scrotal skin needs to be shaved, high DHT levels
Buccal T (Striant)	Gum region	30 mg bid		Gum-related adverse events in 16% of treated men
T pellets (Testopel)	SC	4–10 75-mg pellets implanted SC	Infrequent dosing	Requires surgical incision for insertions, pellets may extrude spontaneously
Oral T undecanoate (Andriol, Androxon, Understor, Restandol, Restinsol)	Oral	40–80 mg 2–3 ×/day with meals	Convenience of oral administration	Not approved in the United States, variable clinical responses, variable serum T levels, high DHT:T ratio

DHT = dehydrotestosterone; IM = intramuscular; SC = subcutaneous; T = testosterone.

Adapted from Bhasin S, Cunningham GR, Hayes FJ, et al. Testosterone therapy in men with androgen deficiency syndromes: an endocrine society clinical practice guideline. J Clin Endocrinol Metab. 2010;95:2536–2559.

attempt to reduce this has been the introduction in 2011 of three high-potency, low-volume T gels/solution. Testosterone can also be mixed to individual specifications into a cream base for topical use by a compounding pharmacy. A long-acting injection formulation (T undecanoate) is dosed every 10 to 12 weeks and is available internationally but has not yet been approved for use in the United States. T pellets provide 3 to 6 months of normal serum T and are placed subcutaneously in the gluteal region via an in-office surgical implantation procedure under local anesthesia. This formulation also has some disadvantages such as extrusion of pellets after the surgical procedure and risk of infection.

In addition, the genetic background relating to patient responsiveness to androgens, hence, androgen receptor polymorphisms, are likely to play an interindividual role (Lakshman and Basaria, 2009). Furthermore, considerable uncertainty exists regarding (a) the accuracy of T assays, (b) the application of total or free T to clinical assessment of TD, and (c) the subject of age stratification. Such considerations have to be taken into account when managing patients with TD who definitely need diagnosis and treatment. Physicians have to use their clinical judgment and experience in such cases. For a practicing primary care clinician, we suggest the following approach to men with symptoms of TD.

DIAGNOSIS OF TESTOSTERONE DEFICIENCY AND TESTOSTERONE REPLACEMENT THERAPY TO MAINTAIN THRESHOLD LEVELS

The goal of TRT is to safely restore testosterone to normal physiologic levels, thereby ameliorating symptoms associated with TD and improving patient health and well-being. At the biochemical level, the goal is to raise total testosterone to a range considered normal for healthy young men, 300 to 1,050 ng/dl (Bhasin et al., 2006; Dandona and Rosenberg, 2010; Miner and Sadofsky, 2007). Note that these are *physiologic* (or eugonadal) testosterone levels, not *supraphysiologic* levels; there is no basis for recommending TRT dose escalations in pursuit of greater efficacy, and the practice may increase the risk of treatment side effects. TRT should also achieve physiologic levels of key testosterone metabolites, including estradiol, a sex hormone with major influence on male bone density (Lunenfeld and Nieschlag, 2007; Practice Committee of American Society for Reproductive Medicine, 2008).

The level of total testosterone at which TRT should be considered for the individual patient is not clear from research and is not consistent across published guidelines for TD management (Bhasin et al., 2006; Wang et al., 2009). Clinical judgment is essential to decision making about treatment, and judgment should be guided by these basic principles: (a) total testosterone levels greater than 350 ng/dl do not require repletion, and (b) a trial of TRT is appropriate to consider for men with unquestionably low or borderline low testosterone levels, a consistent clinical picture of TD, and no contraindications to TRT. This trial should be no shorter than 3 months.

LIFESTYLE INTERVENTIONS

TRT is only the pharmacologic component of TD therapy. All TRT is bioidentical, unlike the hormonal replacement used in the Women's Health Initiative (WHI). Another difference from the WHI is that positive health behaviors, such as exercise, diet, and avoidance of smoking, are considered a means of preventing TD, and they correlate significantly with higher testosterone levels over time in population-based research (Yeap et al., 2009).

CURRENT TREATMENT MODALITIES

Current treatment modalities appear relatively safe, and those adverse events that have been definitively associated with treatment are reversible with cessation of treatment. These include acne, gynecomastia, erythrocytosis, and edema. A number of additional risks have appeared in the literature, but their relationship to TRT is less well established. These include sleep apnea, worsening of urinary voiding symptoms, and prostate cancer. Standard forms of TRT do not appear to adversely affect lipid profiles (Saad et al., 2008; Traish, Abdou, and Kypreos, 2009; Zitzmann and Nieschlag, 2007), or renal function. TRT does not appear to cause liver toxicity, with the exception of oral alkylated T preparations (e.g., methyltestosterone), which should not be used for TRT for this reason.

Areas of Concerns and Uncertainty in the Management of Testosterone Replacement Therapy

LACK OF CONSENSUS REGARDING BIOCHEMICAL IDENTIFICATION OF MEN WITH TESTOSTERONE DEFICIENCY

A key area of controversy relates to the biochemical determination of TD. There is no defined serum threshold for T that clearly distinguishes men who are T deficient from those who are not. Yet all published guidelines recommend one arbitrary threshold or another, generally ranging from 200 to 350 ng/dl (6.94 to 12.15 nmol/L). Variation in SHBG levels also confounds the interpretation of bioavailable T levels. There is general agreement that free or bioavailable T provides a better estimation of T status, but there is uncertainty regarding the reliability of those assays. In addition, genetic variation may influence response to circulating T. For these reasons, we believe clinical presentation that permits assessment of the signs and symptoms of TD plays a critical role in the diagnosis of TD, with blood tests providing additional diagnostic support.

TESTOSTERONE REPLACEMENT THERAPY AND PROSTATE CANCER RISK

An international study identified that the greatest concern of physicians with regard to T therapy is potentially stimulating PCa (Gooren et al., 2007). This concern stems from the use of androgen deprivation for the treatment of advanced prostate cancer. However, current data fail to demonstrate a significant association between serum androgen concentrations and prostate cancer. A large international study comprising 3,886 men with PCa and 6,438 age-matched controls found no associations between PCa risk and serum concentrations of T, calculated free T, or dihydrotestosterone (Carpenter et al., 2008; Endogenous Hormones and Prostate Cancer Collaborative Group, 2008).

A meta-analysis of 19 studies revealed no greater risk of PCa in men diagnosed with TD who received placebo versus men who received T therapy (Calof et al., 2005). Although no long-term, large-scale studies on the safety of T therapy have been performed, evidence accumulated over the last 15 years strongly indicates that beyond the near-castrate range there is little, if any, impact of changes in serum T on PCa growth (Morgentaler and Traish, 2009).

Recommendations for Surveillance on Testosterone Replacement Therapy

TRT offers benefits that can extend to sexual and physical domains, psychological health, and restored vigor for life and positive metabolic changes (Cunningham and Toma, 2011; Morgentaler, 2007), and it has never been proved to cause the development or progression of prostate cancer. Therapy even for men with a history of treated prostate cancer is no longer ruled out (Morgentaler, 2011; Morgentaler et al., 2011). For physicians to deny hypogonadal men the possibility of TRT benefits out of fear of prostate or other potential safety issues may be excessively cautious. However, if providers remain uncomfortable with management of TRT, then referral to a specialist should be considered. It is at least the responsibility of the primary care provider to make the diagnosis of testosterone deficiency.

The solution lies in monitoring TRT to ensure safety while achieving benefits (Table 13.3). In both the near term and throughout the patient's course of care, which may be lifelong, a sustained monitoring program offers the best path to successful outcomes. More than just an option, monitoring TRT should be considered an indispensable corollary to the decision to treat. It requires commitment and collaboration by all parties—primary care practitioner, patient, other health office personnel, and specialists who may be consulted—and an understanding of how to proceed over time. Lunenfeld and Nieschlag (2007) noted that monitoring of TRT "is a shared responsibility that cannot be taken lightly." That said, monitoring of testosterone therapy is not a prohibitive task for either the physician or patient. Many of the recommended elements of TRT monitoring coincide with standard medical guidelines for older men generally, and even the more intensive first-year monitoring schedule does not place extreme demands on resources or time. Published guidelines, including those from the Endocrine Society (Bhasin et al., 2010), the American Society for Reproductive Medicine (2008), the European Association of Urology and the International Society of Andrology (Nieschlag et al., 2005), and others, are based on evolving principles for TRT monitoring:

- The monitoring program should be planned at the outset of TRT; specific goals, follow-up visits, and parameters for surveillance must be delineated.
- Patient education and counseling are essential components.
- Monitoring includes regular assessment of both biochemical and clinical changes.
- The patient's clinical presentation at monitoring visits may be a better guide to TRT efficacy and adjustments to treatment than serum testosterone levels, and levels should never be solely targeted without clinical response.
- The health of the prostate and the production of red blood cells are the primary targets of TRT safety evaluations.
- The type of TRT formulation in use will influence the monitoring schedule and the nature of potential adverse events.
- Treatment should begin as a trial of 3 to 6 months, with continuation predicated on evidence of safety and efficacy.

Table 13.3: Guide to Monitoring Testosterone Replacement Therapy

Target of Monitoring	When to Monitor	Actions to Consider
Symptomatic response: clinical improvements and side effects (general and formulation specific)	1–3 months after initiation, then annually	If suboptimal response, consider dosage change, switch TRT formulation, discontinue, refer
Testosterone level	All formulations: BaselineGel: 1–2 weeks after initiation Injectable: midway between injections Patch: 3–12 hr after application Pellets: at end of dosing interval Buccal tablet: immediately after application of new tablet	If TT >700 ng/dl or <400 mg/dl (as low as 350 ng/dl in older men), adjust dose or dosing interval to achieve physiologic (midnormal) testosterone range
Hematocrit	Baseline, 3–6 months, then annually	If hematocrit >52%–55%, suspend therapy while level declines, evaluate for hypoxia and sleep apnea. Have patient consider blood donation if long-acting preparations are used and testosterone cannot be held. Restart TRT at reduced dose
Prostate: PSA	Baseline, 3–6 months, then per routine guidelines	Consult on biopsy/withdrawal of TRT if PSA increases >1.4 ng/ml in any 12 months, or if PSA velocity is >0.4 ng/ml/year. Most would use 0.75 ng/ml/year. There are many thresholds out there
Prostate: DRE	Baseline, 3–6 months, then per routine guidelines	Consult on biopsy/withdrawal of TRT if abnormal (palpatory nodule, induration)

(continued)

Table 13.3: (continued)

Target of Monitoring	When to Monitor	Actions to Consider
BMD	Baseline, 1–2 years	Measure BMD of lumbar spine and/or femoral neck in patients with osteoporosis or low trauma fracture
Lipids	Baseline, 6–12 months, then annually	More frequent measurements if specific reductions targeted
Adherence to therapy	Each visit	Address adherence history at baseline; plan monitoring schedule, education, and TRT regimen accordingly

BMD = bone mineral density; DRE = digital rectal examination; PSA = prostate-specific antigen; TRT = testosterone replacement therapy; TT = total testosterone.
From Wang et al., 2009; Bhasin et al., 2010; Dandona & Rosenberg, 2010; Rhoden & Morgentaler, 2004; Miner & Sadofsky, 2007 and Guay & Traish, 2009.

- Referral to a urologist or other specialist may be appropriate in some cases where safety or efficacy is a concern.

These principles are thorough and cautious and they allow for tailoring to meet the indications and needs of the individual patient.

FREQUENCY OF FOLLOW-UP EVALUATIONS

Use of TRT mandates baseline assessment and regular follow-up of the hypogonadal patient (Table 13.3). Although general schedules for follow-up monitoring have been proposed, the optimum schedule for each patient remains a matter of clinical judgment and should be derived based on such factors as the severity of TD and related symptoms, anticipated benefits of therapy, concerns about specific side effects, coexisting health problems (e.g., metabolic syndrome, osteoporosis), patient age and race, type of TRT formulation in use, concerns about adherence, and patient preferences and constraints (e.g., access or cost issues). Biochemical and symptomatic effects of T occur in relationship to the type of therapy (Morales et al., 2010; Saad et al., 2011), but the most intensive period of change, and thus the most intensive period of monitoring, is during the first 6 months of therapy. Guidelines generally suggest at least one visit in this period, as early as 1 month but no later than 3 months after baseline evaluations (Bhasin et al., 2010). Many experts recommend a second visit at 6 months to repeat tests and examination (Wang et al., 2009; Morales et al., 2010; Practice Committee of American Society for Reproductive Medicine, 2008).

The earlier evaluations in TRT monitoring are opportunities for dose adjustments, switching TRT formulations, or referral to a specialist if clinical improvements are suboptimal or side effects are a concern (Miner and Sadofsky, 2007). Findings of safety and efficacy by 6 months are crucial to the decision to continue TRT; although some anthropomorphic benefits may take at least 12 to 15 months to appear, improvements in libido, emotional well-being, energy, and erectile function typically occur earlier, as do changes in hematocrit and prostate-specific antigen (PSA) (Miner and Sadofsky, 2007). If the decision is made to continue treatment, monitoring should be scheduled on at least an annual basis or in accord with routine, age- and race-appropriate screening guidelines for men.

Problematic or persistent side effects or a lack of clinical response to TRT call for discontinuation of treatment after 3 to 6 months (recall, longer term goals such as increased bone mineral density [BMD] may require extended therapy). A poor response may indicate inadequate TRT dose or an unsuitable formulation, but it may also reflect problems with patient adherence, and this should be discussed both at the outset of therapy and over its course. Patient education is key in this area, including counseling about realistic expectations of TRT and the importance of follow-up visits. If the patient misses appointments, therapy should be stopped.

The primary care provider should be prepared to search for other causes of the patient's symptoms if TRT is unhelpful. This may require a urology, endocrinology, psychiatric, or other specialist consultation. Further, referral to a urologist is warranted when PSA increases significantly or if induration or nodule of the prostate is detected. Other conditions meriting specialist involvement are pituitary disease, testicular abnormalities, genetic history, or the need for fertility-sparing treatment for patients desiring paternity.

MEASUREMENTS USED IN TESTOSTERONE REPLACEMENT THERAPY SURVEILLANCE

Measurements during TRT monitoring are intended to ascertain treatment impact on testosterone level, the prostate, red blood cell production, and parameters such as lipid profile and BMD that may be of particular interest because of patient comorbidities (e.g., metabolic syndrome, diabetes, or osteoporosis).

Serum Testosterone

Measurement of serum testosterone level is fundamental to TRT monitoring. The goal for total testosterone is typically 400 to 500 ng/dl, considered a midnormal physiologic range (Bhasin et al., 2010), though we suggest testing free hormone levels and treating patients individually and to symptom relief as long as this is within physiologic ranges. The recommended testosterone measurement schedule is at baseline and 3 to 6 months, then annually. Within that schedule, however, the appropriate timing of testosterone measurement depends to a large extent on the pharmacokinetics of the TRT formulation in use. Measurements in patients using injectable testosterone enanthate or cypionate should be made midway in the dosing interval. With topical gels, testosterone should be measured any time after 1 to 2 weeks of therapy, ideally in the morning prior to the next application. Patch users should be tested 3 to 12 hours after application. With implanted pellets, measurement is appropriate at the end of the dosing interval, and with buccal tablets, immediately after application of a new system (Cunningham and Toma, 2011). If total testosterone remains less than 350 ng/dl or has increased to greater than 700 ng/dl, adjustments to the dosage, frequency, or formulation of TRT are needed.

Even if testosterone levels are maintained in a physiologic range, testosterone repletion is an empiric therapy. There is no consensus on the optimum testosterone levels for achieving desired outcomes and safety with TRT. Some men may respond better at low-normal than midnormal range. As stated earlier, given the uncertainties of testosterone interpretation, the patient's clinical presentation becomes equally or more important than testosterone level as a guide to ongoing treatment decisions.

PSA and Digital Rectal Examination (DRE)

Because of concerns regarding TRT and prostate cancer risk or an exacerbation of lower urinary tract symptoms (LUTSs), the health of the prostate must be assessed by PSA measurement and DRE at baseline, during the first year of follow-up, and thereafter in compliance with general guidelines for prostate cancer screening. The Endocrine Society recommends these tests for men older than 40 years with a baseline PSA greater than 0.6 ng/ml (median for patients this age) (Bhasin et al., 2010).

A rise in PSA from baseline to a level seen in eugonadal men occurs commonly in hypogonadal men by 3 to 6 months after TRT commencement. This level should represent a plateau, and after a year or so, further increases in PSA should occur slowly and only as a result of aging (Saad et al., 2011). An increase of greater than 1.4 ng/ml in any 12-month period should prompt referral to a urologist for consideration of prostate biopsy, according to guidelines of the Endocrine Society (Bhasin et al., 2010). To detect any rapid PSA increases as TRT continues, estimation of the velocity of PSA change is an important step, as a rapid rise may indicate pre-existing undiagnosed cancer. Estimation of velocity requires multiple measurements of PSA over time; it is calculated as the change from baseline PSA divided by years since that measurement. For example, a PSA of 2.4 ng/ml that has increased to 3.0 ng/ml after 2 years of TRT, for an absolute change of 0.6 ng/ml, translates to a PSA velocity of 0.3 ng/ml/year (Bhasin et al., 2003). The Endocrine Society notes that a velocity of greater than 0.4 ng/ml/year (with the 6-month reading as reference) justifies urology consultation, as do suspicious findings on any DRE (Bhasin et al., 2010).

Hematocrit

Regardless of the TRT formulation in use, hematocrit should be measured at baseline and each first-year follow-up visit, and annually thereafter (Bhasin et al., 2010; Wang et al., 2009). Although the increased oxygen-carrying capacity of the blood may boost the patient's energy, an elevated hematocrit increases the risk of a thromboembolic event and cannot go unaddressed (no such events have been reported in association with TRT).

Rises in hematocrit and hemoglobin may be evident in some patients early after TRT initiation as a result of the stimulatory effect of testosterone on erythropoiesis. Increases of 10% to 15% in hematocrit (Cunningham and Toma, 2011) may occur and raise this parameter to the point of possible erythrocytosis. In fact, hematocrit greater than 50% has been the most frequent testosterone-related adverse event seen in clinical trials, especially among older men. A meta-analysis of 19 randomized controlled trials found that testosterone-treated men age 45 years or older were almost four times more likely to reach this level than placebo-treated men (Calof et al., 2005). Elevated hematocrit is testosterone dose related and observed less often with transdermal gels and patches than with intramuscular injections or implantable pellets, possibly as a result of the rapid stimulation of bone marrow by the high dose quickly available from the last two preparations.

Patients with hematocrit values above 52% to 54% (Bhasin et al., 2010) should receive a dose adjustment or a change in TRT formulation to maintain safe hematologic values. Blood donation is another effective remedy. On rare occasions, therapy needs to be stopped until the hematocrit returns to normal.

BMD

Testosterone plays a vital role in maintenance of bone health, chiefly through its aromatization to estradiol (Isidori et al., 2005). Testosterone deficiency is a known cause of decreased BMD and male osteoporosis, and testosterone repletion has been shown in meta-analyses to significantly improve BMD in the lumbar spine (Tracz et al., 2006). Improvements in femoral neck BMD are less certain (Tracz et al., 2006), and there is no clear evidence that TRT can prevent fractures. Nevertheless, measurement of BMD in the lumbar spine and/or femoral neck should take place at the initiation of TRT. For men who have osteopenia, osteoporosis, or low-trauma fracture, BMD testing should be repeated after 1 to 2 years of TRT (Bhasin et al., 2010).

Lipid Profile

The effects of TRT on lipids are incompletely understood, but there is little evidence of an adverse impact. Meta-analyses have noted small reductions in high-density lipoprotein (HDL) cholesterol, as well as in total cholesterol (Fernández-Balsells et al., 2011; Isidori et al., 2005). Such changes have not been connected to cardiovascular outcomes in TRT treatment trials. However, lipid status, particularly triglyceride level, is highly relevant to metabolic syndrome, and TRT has been noted to reduce triglycerides in patients with this syndrome (Corona et al., 2011). For hypogonadal men receiving TRT, lipid profile should be measured at baseline, at 6 to 12 months, and then annually. When specific lipid goals are targeted, more frequent monitoring may be needed; reductions in total cholesterol and triglycerides may be evident as early as 4 weeks after the start of TRT (Saad et al., 2011).

Conclusion: The Broader Health Implications of Testosterone Deficiency

We therefore recommend a 3- to 6-month trial of TRT, with appropriate monitoring to ensure that adequate serum T levels are achieved. At the end of this period the patient will be assessed for resolution of his symptoms and for physical and biochemical changes, including sexual function, waist circumference, fasting glucose, and lipid profile. Some evidence exists that a 3-month trial showed improvement in several parameters, including energy, mood, and sexual function. Our recommendations here are in general agreement with most published guidelines, with two primary sources of disagreement: one is that we emphasize clinical presentation over biochemical thresholds in the diagnosis of TD, and the second is that we believe there is adequate evidence to support the use of TRT in selected cases for metabolic and general health indications. It should be noted that although some parameters will be improved during a 3-month trial, anthropomorphic changes are unlikely to change during this short period. If ED persists, a PDE5 inhibitor will be prescribed. Diet and exercise recommendations will be encouraged and reinforced.

Complementary and Alternative Medicine and Testosterone Replacement Therapy: What Is the Connection?

There has been much enthusiasm for the discovery of a "hormonal fountain of youth." The levels of many hormones decline with aging; however, it is uncertain whether replacement of these hormones will extend life and improve its quality or increase life span. In a literature search of the following compounds, many of the articles (~75%) were of newspaper or magazine origin. There is a paucity of structured clinical trials involving these agents to validate perceived claims by strategic marketing.

DHEA/PREGNENOLONE

Individuals pursuing antiaging compounds have a major interest in two steroid precursor hormones, dehydroepiandrosterone (DHEA) and pregnenolone. Both of these hormones decline dramatically with aging (Corona et al., 2011). A number of studies have examined the effects of DHEA replacement with aging. In low doses, DHEA has minimal effects in older persons (Baulieu et al., 2000). In doses of 100 mg daily, Morales and colleagues (1998) found an increase in muscle mass in men. Pregnenolone is the true "mother hormone," being made from cholesterol and being the precursor of all steroid hormones. In mice, pregnenolone is the most potent known memory enhancer (Flood et al., 1992; Flood et al., 1995). In humans, pregnenolone improves attention and decreases arthritic pain but fails to improve memory (Sih et al., 1999). At present, there is no evidence to support the use of DHEA or pregnenolone as antiaging hormones.

GROWTH HORMONE

Both growth hormone and insulin-like growth factor 1 levels decline with aging. These declines are more dramatic in malnourished persons (Anawalt and Merriam, 2001; Ravalgia et al., 2000). Rudman and colleagues suggested the existence of a growth hormone "menopause." (Rudman et al., 1990). Studies on growth hormone replacement have unfortunately provided minimal positive effects and a plethora of unpleasant side effects (Rudman et al., 1990; Johannsson et al., 2000). A study did find positive effects of a combination of growth hormone and testosterone (von Werder, 1999). However, animal and epidemiological studies have failed to support a role for growth hormone as an antiaging hormone (Christmas et al., 2002). A recent animal study found that growth hormone excess resulted in a decline in superoxide dismutase and glutathione peroxidase (Bartke et al., 2001). These findings of a decline in free radical defenses were suggested as one of the mechanisms of early mortality produced by growth hormone excess.

EXERCISE

Perhaps the best antiaging medicine is exercise (Evans, 2000; Fiatarone-Singh, 2002). Resistance exercise seems to be particularly useful because it not only improves strength (Hortobagyi et al., 2001; Westerterp and Meijer, 2001) but also enhances cognition (Etnier et al., 1997; Kramer et al., 2000) and decreases depression (Keysor and Jette, 2001). Despite these positive effects, Keysor and

Jette (2001) have pointed out that it is very difficult to demonstrate long-term functional effects of exercise programs.

Although the concept of antiaging therapies is intriguing, there is clearly little evidence-based medicine to support most of the generally touted approaches. Research does need to go forward, but it is important that clinicians do not provide support for the large number of inappropriate antiaging therapies (Olshansky et al., 2002; Smith and Olshansky, 2002).

MACA ROOT

"Meet maca. This hot Peruvian herb is thought to help boost libido and fertility in men, and offers multiple benefits for women, too."

These claims are among the ads for maca root products. Having been consumed by indigenous Peruvians for centuries (Cicero et al., 2001), the rumored energy-enhancing properties of the root of the maca plant have recently gained notoriety (Grunewald and Bailey, 1993), and its use has grown in popularity among athletes. Previous research exploring the scientific efficacy of maca supplementation on exercise performance has shown that consumption of maca improves various markers associated with sports performance (Milasius et al., 2008); however, the trial was not placebo controlled.

In one study, time to complete a 40-km bicycle time trial was significantly improved following 14 days of supplementation with maca. All eight cyclists improved their performance time from baseline in the Maca excluded (ME) trial. Following the placebo supplementation, there was no change in 40-km time trial performance. This study was a randomized crossover, double-blind design; therefore, any potential learning effects can be ruled out. Given that no changes in heart rate were observed, it is likely that any change in performance was not related to increased effort but rather that other mediating physiological variables were responsible.

Consumption of maca has tentatively been linked with an increase in testosterone in some (Milasius et al., 2008) but not all studies (Gonzales et al., 2002).

In the Spector study, 14 days of supplementation of maca significantly increased self-rated sexual desire (Spector et al., 1996), with no changes being observed in the placebo trial. These findings support previous in vivo investigations into the effect of maca consumption on sexual desire in humans and rats (Cicero et al., 2001; Gonzales et al., 2002). However, in this study (Gonzales et al., 2002), researchers did not encounter an increase in sexual desire until 8 weeks of treatment. And methodology at best was flawed; participants were subjectively asked to simply report if treatment diminished, did not change, increased mildly, or increased moderately to highly sexual desire. In the Spector study 14 days proved sufficient to elucidate a response in sexual desire (Spector et al., 1996).

TRIBULUS TERRESTRIS

The *Tribulus terrestris* (TT) herb has been commonly used in folk medicine to energize, vitalize, and improve sexual function and physical performance in men. Although different effects of TT on animals (Gauthaman, Adaikan and Prasad, 2002; Gauthaman, Ganesan and Prasad, 2003) and men (Brown et al., 2001; Kohut et al., 2003) have been evaluated and many active compounds from TT extract have been established (Cai et al., 2001; Huang et al., 2003), the mode of its action and efficacy remains uncertain and controversial. It is widely believed that TT strongly affects androgen metabolism, increasing testosterone or testosterone precursor levels significantly.

ANDROSTENEDIONE

In men, serum androstenedione concentrations are increased up to sevenfold above baseline and remain elevated for more than 6 hours after ingesting 100 to 300 mg of androstenedione (Beckham and Earnest, 2003; Earnest et al., 2000; King et al., 1999; Leder et al., 2000), indicating that a considerable amount of the ingested androstenedione escapes hepatic catabolism. Interestingly, Beckham and Earnest (2003) observed that the acute serum androstenedione response to ingesting 200 mg of androstenedione is markedly attenuated after 28 days of androstenedione ingestion, suggesting that chronic intake of androstenedione results in either reduced absorption, enhanced clearance, or enhanced catabolism of the ingested androstenedione with prolonged androstenedione intake.

One of the primary marketing claims for androstenedione, based on a German patent application (Hacker and Mattern, 1995), is that 50 mg of androstenedione increases serum testosterone concentrations by 40% to 83% within 15 minutes of intake, whereas 100 mg increases serum testosterone by 111% to 237%. These claims, however, have been invalidated by numerous scientific investigations.

In the first systematic investigation on the effects of androstenedione ingestion in men (aged 19 to 29 years; mean = 23 years), a single 100-mg dose of androstenedione did not increase serum free or total testosterone concentrations during the 6 hours after intake (King et al., 1999). Others have also reported that serum testosterone concentrations are not increased in men.

Although 100 mg of androstenedione is the dose frequently suggested by manufacturers, it is likely that athletes are using much larger doses. Earnest et al. (2000) reported that 200 mg of androstenedione in men aged approximately 24 years increases the serum testosterone area under the curve by approximately 15% during the 90 minutes after ingestion. The serum testosterone concentrations in this investigation, however, were not significantly higher at any time point following ingestion of androstenedione. It appears that the values reported for the area under the curve apparently included the area attributable to baseline serum testosterone concentrations, which were slightly higher in the group of subjects ingesting androstenedione. Furthermore, those investigators (Beckham and Earnest, 2003) later reported that a 200-mg dose of androstenedione does not acutely raise serum testosterone concentrations in men.

Leder et al. (2000) observed that a single 300-mg dose of androstenedione increased serum testosterone concentrations by approximately 34% during the 8 hours after intake in men aged 20 to 40 years. Considerable variations were seen in these data, however, and two subjects exhibited large increases in serum testosterone after intake of 300 mg of androstenedione, whereas the remaining 12 men had only a very small increase in serum testosterone. The causative factors determining why some people are androstenedione "responders" and some "nonresponders" are unknown.

All of these compounds have received much "lay press" attention in the discussions surrounding the use of "performance-enhancing steroids" in athletes, with public opinion swaying scientific study. It is strikingly clear from the evidence presented earlier that consequences and efficacy from both short-term and long-term use of these compounds remain largely unknown.

EFFECT OF SOY PROTEIN ON TESTOSTERONE LEVELS

A search of soy protein and testosterone levels revealed 37 studies performed from 1995 to 2010. Most of these studies were performed in animal subjects, and the results varied greatly in the few studies in human subjects. One such study showed a 19% decrease in testosterone levels for 13 men ranging from ages 25 to 47 years who took 56 g of soy protein isolate daily for 4 weeks (Goodin et al., 2007). Yet, another study, which randomized 24 men (mean age 58.6 years) to a high- or low-soy diet for 3 months (Maskarinec et al., 2006), showed no difference in T levels after ingestion of soy. This was a crossover study following a 1-month washout period, with the men entering the other treatment group. In the high-soy diet the men consumed two daily soy servings, whereas they followed their usual diet in the low-soy diet.

Dietary compliance was assessed by soy calendars, 24-hour dietary recalls, and urinary soy isoflavone excretion measured by liquid chromatography. Serum samples were analyzed for serum testosterone levels and PSA by radioimmunoassay. No significant between-group and within-group differences were detected. A 14% decline in serum PSA levels (p = 0.10), but no change in testosterone (p = 0.70), was observed during the high-soy diet in contrast to the low-soy diet.

The Goodin study was highly criticized in a letter to the editor in the same journal for the following concerns (Messina et al., 2007): (a) Testosterone levels were measured only three times in the 4 weeks of the intervention, at baseline, after 2 weeks of the intervention, and then at completion (e.g., 4 weeks). More importantly, the 19% drop in T levels was later recalculated to be 4%, within chance during the course of such a small trial. (b) One of the study subjects had T levels over 200% higher than the mean of the 12 subjects, and this level continued to drop even after stopping the high-soy diet, therefore suggesting this individual subject could have altered the researchers' data significantly (the letter proposed that the individual described might have been using some form of testosterone supplementation prior to entering the study). (c) Lastly, this single study contradicts the findings of 15 investigations prior to 2007 that showed the consumption of soy protein had no effect on testosterone levels. Most, if not all, of these studies showed that soy protein consumption led to a similar gain in muscle mass to whey protein intake. In another letter to the editor (Goodin et al., 2007), the authors countered that the statistically significant reduction in serum testosterone of 19% +/− 22% from baseline to day 28 was correct. The mean testosterone level and luteinizing hormone level should be clarified correctly in the text to represent that baseline levels are drawn on an average of days −7 to 0, as it is a common practice to use more observations before treatment to decease variation. And lastly, the authors stated that they chose a commonly used soy protein supplement widely available but did not evaluate the isoflavone content, as a correlation between content and effects on testosterone has not been consistent. They suggest that such assays be included in studies of soy in the future because of the power of the assay to detect the many different estrogen compounds.

Thus, the debate continues. Phytoestrogens have been extensively studied for their potential beneficial effects against hormone-dependent and age-related diseases. We continue to seek the biological effects of phytoestrogens on male reproductive endocrinology and insights into the potential protective effects of an Eastern diet high in these phytoestrogens in male disorders such as benign prostatic hypertrophy and prostate cancer incidence.

CONCLUSION

Despite nearly a half-century of research on aging and sex steroids in men, answers to key questions that would allow us to confidently assess risk/benefit ratios for androgen replacement in older men with the partial androgen deficiency of aging men (PADAM) syndrome remain uncertain. Although it is now reasonably clear that a significant percentage of otherwise healthy older men have decreases in testosterone and bioavailable testosterone to levels consistent with hypogonadism, the clinical implications of this change remain uncertain. Data suggest that low testosterone in older men is correlated to varying degrees with loss of lean body mass and muscle strength, and increased total and central body fat. Less certain, but suggestive, are data relating low testosterone levels to decreased bone density, loss of insulin sensitivity, and cognitive and affective deterioration, as well as reduced sexual function. Replacement of testosterone in older men has shown some positive effects on each of these variables, but findings have been inconsistent, perhaps because studies have employed different preparations and doses of androgens, treated for various durations, and defined their target populations in different ways.

I wish to end this chapter with an excerpt from one of the most highly respected "testosterone thinkers," Dr. Stan M. Harman, in his thoughtful analysis "Testosterone in Older Men after the Institute of Medicine Report: Where do we go from here?" (Harman, 2005)

Treatment and prevention are different strategies and frequently require different approaches and agents. It is the failure to differentiate between prevention and treatment with regard to atherosclerosis that has led to the widespread misinterpretation of the results of the now discontinued Women's Health Initiative (WHI) hormone trial. In the WHI trials, women long enough past menopause for substantial accumulation of atherosclerotic plaque to have occurred were started on female hormone replacement with the aim of investigating prevention of cardiovascular disease. However, one cannot "prevent" currently incident disease, only the development of disease not yet present. Thus, the failure of the WHI hormone trials to demonstrate cardioprotection in women averaging 63 years of age at randomization during only 5 years of treatment should not have been a surprise.

Most middle-aged and older men currently embarking on a regimen of testosterone treatment are doing so in order to slow progression or avoid onset of perceived age-related debilities such as diminished sexual capacity, loss of muscle mass and strength and bone loss. Only trials large enough and carried out for long enough to determine with confidence the adverse outcomes and benefits from testosterone initiated before the "aging phenotype" is fully expressed will provide the data required for physicians to credibly counsel men with regard to the advisability of male hormone replacement (Harman, 2005).

REFERENCES

Akishita M, Hashimoto M, Ohike Y, et al. Low testosterone level as a predictor of cardiovascular events in Japanese men with coronary risk factors. Atherosclerosis. 2009;210:232–236.

Akishita M, Hashimoto M, Ohike Y, et al. Low testosterone level is an independent determinant of endothelial dysfunction in men. Hypertens Res. 2007;30:1029–1034.

Allan CA, McLachan RI. Age related changes in testosterone and the role of replacement therapy in older men. Clin Endocrinol. 2004;60:653–670.

Allan CA, Strauss BJ, Burger HG, Forbes EA, McLachlan RI. Testosterone therapy prevents gain in visceral adipose tissue and loss of skeletal muscle in nonobese aging men. J Clin Endocrinol Metab. 2008;93:139–146.

Anawalt BD, Merriam GR. Neuroendocrine aging in men. Andropause and somatopause. Endocrinol Metab Clin North Am. 2001;30:647–669.

Anderson RA, Bancroft J, Wu FC. The effects of exogenous testosterone on sexuality and mood of normal men. J Clin Endocrinol Metab. 1992;75:1503–1507.

Araujo AB, Esche GR, Kupelian V, et al. Prevalence of symptomatic androgen deficiency in men. J Clin Endocrinol Metab. 2007;92:4241–4247.

Aversa A, Bruzziches R, Francomano D, Rosano G, Lenzi A, Spera G. Effects of testosterone undecanoate on cardiovascular risk factors and atherosclerosis in middle-aged men with late onset hypogonadism and metabolic syndrome: results from a 24-months, randomized double blind placebo-controlled study. J Sex Med. 2010;7:3495–3503.

Aversa A, Bruzziches R, Francomano D, Spera G. Efficacy and safety of two different testosterone undecanoate formulations in hypogonadal men with metabolic syndrome. J Endocrinol Invest. 2010;33:776–783.

Aversa A, Isidori AM, Spera G, Lenzi A, Fabbri A. Androgens improve cavernous vasodilation and response to sildenafil in patients with erectile dysfunction. Clin Endocrinol. 2003;58:632–638.

Bartke A, Coshigano K, Kopchick J, et al. Genes that prolong life: relationships of growth hormone and growth to aging and life span. J Gerontol Biol Sci. 2001;56A:B340–B349.

Basaria S, Coviello AD, Travison TG, et al. Adverse events associated with testosterone administration. N Engl J Med. 2010;363:109–122.

Basaria S, Muller DC, Carducci MA, Egan J, Dobs AS. Hyperglycemia and insulin resistance in men with prostate carcinoma who receive androgen-deprivation therapy. Cancer. 2006;106:581–588.

Baulieu EE, Thomas G, Legrain S, et al. Dehydroepiandrosterone (DHEA), DHEA sulfate, and aging: contribution of the DHEAge Study to a sociobio-medical issue. Proc Natl Acad Sci USA. 2000;97:4279–4284.

Beckham SG, Earnest CP. Four weeks of androstenedione supplementation diminishes the treatment response in middle-aged men. Br J Sports Med. 2003;37:212–218.

Benkert O, Witt W, Adam W, Leitz A. Effects of testosterone undecanoate on sexual potency and the hypothalamic-pituitary-gonadal axis of impotent males. Arch Sex Behav. 1979;8:471–479.

Bhasin S, Cunningham GR, Hayes FJ, et al. Testosterone therapy in adult men with androgen deficiency syndromes: an Endocrine Society clinical practice guideline. J Clin Endocrinol Metab. 2006;91:1995–2010.

Bhasin S, Cunningham GR, Hayes FJ, et al. Testosterone therapy in men with androgen deficiency syndromes: an endocrine society clinical practice guideline. J Clin Endocrinol Metab. 2010;95:2536–2559.

Bhasin S, Singh AB, Mac RP, Carter B, Lee MI, Cunningham GR. Managing the risks of prostate disease during testosterone replacement therapy in older men: recommendations for a standardized monitoring plan. J Androl. 2003;24:299–311.

Bolona ER, Uraga MV, Haddad RM, et al. Testosterone use in men with sexual dysfunction: a systematic review and meta-analysis of randomized placebo-controlled trials. Mayo Clin Proc. 2007;82(1):20–28.

Brown GA, Vukovich MD, Martini ER, et al. Effects of androstenedione-herbal supplementation on serum sex hormone concentrations in 30–59 years old men. Int J Vitamin Nutr Res. 2001;71:293–301.

Brunton SA, Sadovsky R. Late-onset male hypogonadism and testosterone replacement therapy in primary care. J Fam Pract. 2010;59(7 Suppl):S1–8.

Cai L, Wu Y, Zhang J, et al. Steroidal saponins from Tribulus terrestris. Planta Med. 2001;67:196–198.

Calof OM, Singh AB, Lee ML, et al. Adverse events associated with testosterone replacement in middle-aged and older men: a meta-analysis of randomized, placebo-controlled trials. J Gerontol A Biol Sci Med Sci. 2005;60:1451–1457.

Caminiti G, Volterrani M, Iellamo F, et al. Effect of long-acting testosterone treatment on functional exercise capacity, skeletal muscle performance, insulin resistance, and baroreflex sensitivity in elderly patients with chronic heart failure a double-blind, placebo-controlled, randomized study. JAm Coll Cardiol. 2009;54:919–927.

Carpenter WR, Whitney RR, Godley PA. Getting over testosterone: postulating a fresh start for etiologic studies of prostate cancer [Editorial]. J Natl Cancer Inst. 2008;100:158–159.

Cavallini G, Caracciolo S, Vitali G, Modenini F, Biagiotti G. Carnitine versus androgen administration in the treatment of sexual dysfunction, depressed mood, and fatigue associated with male aging. Urology. 2004;63:641–646.

Christmas C, O'Connor KG, Harman SM, et al. Growth hormone and sex steroid effects on bone metabolism and bone mineral density in healthy aged women and men. J Gerontol Med Sci. 2002;57A:M12–18.

Cicero AF, Bandieri E, Arletti R. Lepidium meyenii Walp. improves sexual behaviour in male rats independently from its action on spontaneous locomotor activity. J Ethopharmacol. 2001;75:225–229.

Corona G, Maggi M. The role of testosterone in erectile dysfunction. Nat Rev Urol. 2010;7:46–56.

Corona G, Monami M, Rastrelli G, et al. Testosterone and metabolic syndrome: a meta-analysis study. J Sex Med. 2011;8(1):272–283.

Cunningham GR, Toma SM. Why is androgen replacement in males controversial? Clin Endocrinol Metab. 2011;96:38–52.

Dandona P, Rosenberg MT. A practical guide to male hypogonadism in the primary care setting. Int J Clin Pract. 2010;64:682–696.

Earnest CP, Olson MA, Broeder CE, Breuel KF, Beckham SG. In vivo 4-androstene-3, 17-dione and 4-androstene-3 beta, 17 beta-diol supplementation in young men. Eur J Appl Physiol. 2000;81:229–232.

Endogenous Hormones and Prostate Cancer Collaborative Group. Endogenous sex hormones and prostate cancer: a collaborative analysis of 18 prospective studies. J Natl Cancer Inst. 2008;100:170–183.

Esposito K, Giugliano F, Martedi E, et al. High proportions of erectile dysfunction in men with metabolic syndrome. Diabetes Care. 2005;28:1201–1203.

Etnier JL, Salazar W, Landers DM, Petruzzello SJ, Han M, Nowell P. The influence of physical fitness and exercise upon cognitive functioning—a meta-analysis. J Sport Exercise Psychology. 1997;19:249–277.

Evans WJ. Exercise strategies should be designed to increase muscle power. J Gerontol Med Sci. 2000;55A:M309–M310.

Fernández-Balsells MM, Murad MH, Barwise A, et al. Adverse effects of testosterone therapy in adult men: a systematic review and meta-analysis. J Clin Endocrinol Metab. 2011;96:905–912.

Fernández-Balsells MM, Murad MH, Lane M, et al. Clinical review 1: adverse effects of testosterone therapy in adult men: a systematic review and meta-analysis. J Clin Endocrinol Metab. 2010;95:2560–2575.

Fiatarone-Singh MA. Exercise comes of age: rationale and recommendations for a geriatric exercise prescription. J Gerontol Med Sci. 2002;57A:M262–M282.

Flood JF, Morley JE, Roberts E. Memory-enhancing effects in male mice of pregnenolone and steroids metabolically derived from it. Proc Natl Acad Sci USA. 1992;89:1567–1571.

Flood JF, Morley JE, Roberts E. Pregnenolone sulfate enhances post-training memory processes when injected in very low doses into limbic system structures: the amygdala is by far the most sensitive. Proc Natl Acad Sci USA. 1995;92:10806–10810.

Fukui M, Kitagawa Y, Ose H, Hasegawa G, Yoshikawa T, Nakamura N. Role of endogenous androgen against insulin resistance and atherosclerosis in men with type 2 diabetes. Curr Diabetes Rev. 2007;3:25–31.

Gauthaman K, Adaikan PG, Prasad RN. Aphrodisiac properties of Tribulus *Terrestris extract* (Protodioscin) in normal and castrated rats. Life Sci. 2002;71:1385–1396.

Gauthaman K, Ganesan AP, Prasad RN. Sexual effects of puncturevine (*Tribulus terrestris*) extract (protodioscin): an evaluation using a rat model. J Altern Complement Med. 2003;9:257–265.

Gonzales GF, Córdova A, Vega K, et al. Effect of Lepidium meyenii (MACA) on sexual desire and its absent relationship with serum testosterone levels in adult healthy men. Andrologia. 2002;34:367–372.

Goodin S, Shih WJ, Gallo M, et al. Effect of soy protein on testosterone levels. Cancer Epidemiol Biomarkers Prev. 2007;16:829–883.

Goodin S, Shih WJ, Gallo M, et al. Effect of soy protein on testosterone levels (Letter to the Editor). Cancer Epidemiol Biomarkers Prev. 2007;16(12):2796.

Gooren LJ, Behre HM, Saad F, Frank A, Schwerdt S. Diagnosing and treating testosterone deficiency in different parts of the world. Results from global market research. Aging Male. 2007;10:173–181.

Gray A, Feldman HA, McKinlay JB, Longcope C. Age, disease, and changing sex hormone levels in middle-aged men: results of the Massachusetts Male Aging Study. J Clin Endocrinol Metab. 1991;73:1016–1025.

Grunewald KK, Bailey RS. Commercially marketed supplements for body-building athletes. Sports Med. 1993;15:90–103.

Guay AT, Traish AM. The clinical picture of adult male hypogonadism: a case-based approach. 2009. MedscapeCME Urology. Available at: http://www.medscape.org/viewarticle/710122. Accessed October 15, 2011.

Guembe MJ, Toledo E, Barba J, et al. Association between metabolic syndrome or its components and asymptomatic cardiovascular disease in the RIVANA study. Atherosclerosis. 2010;211:612–617.

Hacker R, Mattern C. Androstenedione Patent Application (Germany). Arrowdeen Ltd. DE 1995;42:14953.

Haddad RM, Kennedy CC, Caples SM, et al. Testosterone and cardiovascular risk in men: a systematic review and meta-analysis of randomized placebo-controlled trials. Mayo Clin Proc. 2007;82:29–39.

Haidar A, Yassin A, Saad F, Shabsigh R. Effects of androgen deprivation on glycaemic control and on cardiovascular biochemical risk factors in men with advanced prostate cancer with diabetes. Aging Male. 2007;10:189–196.

Hak AE, Witteman JCM, de Jong FH, Geerlings MI, Hofman A, Pols HAP. Low levels of endogenous androgens increase the risk of atherosclerosis in elderly men: the Rotterdam Study. J Clin Endocrinol Metab. 2002;87:3632–3639.

Harman SM, Metter EJ, Tobin JD, Pearson J, Blackman MR. Longitudinal effects of aging on serum total and free testosterone levels in healthy men. J Clin Endocrinol Metab. 2001;86:724–731.

Harman SM. Testosterone in older men after the Institute of Medicine Report. Climacteric. 2005;8:124–135.

Heufelder AE, Saad F, Bunck MC, Gooren L. Fifty-two-week treatment with diet and exercise plus transdermal testosterone reverses the metabolic syndrome and improves glycemic control in men with newly diagnosed type 2 diabetes and subnormal plasma testosterone. J Androl. 2009;30:726–733.

Hobbs CJ, Plymate SR, Rosen CJ, Adler RA. Testosterone administration increases insulin-like growth factor-I levels in normal men. J Clin Endocrinol Metab. 1993;77:776–779.

Hortobagyi T, Tunnerl D, Moody J, Beam S, DeVita P. Low- or high- intensity strength training partially restores impaired quadriceps force accuracy and steadiness in aged adults. J Gerontol Med Sci. 2001;56A:B38–47.

Huang JW, Tan CH, Jiang SH, Zhu DY. Terrestrinins A and B, two new steroid saponins from *Tribulus terrestris*. J Asian Natural Products Res. 2003;5:285–290.

Isidori AM, Giannetta E, Gianfrilli D, et al. Effects of testosterone on sexual function in men: results of a meta-analysis. Clin Endocrinol (Oxf). 2005;63:381–394.

Isidori AM, Giannetta E, Greco EZ, et al. Effects of testosterone on body composition, bone metabolism and serum lipid profile in middle-aged men: a meta-analysis. J Clin Endocrinol (Oxf). 2005;63(3):280–293.

Johannsson G, Svensson J, Bengtsson BA. Growth hormone and ageing. Growth Hormone Igf Res. 2000;10(suppl B):S25–30.

Kalinchenko SY, Tishova YA, Mskhalaya GJ, Gooren LJ, Giltay EJ, Saad F. Effects of testosterone supplementation on markers of the metabolic syndrome and inflammation in hypogonadal men with the metabolic syndrome: the double-blinded placebo-controlled Moscow study. Clin Endocrinol (Oxf). 2010;73:602–612.

Kapoor D, Channer KS, Jones TH. Rosiglitazone increases bioactive testosterone and reduces waist circumference in hypogonadal men with type 2 diabetes. Diab Vasc Dis Res. 2008;5(2):135–137.

Kapoor D, Goodwin E, Channer KS, Jones TH. Testosterone replacement therapy improves insulin resistance, glycaemic control, visceral diposity and hypercholesterolaemia in hypogonadal men with type 2 diabetes. Eur J Endocrinol. 2006;154:899–1006.

Kaufman JM, Vermeulen A. The decline of androgen levels in elderly men and its clinical and therapeutic implications. Endocr Rev. 2005;26:833–876.

Keysor JJ, Jette AM. Have we oversold the benefit of late-life exercise? J Gerontol Med Sci. 2001;56A:M412–M423.

Khaw K-T, Dowsett M, Folkerd E, et al. Endogenous testosterone and mortality due to all causes, cardiovascular disease, and cancer in men: European Prospective Investigation Into Cancer in Norfolk (EPIC-Norfolk) Prospective Population Study. Circulation. 2007;116:2694–2701.

King DS, Sharp RL, Vukovich MD, et al. Effect of oral androstenedione on serum testosterone and adaptations to resistance training in young men: a randomized controlled trial. JAMA. 1999;281:2020–2028.

Kohut ML, Thompson JR, Campbell J, et al. Ingestion of a dietary supplement containing dehydroepiandrosterone (DHEA) and androstenedione has minimal effect on immune function in middle-aged men. J Am Coll Nutr. 2003;22:363–371.

Kramer AF, Hahn S, McAuley E. Influence of aerobic fitness on the neurocognitive function of older adults. J Aging Physical Activity. 2000;8:379–385.

Kunelius P, Lukkarinen O, Hannuksela ML, Itkonen O, Tapanainen JS. The effects of transdermal dihydrotestosterone in the aging male: a prospective, randomized, double blind study. J Clin Endocrinol Metab. 2002;87:1467–1472.

Kupelian V, Page St, Araujo AB, et al. Low sex hormone-binding globulin, total testosterone, and symptomatic androgen deficiency are associated with development of the MetS in non-obese men. J Clin Endocrinol Metab. 2006;91:843–850.

La Vignera S, Calogero AE, D'Agata R, et al. Testosterone therapy improves the clinical response to conventional treatment for male patients with metabolic syndrome associated to late onset hypogonadism. Minerva Endocrinol. 2008;33:159–167.

Laaksonen DE, Niskanen L, Punnonen K, et al. Sex hormones, inflammation and the metabolic syndrome: a population-based study. Eur J Endocrinol. 2003;149:601–608.

Laaksonen DE, Niskanen L, Punnonen K, et al. Testosterone and sex hormone-binding globulin predict the metabolic syndrome and diabetes in middle-aged men. Diabetes Care. 2004;27:1036–1041.

Lakshman KM, Basaria S. Safety and efficacy of testosterone gel in the treatment of male hypogonadism. Clin Interv Aging. 2009;4:397–412.

Laughlin GA, Barrett-Connor E, Bergstrom J. Low serum testosterone and mortality in older men. J Clin Endocrinol Metab. 2008;93:68–75.

Leder BZ, Longcope C, Catlin DH, Ahrens B, Schoenfeld DA, Finklestein JS. Oral androstenedione administration and serum testosterone concentrations in young men. JAMA. 2000;283:779–782.

Lorenzo C, Williams K, Hunt KJ, Haffner SM. The National Cholesterol Education program—Adult Treatment Panel III, International Diabetes Federation, and World Health Organization definitions of the metabolic syndrome as predictors of incident cardiovascular disease and diabetes. Diabetes Care. 2007;30:8–13.

Lunenfeld B, Nieschlag E. Testosterone therapy in the aging male. Aging Male. 2007;10:139–153.

Lunenfeld B, Nieschlag E. Testosterone therapy in the aging male. Aging Male. 2007;10:139–153.

Makinen J, Jarvisalo M, Pollanen P, et al. Increased carotid atherosclerosis in andropausal middle-aged men. J Am Coll Cardiol. 2005;45:1603–1608.

Makinen JI, Perheentupa A, Irjala K, et al. Endogenous testosterone and serum lipids in middle-aged men. Atherosclerosis. 2008;197:688–693.

Malkin CJ, Pugh PJ, Jones RD, Kapoor D, Channer KS, Jones TH. The effect of testosterone replacement on endogenous inflammatory cytokines and lipid profiles in hypogonadal men. J Clin Endocrinol Metab. 2004;89:3313–3318.

Maskarinec G, Morimoto Y, Hebshi S, Franke AA, Stanczyk FZ. Serum prostate-specific antigen but not testosterone levels decrease in a randomized soy intervention among men. Eur J Clin Nutr. 2006;60:1423–1429.

Messina M, Hamilton-Reeves J, Kurzer M, Phipps W. Effect of soy on testosterone levels (Letter to the Editor). Cancer Epidemiol Biomarkers Prev. 2007;16(12):2795.

Milasius K, Dadelien R, Tubelis L, Raslanas A. Effects of a maca booster food supplement on sportsmen's bodily adaption to physical loads. In: 13th Annual Congress of the European College of Sports Sciences, Estoril, Portugal, 2008, p. 226.

Miner MM, Kuritzky L. Erectile dysfunction: a sentinel marker for cardiovascular disease in primary care. Cleve Clin J Med. 2007;74(Suppl 3):S30–S37.

Miner MM, Sadofsky R. Evolving issues in male hypogonadism: evaluation, management, and related comorbidities. Cleveland Clin J Med. 2007;74(Suppl 3):S38–S46.

Morales A, Bella AJ, Chun S, et al. A practical guide to diagnosis, management and treatment of testosterone deficiency for Canadian physicians. *Can Urol Assoc J.* 2010;4(4):269–275.

Morales AJ, Haubrich RH, Hwang JY, Asakura H, Yen SSC. The effect of six months treatment with a 100 mg daily dose of dehydroepiandrosterone (DHEA) on circulating sex steroids, body composition and muscle strength in age-advanced men and women. Clin Endocrinol. 1998;49:421–432.

Morgentaler A, Lipshultz LI, Bennett R, Sweeney M, Avila D Jr, Khera M. Testosterone therapy in men with untreated prostate cancer. J Urol. 2011;185:1256–1261.

Morgentaler A, Traish AM. Shifting the paradigm of testosterone and prostate cancer: the saturation model and the limits of androgen- dependent growth. Eur Urol. 2009;55:310–320.

Morgentaler A. Commentary: guideline for male testosterone therapy: a clinician's perspective. J Clin Endocrinol Metab. 2007;92:416–417.

Morgentaler A. Testosterone and prostate cancer: what are the risks for middle-aged men? Urol Clin North Am. 2011;38:119–124.

Muller M, Grobbee DE, den Tonkelaar I, Lamberts SWJ, van der Schouw YT. Endogenous sex hormones and metabolic syndrome in aging men. J Clin Endocrinol Metab. 2005;90:2618–2623.

Mulligan T, Frick MF, Zuraw QC, Stemhagen A, McWhirter C. Prevalence of hypogonadism in males aged at least 45 years: the HIM study. Int J Clin Pract. 2006;60:762–769.

Mulligan T, Frick MF, Zuraw QC, Stemhagen A, McWhirter C. Prevalence of hypogonadism in males aged at least 45 years: the HIM Study. Int J Clin Pract. 2006;60:762–769.

Nettleship JE, Pugh PJ, Channer KS, Jones T, Jones RD. Inverse relationship between serum levels of interleukin-1beta and testosterone in men with stable coronary artery disease. Horm Metab Res. 2007;39:366–371.

Nieschlag E, Swerdloff R, Behre HM, et al.; International Society of Andrology (ISA); International Society for the Study of the Aging Male (ISSAM); European Association of Urology (EAU). Investigation, treatment and monitoring of late-onset hypogonadism in males. ISA, ISSAM, and EAU recommendations. Eur Urol. 2005;48:1–4.

Oh JY, Barrett-Connor E, Wedick NM, Wingard DL. Endogenous sex hormones and the development of type 2 diabetes in older men and women; the Rancho Bernardo study. Diabetes Care. 2002;25:55–60.

Olshansky SJ, Hayflick L, Carnes BA. Position on human aging. J Gerontol Biol Sci. 2002;57A:B292–297.

Osuna JA, Gómez-Pérez R, Arata-Bellabarba G, Villaroel V. Relationship between BMI, total testosterone, sex hormone-binding-globulin, leptin, insulin and insulin resistance in obese men. Arch Androl. 2006;52:355–361.

Park NC, Yan BQ, Chung JM, Lee KM. Oral testosterone undecanoate (Andriol) supplement therapy improves the quality of life for men with testosterone deficiency. Aging Male. 2003;6:86–93.

Phillips G, Pinkernell B, Jing T. The association of hypotestosteronemia with coronary artery disease in men. Arterioscler Thromb. 1994;14:701–706.

Pitteloud N, Hardin M, Dwyer AA, et al. Increasing insulin resistance is associated with a decrease in Leydig cell testosterone secretion in men. J Clin Endocrinol Metab. 2005;90:2636–2641.

Pitteloud N, Mootha VK, Dwyer AA, et al. Relationship between testosterone levels, insulin sensitivity, and mitochondrial function in men. Diabetes Care. 2005;28:1636–1642.

Practice Committee of American Society for Reproductive Medicine in collaboration with Society for Male Reproduction and Urology. Androgen deficiency in the aging male. Fertil Steril. 2008;90(5 Suppl):S83–87.

Ravalgia G, Forti P, Maioli F, et al. Body composition, sex steroids, IGF-1, and bone mineral status in aging men. J Gerontol Med Sci. 2000;55A:M516–521.

Rhoden EL, Morgentaler A. Risks of testosterone-replacement therapy and recommendations for monitoring. N Engl J Med. 2004;350:482–492.

Rudman D, Feller AG, Nagraj HS, et al. Effects of human growth hormone in men over 60 years old. N Engl J Med. 1990;323:1–6.

Saad F. Effects of testosterone supplementation on markers of the metabolic syndrome and inflammation in hypogonadal men with the metabolic syndrome: the double-blinded placebo-controlled Moscow study. Clin Endocrinol (Oxf). 2010;73:602–612.

Saad F, Aversa A, Isidori AM, Zafalon L, Zitzmann M, Gooren L. Onset of effects of testosterone treatment and time span until maximum effects are achieved. Eur J Endocrinol. 2011;165:675–685.

Saad F, Gooren LJ, Haider A, Yassin A. A dose-response study of testosterone on sexual dysfunction and features of the metabolic syndrome using testosterone gel and parenteral testosterone undecanoate. J Androl. 2008;29:102–105.

Schiavi RC, White D, Mandeli J, Levine AC. Effect of testosterone administration on sexual behavior and mood in men with erectile dysfunction. Arch Sex Behav. 1997;26:231–241.

Selvin E, Feinleib M, Zhang L, et al. Androgens and diabetes in men. Diabetes Care. 2007;30:234–238.

Seyrek M, Yildiz O, Ulusoy HB, Yildirim V. Testosterone relaxes isolated human radial artery by potassium channel opening action. J Pharmacol Sci. 2007;103:309–316.

Shabsigh R, Kaufman JM, Steidle C, Padma-Nathan H. Randomized study of testosterone gel as adjunctive therapy to sildenafil in hypogonadal men with erectile dysfunction who do not respond to sildenafil alone. J Urol. 2004;172:658–663.

Shabsigh R. Testosterone therapy in erectile dysfunction and hypogonadism. J Sex Med. 2005;2:785–792.

Shores MM, Matsumoto AM, Sloan KL, Kivlahan DR. Low serum testosterone and mortality in male veterans. Arch Intern Med. 2006;166:1660–1665.

Sih R, Kamel H, Horani H, Morley JE. Dehydroepiandrosterone and pregenolone. In: Meikle AW, ed. *Hormone Replacement Therapy*. Totowa, NJ: Humana Press; 1999:241–262.

Simon D, Charles MA, Nahoul K, et al. Association between plasma testosterone and cardiovascular risk factors in healthy adult men: the Telecom study. J Clin Endocrinol Metab. 1997;82:682–685.

Singh R, Artaza JN, Taylor WE, et al. Testosterone inhibits adipogenic differentiation in 3T3-L1 cells: nuclear translocation of androgen receptor complex with beta-catenin and T-cell factor 4 may bypass canonical Wnt signaling to down-regulate adipogenic transcription factors. Endocrinology. 2006;147:141–154.

Smith JR, Olshansky SJ. Position statement on human aging [editorial]. J Gerontol Biol Sci. 2002;57A:B291.

Spector IP, Carey MP, Steinberg L. The sexual desire inventory: development, factor structure, and evidence of reliability. J Sex Marital Ther. 1996;22:175–190.

Srinivas-Shankar U, Roberts SA, Connolly MJ, et al. Effects of testosterone on muscle strength, physical function, body composition, and quality of life in intermediate-frail and frail elderly men: a randomized, double-blind, placebo-controlled study. J Clin Endocrinol Metab. 2010;95:639–650.

Stanworth RD, Kapoor D, Channer KS, Jones TH. Statin therapy is associated with lower total but not bioavailable or free testosterone in men with type 2 diabetes. Diabetes Care. 2009;32:541–546.

Stellato RK, Feldman HA, Hamdy O, Horton ES, McKinlay JB. Testosterone, sex hormone-binding globulin, and the development of type 2 diabetes in middle-aged men: prospective results from the Massachusetts male aging study. Diabetes Care. 2000;23:490–494.

Svartberg J, Aasebo U, Hjalmarsen A, Sundsfjord J, Jorde R. Testosterone treatment improves body composition and sexual function in men with COPD, in a 6 month randomized controlled trial. Resp Med. 2004;98:906–913.

Tajar A, Forti G, O'Neill TW, et al. European Male Aging Study Group. Characteristics of secondary, primary, and compensated hypogonadism in aging men: evidence from the European Male Aging Study. J Clin Endocrinol Metab. 2010;95:1810–1818.

Tracz MJ, Sideras K, Boloña ER, et al. Clinical review: testosterone use in men and its effects on bone health. A systematic review and meta-analysis of randomized placebo-controlled trials. J Clin Endocrinol Metab. 2006;91:2011–2016.

Traish AM, Abdou R, Kypreos KE. Androgen deficiency and atherosclerosis: the lipid link. Vascul Pharmacol. 2009;51:303–313.

Traish AM, Feeley RJ, Guay A. Mechanisms of obesity and related pathologies: androgen deficiency and endothelial dysfunction may be the link between obesity and erectile dysfunction. FEBS J. 2009;276:5755–5767.

Traish AM, Guay A, Feeley R, Saad F. The dark side of testosterone deficiency: I. Metabolic syndrome and erectile dysfunction. J Androl. 2009;30:10–22.

Traish AM, Saad F, Feeley RJ, Guay A. The dark side of testosterone deficiency: III. Cardiovascular disease. J Androl. 2009;30:477–494.

Traish AM, Saad F, Guay A. The dark side of testosterone deficiency: II. Type 2 diabetes and insulin resistance. J Androl. 2009;30:23–32.

Travison TG, Araujo AB, O'Donnell AB, Kupelian V, McKinlay JB. A population-level decline in serum testosterone levels in American men. J Clin Endocrinol Metab. 2007;92:196–202.

van Pottelbergh I, Braeckman L, De Bacquer D, De Backer G, Kaufman J. Potential contribution of testosterone and estradiol in the determination of cholesterol and lipoprotein profile in healthy middle-aged men. Atherosclerosis. 2003;166:95–102.

von Werder K. The somatopause is no indication for growth hormone therapy. J Endocrinol Invest. 1999;22(suppl 5):137–141.

Wang C, Nieschlag E, Swerdloff R, et al. ISA, ISSAM, EAU, EAA and ASA recommendations: investigation, treatment, and monitoring of late-onset hypogonadism in males. Aging Male. 2009;12:5–1.

Wang C, Nieschlag E, Swerdloff R, et al. ISA, ISSAM, EAU, EAA and ASA recommendations: investigation, treatment and monitoring of late-onset hypogonadism in males. Int J Impot Res. 2009;21:1–8.

Wang C, Swerdloff RS, Iranmanesh A, et al. Transdermal testosterone gel improves sexual function, mood, muscle strength, and body composition parameters in hypogonadal men. J Clin Endocrinol Metab. 2000;85:2839–2853.

Westerterp KR, Meijer EP. Physical activity and parameters of aging: a physiological perspective. J Gerontol Biol Sci Med Sci. 2001;56A(Special Issue II):7–12.

Wu FC, Tajar A, Pye SR, et al.; European Male Aging Study Group. Hypothalamic-pituitary testicular axis disruptions in older men are differentially linked to age and modifiable risk factors: the European Male Aging Study. J Clin Endocrinol Metab. 2008;93:2737–2745.

Wu FCW, Tajar A, Beynon J, et al. Identification of late-onset hypogonadism in middle-aged and elderly men. N Engl J Med. 2010;363:123–135.

Yeap BB, Chubb SA, Hyde Z, et al. Lower serum testosterone is independently associated with insulin resistance in non-diabetic older men: the Health in Men Study. Eur J Endocrinol. 2009;161:591–598.

Yialamas MA, Dwyer AA, Hanley E, Lee H, Pitteloud N, Hayes FJ. Acute sex steroid withdrawal reduces insulin sensitivity in healthy men with idiopathic hypogonadotropic hypogonadism. J Clin Endocrinol Metab. 2007;92:4254–4259.

Yildiz O, Seyrek M. Vasodilating mechanisms of testosterone. Exp Clin Endocrinol Diabetes. 2007;115:1–6.

Zitzmann M, Faber S, Nieschlag E. Association of specific symptoms and metabolic risks with serum testosterone in older men. J Clin Endocrinol Metab. 2006;91:4335–4343.

Zitzmann M, Nieschlag E. Androgen receptor gene CAG repeat length and body mass index modulate the safety of long-term intra-muscular testosterone undecanoate therapy in hypogonadal men. J Clin Endocrinol Metab. 2007;92:3844–3853.

Zitzmann M. Testosterone deficiency and treatment in older men: definition, treatment, pitfalls. Asian J Androl. 2010;12:623–625.

Zitzmann M. Testosterone deficiency, insulin resistance and the metabolic syndrome. Nat Rev Endocrinol. 2009;5:673–681.

14

Bone Health

GEORGE E. MUÑOZ

Arthritis and Osteoporosis Prevention and Treatment Strategies

As an integrative rheumatologist with almost 30 years of clinical practice treating patients with arthritis and rheumatic diseases, I request some latitude and license to distill this significant clinical experience into some usable simplified constructs for both the health professional and the lay reader. This chapter will focus on the most common maladies vis-à-vis osteoarthritis and the less common but potentially more debilitating types of inflammatory arthritides such as rheumatoid arthritis and its variants. Because this book is focused on men's health, I will discuss arthritis prevention in the context of a "man's world" but by no means exclude women from the implications of activities prone to increase the incidence of bone or joint damage. This is especially true with the advent of Title 5 in collegiate sports where the marked increase in the number of female athletes has led to an increase in sports-related injuries and the arthritic sequelae formerly more reserved for male athletes. Finally, this chapter will delve into a less frequently recognized or unrecognized condition in men, namely, male osteoporosis. The condition has "suffered" lack of recognition in both the medical and nonmedical spheres, and there has not really been a formal policy or recommendation by specialty medical societies on how men should be screened, evaluated, and treated for bone health; these recommendations exist only for postmenopausal women. Consequently, men have been "cast to the side" in this respect to the point that as recently as 12 years ago, I was personally challenged by a specialist colleague as to why I was performing dual-energy X-ray absorptiometry (DEXA) scans on men! I provided him with literature justifying the need for bone density measurements in men (A. Chapters 1 and 25) as well as postmenopausal women, and he also began performing them after this "educational encounter." So it is with a measure of perspective focusing on where we *were*, where we currently *are*, and where we *are headed* in these realms that this chapter on men's bone health is written.

Osteoarthritis and Back Pain

Osteoarthritis is the most common type of arthritis affecting men. This type of arthritis includes degeneration of joint cartilage or of the intervertebral disc structures, both of which act as biomechanical cushions reducing physical forces and allowing ease of movement for their respective bone structures. For both joint cartilage and vertebral discs, the loss of structural matrix (important glycoproteins) and loss of water content contribute to loss of stability, flexibility, and thickness and subsequent loss of biomechanical properties. These attributes are needed in joints, especially large weight-bearing ones such as the hips and knees for normal function and for extremes required in sports. In the spine, this degeneration translates to disc narrowing with the potential for herniations and pinched nerves (e.g., sciatica) or tightening of the spinal canal due to arthritis bone spurs (central spinal stenosis) or impingement of nerve openings or foramina (foraminal stenosis), which results in burning neuropathic (nerve) pain of the extremities. In more advanced cases neuromuscular deficits with weakness or atrophy of the arms or legs can occur.

Low back pain is clearly one of the most prevalent maladies affecting both men and women globally. Common causes of low back pain in most younger individuals tend to be less associated with osteoarthritis and more with lack of flexibility, tendonitis, or inflammation, such as in sacroiliitis or ankylosing spondylitis, and the variants of these inflammatory rheumatic conditions. The amount of disability and loss of work-days related to low back pain and its related conditions is staggering. For an aging man, this condition may signal the mindset of "I'm getting old." The possible causes of low back pain are numerous, but we will focus on the benign causes primarily. Most of the time, there is a history of lifting, bending, moving inappropriately, or frank trauma. Typical descriptions of symptoms include "feeling locked up" or "shooting pains up and down the spine" with exacerbations even with breathing. Many individuals have had at least one version of these scenarios in their lives. The acute pain is usually due to abrupt muscle spasm, which is initiated usually by some form of microtear along the tendinous insertions of the paraspinal muscles at their attachments. In a minority of cases, acute back pain, especially if it radiates or travels down one or both legs, suggests nerve roots being involved with inflammation, swelling, or acute impingement. This leads to the classical clinical picture of the well-known case of sciatica. The more acute the case, in general, the better the prognosis for complete resolution, but the longer or more chronic the situation, the poorer the general prognosis for obtaining total resolution. Equally uncommon is the case of the unstable spine (spondylolisthesis) where a vertebra can shift with flexion or extension movements. A comprehensive evaluation including physical examination, x-rays (supine and flexion and extension views), and appropriate imaging techniques (magnetic resonance imaging [MRI], computed tomography [CT], etc.) are needed in those cases not responding to simple measures or basic diagnostics or where the examination points toward a neurologic deficit.

Aside from these situations, the proverbial existence and recurrence of "back problems" in men may be attributed to a man's role, generally speaking, as the one who traditionally will do more physical labor around the house or who believes he can still lift heavy objects. Proper body mechanics, maintenance of spinal and general body flexibility, and intrinsic core strengthening on a consistent basis are long-term solutions for prevention of chronic spinal and back pain of most types. Beginners' yoga for the novice and more advanced classes for the well initiated, tai chi for balance and strength, and Pilates for lengthening and strengthening of muscles are all excellent recommendations for preventing back pain. Acute episodes should be managed under medical supervision, many times involving physical therapy including modalities (such as ice for acute spasm and heat for more chronic conditions), lumbar or spinal traction (when spinal decompression is needed to reduce nerve entrapment or radicular pain), and back strengthening and stretching programs with education on how to move, lift, and get up properly (biomechanical education). To this end, "back schools" have become popular, which may include water aerobics, water tai chi, and yoga.

From an integrative medicine perspective I would like to offer some additional options to the usual and customary approach of using nonsteroidal anti-inflammatory drugs (NSAIDs) and muscle relaxants with or without narcotics as the acute pharmacotherapeutic approach for both acute and chronic back pain. These approaches could include traditional Chinese medicine (TCM) and acupuncture for acute pain (see acupuncture chapter). Homeopathic approaches (Kremer et al., 1995) including Arnica montana 9 C and Nux vomica 9 C or 30 C, 5 pellets sublingually every hour in the acute phase, then tapering to three times daily, are very safe. If the back pain is worse with awakening and movement, use Rhus toxicodendron 9 C 5 pellets hourly during the acute phase, then three times daily. Many pharmacies and healthy grocery stores carry these over-the-counter homeopathic remedies, which are U.S. Food and Drug Administration (FDA) regulated. (For more information see the homeopathy chapter). Back pain associated with or worsened by tension, stress, or life situations is another area to explore both for the practitioner and the patient. The energetics of "body speak" have been explored and written about by Carolyn Myss and others. The language of the body, formerly known exclusively as "somatization" in conventional medicine and psychiatric disciplines, appears to be much more descriptive, complex, and on a deeper psychic level than generally gleaned. Sometimes a situation that an individual can't or won't change manifests itself as low back pain, which is inexplicably relieved or "cured" by addressing the solution of the conscious or subconscious conflict. I find that in my practice asking individuals to draw their pain anatomically on a chart and then to draw a pictorial of their pain helps free their subconscious in this regard. *Art therapy* is a useful and effective adjunct in approaching recurrent or chronic pain of any type. In fact, engaging the *senses* through *sound, smell,* and *vision* becomes part of the integrative approach to helping back pain and any chronic pain or arthritic condition. My patients regularly comment that our facility "feels relaxing" or "has good energy," or they say, "What is going on here? I came in stressed but now feel better!" So, our environments where we work as healers and our own mindsets and those of the staff all impact the energetics and the psyche of the people entering a healing space. To this end, my own personal *intention* set for the clinic, those who enter, and the staff is all consciously directed. As a shamanic healer, I had the privilege of learning ceremonial indigenous techniques. These are readily done irrespective of one's personal religious beliefs and are simply about *intention* and having a *clear energy space* for the healing work carried out in a clinic, hospital, intensive care unit, and so forth. From a practical standpoint, I ask my patients questions such as "What does this pain mean to you?" In an era of evaluations of cost and evidence-based practices, one could make arguments that back pain for men and women will get better no matter what one does, either with strict bedrest or more intensive interventions, physical therapy, and the approaches discussed earlier. What I ask myself, however, is what is the individual person seeking when he or she comes to me for help? Is he or she waiting to be told, "It doesn't matter what we do; either go to bed for 7 to 10 days or start physical therapy and aggressive back school and take these two to three medications and call me if you don't get better."

As an integrative physician, I look for the opportunity to help my patients at multiple levels, physically, emotionally, and spiritually if requested. This paradigm shift for a man's health I feel is unique and different now. The prior generations of men were told to "tough it out" or "deal with it." Is this truly a healing approach for anyone? *"Simple back pain" for men then becomes an entry point to engage men in the integrative model for overall health, because this condition is common and allows for trust formation with their physicians or health care providers.* Molding an integrated back program could include topics of prevention that have positive impacts for overall health. These could include a healthy diet, one that is low in processed sugars and anti-inflammatory to keep excessive body fat and inflammation to a minimum. A balanced exercise program with back and core strengthening and flexibility training are recommended for a healthy spine, as well as for injury and fall prevention, and may allow one to age gracefully. I recommend one try various forms of yoga to see what resonates with the individual. The same holds true for other martial art disciplines as there are various styles of tai qi and qigong. As long as the intent is there and the dynamic of a positive environment exists, the benefit of performing these practices and incorporating them into one's lifestyle is immense.

Additionally, it is appropriate to discuss the role of *manual therapies* in the context of an integrative approach. There are a variety of options in this regard. Manual therapies can be powerful tools for diagnosis and treatment of painful conditions. Restrictions in movement of the spine lead not only to pain in the back but also to pathologies in corresponding muscles and visceral organs. There is a long-standing tradition of manual therapies, dating back to the days of Hippocrates. Chiropractic manipulation, physical therapy, McKenzie spinal practitioners, massage, and osteopathy all have important roles to play in the assessment and treatment of musculoskeletal conditions. Their modalities are diverse; thus, an extensive description of their use is beyond the scope of this book, but given the prevalence of musculoskeletal disorders in men, it behooves the health care provider to take full advantage of the expertise of such manual therapy providers when treating men with pain conditions. Neuromuscular therapy, myofascial release, and myriad new and seemingly better techniques are abounding. These include MAT (Muscle Activation Techniques; http://www.muscleactivation.com), CORE myofascial release, active isolated stretching techniques, soft tissue release (STR) craniosacral therapies, deep tissue massage, shiatsu, and many others. I recommend licensed, experienced therapists for whatever discipline is chosen. Athletes, with their specialized needs, may require a different set of hands and skill sets than the sedentary population and may go to sports-specific therapists. Similarly, less active individuals need specialized care as well to help relieve pain, identify imbalances, and encourage them toward a healthier lifestyle. Acupressure techniques applied by both practitioners and patients are effective and powerful modalities to apply during exercise, during competition, or after activities.

Inflammatory and Autoimmune Conditions

Now we will turn to the inflammatory and autoimmune conditions that can affect men. *Rheumatoid arthritis, psoriatic arthritis, spondylitic variants* including *Reiter's syndrome,* and *ankylosing spondylitis* traditionally fall under the autoimmune rubric in conventional medicine and rheumatology training. Their causes or etiopathogeneses are complex, and despite much outstanding and broad research, they are not yet completely defined. Such is the case for many other prevalent conditions, including cancer. The interplay of one's genes with the environment and in some cases infections as possible immune triggers are potential etiologic factors in the conventional paradigm. However, having said this, other than a progressive menu of medication offerings with an increasing potential for toxic side effects and astronomical costs, including biologic agents, little is taught to both physicians and patients about prevention. The effects of lifestyle adaptations to improve conditions or at least minimize the dosing requirements of some of these very potent and costly medical regimens are minimized. Let's review some of what I consider the highlights in these regards.

For the man who develops a sudden onset of incapacitating pain and multiple joint swelling, as in *acute polyarthritis,* fear of permanent disability and pain, dependence, and loss of control become dominant issues for the individual. This fear can actually be a good thing. It creates a more willing individual to accept guidance not only to reduce pain and swelling but also to eliminate the ghastly vision of a wheelchair as the fate for this individual's future. Having said this, I like to introduce my men to the possibility that their lifestyles may be playing some role in their situation. Depending on the history and laboratory analysis, acute infectious, viral, or reactive types of arthritis are ruled in or out. Irrespective of the exact cause, certain recommendations remain fairly universal. These include the need to review one's diet, manage stress levels, improve sleep patterns, and initiate a fully integrated anti-inflammatory lifestyle. Supplements play a huge role in this regard as well. The doses of omega-3 fish oils for treatment tend to be higher than for maintenance of a healthy state in general.

For example, in a perfect world, a male of approximately 70 kg may be recommended 2 to 3 g of a high-potency omega-3 (EPA/DHA) purified fish oil, but a very symptomatic individual of the same body weight might be recommended to take on average 5 to 6 g daily or higher after meals due to the degree of systemic inflammation present. There is no exact science here, but we do have literature that shows that higher doses of omega-3s along with other anti-inflammatory omegas and fats have synergistic benefits (Kremer et al., 1995). Consequently, I like to recommend oleic acid (extra virgin olive oil) 1 to 2 tablespoon daily and black currant seed oil and/or flax seed oil as concurrent anti-inflammatory fatty acids to complement the omega-3 EPA/DHA found in conventional fish oil (C, Chapter 9).

Now, back to our fearful man. The *acute presentation* could signify a temporary arthritis triggered by a viral process (parvovirus, Epstein-Barr virus [EBV], cytomegalovirus [CMV], etc.) or a reactive arthritis due to a bacterial pathogen associated with this clinical course (*Salmonella, Shigella, Campylobacter,* etc.). Irrespective of the cause, the net result is diffuse joint swelling that could be incapacitating. A marked change in lifestyle to include decreasing proinflammatory nutritional, mental, and environmental stressors would be part of this integrative approach. In this regard, many would consider *cow's milk a potential proinflammatory food source.* In fact, what other species on the planet routinely consumes the milk of another species? Beside the lactose intolerance issue, the protein matrix of cow's milk may have its own inherent proinflammatory aspects. Other options including rice milk, almond milk, and coconut milk are better choices. Soy milk may be okay for some but still there is a cross-reactivity and -sensitivity with soy milk in almost one-third of pediatric patients with respect to asthma. What percentage carries over to adults is not definitive, but some percentage clearly does, and this should be taken into account when providing nutritional advice to patients. *Gluten or wheat products* are probably the next biggest category of proinflammatory dietary culprits common in the West. The literature evidence for *anti-inflammatory Mediterranean, vegan, lactovegetarian, and Paleolithic patterned diets* for arthritis inflammatory control is well documented (C, Chapter 7).

Historically, we should realize that wheat was brought over by the Europeans in their zeal and desire to colonize the Americas with their own food staples, so much so that the Spaniards made the indigenous Andean grain, quinoa, illegal due to the significance this food source had both in religious Andean ceremonial stature and as a functional economic grain for the Andean nations (Kolata, 2009). In retrospect, the concept of imposing a food on a people and forcing them to eliminate their own sacred grain was not a way for Europeans to endear themselves to the people of the Americas. Subsequently, it is well chronicled that the slaughter of both North and South American Indians did occur as a result of the European quest to conquer, convert, and impose their respective political, religious, and economic agendas. For the Spanish in South America and the British and French in North America, the results were similar. From an indigenous view, the wheat that was imposed on its people may have been viewed as "cursed" by these Native Americans.

Fast-forwarding to modern times, we now see that wheat and processed foods derived from it are highly proinflammatory, devoid mostly of any nutritional benefit due to the pulverization, dying, and other processing that occurs. Second, gluten and its immunogenic characteristics also are another main issue. Individuals don't have to have full-blown celiac disease to not tolerate gluten or wheat products. Intolerances and sensitivities abound unto themselves as potential manifestations of ingestion of this or any food source. The problem is a combination for the most part of empty calories with very low nutritional value and a high glycemic index and immunogenic characteristics that can manifest in protean ways—rashes, abdominal pain or cramps, indigestion, gastroesophageal reflux disease (GERD), diarrhea with maldigestion or absorption, "leaky gut," and resultant antigen burden exposure to the immune system. Resultant symptoms known to include vasculitis and central nervous system (CNS) symptoms from headaches to cognitive disorders have all been associated with gluten. I routinely recommend a gluten-free diet to my autoimmune patients, especially if they are in an active flare. Elimination of this and substitution to rice products, quinoa, and other nonimmunogenic grains with high fiber density and increased protein matrices are great options. These dietary changes are no longer as difficult as when I was in training as a house officer. Commercial grocery stores of both the generic variety and specialty stores carry gluten-free products. This is the case because the public is now demanding these options as it gains more information and awareness of the issue.

Another topic worthy of mention is *food sensitivities* (D). (Once again, I was not trained in this area during my very excellent medical education, residency, and initial specialty fellowship training, but the topic arises.) As part of my clinical experience, for the past 30 years I have made observations that others too have written about concluding that some people have sensitivities to food. These are not the typical allergic responses with histamine release. These may be vaguer in nature but seem associated mostly by patient dietary logs or food sensitivity testing for immunoglobulin G (IgG). Symptoms including vague rashes, CNS symptoms, fatigue, headaches, migraines, fogginess, and abdominal and vague gastrointestinal (GI) symptoms make up an incomplete list of some food sensitivity symptoms. Formerly nonconventional testing but now much more of a mainstream discipline, functional medicine perspectives may yield further insight into patients' complaints. Causes could include bacterial overgrowth, dysbiosis, leaky gut, and a multitude of micronutrient deficiencies with, many times, profound implications for overall health (D). I was not initially trained in any of these disciplines and frankly was not ready to believe in them. My experiences, driven by patient needs, demands, and requests, have reshaped my thinking and allowed me to have an open mind. My fearful and very willing patient mentioned previously is usually very anxious to hear about any and all options available to help him.

After evaluating one's food log and performing appropriate conventional arthritis autoimmune blood testing for the usual suspects to identify the exact type and cause of polyarthritis, I like to sit and review the patient's lifestyle. Diet has been discussed earlier, so now I will make a brief mention about exercise and stress reduction as essential aspects of the whole-person approach. If one has an acute patient with lots of swelling and pain, exercise will be a challenge. Range of motion and acute splinting should be addressed through formal physical therapy and occupational therapy. In general, aquatic therapies are very well tolerated, safe, and fruitful for both the acute and chronic arthritis individual.

These therapies can include water aerobics, water arthritis programs through the local Arthritis Foundation, and even water yoga and tai chi. For the less acutely involved person, a gradual program incorporating balance, core strengthening, and resistive graduated strengthening that is tailored to the individual and set up after a proper biomechanical evaluation by an experienced physical therapist or advanced athletic trainer who works with medical populations is recommended. I believe that an actual *exercise prescription should be written by the attending physician.* This imparts more significance, follow-up, and adherence by the patient and the practitioner. Similarly, mind–body interventions to include breathing, progressive muscle relaxation, and mindfulness-based meditative practices should be encouraged and prescribed. Yoga, tai chi, formal meditation (TCM), and the like are some options that are generally available.

Pain control in the rheumatic individual, aside from the conventional pharmacotherapy available including prescription opiates and narcotics, as well as NSAIDs with all their potential GI, renal, and cardiovascular risks, is an important issue worth mentioning. Acupuncture, as has been discussed earlier in the book (Chapter 7), is a useful and effective discipline for both acute and chronic pain control in osteoarthritis (OA) and inflammatory polyarthritis (e.g., rheumatoid and variants). High-dose omega-3s and the mind–body interventions mentioned earlier are also important and very useful adjuncts in managing skeletal pain. Conventional rheumatology calls for use of local injections of corticosteroids in recalcitrant joints or for paraspinal nerve entrapment issues (sciatica, cervical radicular syndromes). Other options include homeopathic injections of FDA-regulated homeopathic medications (e.g., Zeel injectable products by Heel) for individuals who do not want to take corticosteroids or cannot tolerate them. Oral homeopathic remedies have already been mentioned. *Botanicals* are another important category of nutraceuticals worthy of mention. NSAID alternatives for individuals in whom use of this class of medication is associated with high risk or is contraindicated allow botanicals a place in arthritis and inflammation management.

I utilize combinations in my practice that include ginger 1 g bid to tid and/or tumeric root (curcumin) extract 0.5 to 1 g bid for inflammatory joint pain in combination with the aforementioned omega-3s. These are easily obtainable at health food stores, through the Internet, or through specialty physician supplement manufacturers. Other options include holy basil and *Boswellia* (*Boswellia serrata*). The latter has both articular and GI anti-inflammatory benefits and inhibits lipoxygenase cytokine pathways. For individuals with inflammatory bowel disorders such as Crohn's and ulcerative colitis, therapies directed toward reduction of bowel inflammation concomitantly tend to improve peripheral joint inflammation (E). This concept is probably true for rheumatoid arthritis with or without overt clinical bowel symptomatology but detectable with functional medicine GI evaluations including intestinal permeability.

Leaky gut in this setting and the attendant micronutrient deficiencies and proinflammatory GI changes are measurable and treatable with an overall functional dietary detoxification and GI mucosal restoration protocol aimed at normalizing GI cellular barrier integrity, columnar epithelial function, and bacterial homeostasis. Tightening of the GI columnar epithelial tight junctions to prevent backwash of antigenic waste materials and loss of vital micronutrients is a key element in this process. Avoidance of foods found to be either allergic, sensitive, or proinflammatory and a high-fiber, probiotic, digestive enzyme– and micronutrient-dense anti-inflammatory Paleo-type diet are essential. Dietary fortification with high omega-3s (as previously outlined) and adequate vitamin D_3 (5,000 units daily on average with serum monitoring for optimal levels 60 to 80 ng/ml), vitamins A and E (400 IU mixed tocopherols), selenium, glutamine, B_{12}, and folic acid (1 to 2 mg/day) intake are other essentials needed to restore the anti-inflammatory GI microenvironments that impact systemic inflammation and the synovial joint milieu.

For conditions including all other autoimmune conditions, including systemic lupus erythematosus (SLE), systemic sclerosis, polymyositis, dermatomyositis, Sjögren's syndrome, vasculitis, and polymyalgia rheumatica, similar approaches apply with some minor adaptations. Once again, my recommendation is to treat patients in a conventional manner as recommended by the American College of Rheumatology but additionally to interface concepts, modalities, and paradigms that address treatment of the whole person. Traditional medications for these conditions have included NSAIDs, corticosteroids, disease-modifying antirheumatic drugs (DMARDs), and immune suppressive drugs such as methotrexate, Imuran or azathioprine, Plaquenil or hydroxychloroquine, sulfasalazine, CellCept, Cytoxan, D-penicillamine, and a myriad of costly biologics. The latter include tumor necrosis factor (TNF) inhibitors (infliximab or etanercept, adalimumab) as well as more recent drugs blocking other immune cell signaling molecule receptors or pathways found to be increased in pathologic inflammatory conditions (e.g., costimulation blockade with abatacept; B-cell depletion with Rituxan; Benlysta as a B-lymphocyte stimulator signal inhibitor). All these medications have helped change the landscape and progression of formerly difficult-to-treat or -control diseases. They in fact have helped revolutionize medicine in a formerly stagnant era, but at a cost. This cost is both financial, as all these medications carry hefty price tags (approximately $1,500 to $2,500/month), and physical, because of the potential short-term and long-term consequences, including risk of atypical infections such as atypical tuberculosis or fungal infections. More serious long-term sequelae besides the immediate types of infusion reactions can be slow CNS viral degenerative infections or a slow CNS degeneration in a minority of individuals. Non-Hodgkin's lymphoma has also been associated with TNF use, but causality is not well established. Nonetheless, for some, these rare but potentially real events may seem worth the financial and potential physical risks, but not for all individuals. Consequently, my patients over the years have demanded options to these agents. Hence, I employ **parallel approaches** in my treatment of these autoimmune rheumatic individuals and evaluate the following parameters on a fairly consistent basis.

The *role of bacterial overgrowth and dysbiosis* in rheumatoid arthritis and scleroderma and autoimmunity in general needs to be addressed. The term *microbiome* now conveys the concept that the human body houses a superorganism. The intestinal microbiota help shape immunity and maintain a balanced environment in ideal healthy states. Perturbation or dysbiosis results in skewed adaptive immune responses to TH17 phenotypes, resulting in pro-inflammatory cascades and autoantibody production (Lee et al., 2010). The intriguing but not new concept that treating rheumatoid arthritis or other autoimmune conditions with broad-spectrum antibiotics and altering dysbiosis has gained popularity (Ogrendk et al., 2011; Tilley et al., 1995). These therapies followed by probiotics and a functional medicine detox protocol may be used. In some cases, prolonged antibiotic therapy has been utilized for treatment of rheumatoid arthritis, especially if biologic or other DMARDs cannot be used. The possibilities of *heavy metal toxicity or subclinical burden* in systemic sclerosis should be investigated. In fact, Cuprimine or D-penicillamine is the only immunosuppressive DMARD other than CellCept routinely prescribed for systemic sclerosis. It is of interest that D-penicillamine is a lathyrogen and eliminates copper. Why would we prescribe a chelator to treat systemic sclerosis? I maintain that other heavy metals including lead, nickel, cadmium, mercury, and antimony should be surveyed through blood, tissue (hair), and urine as well as provocative testing if needed. *Atypical infections* may be explored through GI stool testing as well as serologies associated with viral and bacterial pathogens known to trigger autoimmune dysfunction. Fourfold rises in viral titers for EBV, CMV, or parvovirus for example or IgM elevations are suggestive of either a new infection or reinfection with pathogens not usually associated with these autoimmune conditions primarily. High doses of antioxidants are essential for all of these autoimmune conditions where oxidant stress is high and the constant development of superoxide radicals is bombarding the body's capacity to cope with an excess load of proinflammatory molecules.

Glutathione, B_{12}, folic acid, vitamins C and E, coenzyme Q10, melatonin, and resveratrol are excellent antioxidant support options I utilize in rheumatic active inflammation scenarios. Glutathione is essential if heavy metal burden is detected. Chelating protocols (intravenously or orally) should be considered for these particular individuals by practitioners experienced in this specialized area of care.

Bone Health

Finally, a word about *bone health,* as this is the name of this chapter! This particular topic seems to have come more into focus in the past few years for men. It should be noted that osteoporosis is an important cause of mortality and morbidity among men and highly underpublicized as such (Center et al., 1999). Second, as men get older (i.e., >50 years old), their fracture incidence rises significantly (40%) as a global measure of all fractures, but the mortality of men is higher than that of women after osteoporotic fractures (Haentjens et al., 2010). It is my personal experience and borne out by the literature that men at risk for osteoporosis are commonly not identified or treated (Feldstein, 2005). Originally, the use of bone mass testing via DEXA scans was primarily meant for detection of pathologically low bone density for postmenopausal women. The concept that men could have premature or andropausal abnormal low bone density was at best understated or, in some settings, a completely ignored concept. Men in fact have been a clear far thought with respect to the concept of osteoporosis despite the evidence that they go through a hormonal change with loss of androgens that can clearly affect bone mass in a deleterious fashion. Similar factors that predispose women to osteoporosis affect men as well. These include smoking and genetics. Family history of osteoporosis for either the mother or father are worthy of risk factor categorization for the male patient. Obesity could be a negative factor as it leads to a more sedentary lifestyle and a higher incidence of metabolic syndrome, insulin resistance, and a proinflammatory state associated with low free testosterone. These combinations of events favor a decreased bone mass as well. Finally, aside from the usual endocrinopathies associated with osteoporosis, hyperparathyroidism, or rarer multiple endocrinopathies, vitamins and micronutrients play an important role in prevention. Younger men are less likely to take vitamins in general unless they are highly health conscious or in some form of athletic training. Consequently, unless prompted, men are unlikely to routinely ingest calcium, magnesium, or vitamins D and K. I would like to address the highlights of this grouping of supplements as essential for optimal bone health in men.

Vitamin D, or 25-hydroxyvitamin D_3, is critical to maintaining a healthy bone mass in everyone. For men in particular, the emphasis of taking this supplement early in life cannot be overemphasized. Men tend to have more physical athletic injuries than women and bone and structural healing are affected by a low vitamin D status. Because we can assume that absorption from the sun in sufficient quantities is highly impractical due to time constraints of work, school, and so forth, access to nonpeak hours for 30 minutes per day is difficult if not impossible for some. Therefore, supplementation of vitamin D_3 taken after meals is recommended. How much to take is another issue. The Institute of Medicine (IOM) recommends 600 units daily. I and others feel this is vastly inadequate. The amount of vitamin D required will vary from individual to individual and should be based on a number of factors when bone metabolism and osteoporosis treatment or prevention are the main goals of the therapy. In general, individuals with large body fat mass will require higher doses and longer treatment intervals before serum levels reflect changes. Conventional lab ranges for 25-hydroxyvitamin D_3 levels range from 30 to 100 ng/ml. This represents a huge variability within the proverbial "within normal range" paradigm common in conventional but not optimal medical practice. So, do we want to be "within normal range" or do we want to be "optimal"? Although the exact range is debatable and there lacks a universal consensus in this regard, many considered expert in vitamin D feel that the level in the serum is critical for optimal health, not the individual dose being given at any particular time. Levels between 60 and 80 ng/ml are considered ideal for optimal health. I happen to agree with this concept but would add that because vitamin D_3 is a prohormone steroid, its free level is really the biologically active level and not any measured or bound to transport protein. Once we have determined the serum level, therapeutic decisions can now be made, and most people require 2,000 to 10,000 units daily to achieve optimal levels. Outliers topping these generalizations do exist and customization of individual needs is essential.

I follow urinary or serum bone turnover markers in my osteopenic and osteoporotic patients as a guide in interpreting the response to therapies employed for increasing bone mass. These tests can be done in 3- to 6-month intervals and urine NTX (Osteomark) or serum CTX markers are readily available through commercial labs. The goal is to drive down the bone turnover marker to be consistent with low turnover, which means that bone matrix is not being broken down due to osteoclastic resorptive activity. In fact, I determine my vitamin D supplementation doses according to this level and follow serum calcium, magnesium, and phosphorous to make sure elevations in these mineral ions stay within normal ranges. In higher risk stone-forming patients, 24-hour urine studies for calcium, urate, and oxalate are useful in this determination. For men in particular, andropause may bring an increased loss of bone mass parallel to the situation in women for the postmenopausal period following the climacteric changes. Monitoring of androgen level including free testosterone, dehydroepiandrosterone (DHEA)-sulfate, urine NTX, and serum vitamin D_3 levels is a useful diagnostic guide. It is imperative that low and suboptimal vitamin D_3 levels be corrected in men and all patients with osteoporosis/osteopenia and done *before* ant-resorptive therapies are prescribed, such as bisphosphonates. It is my personal observation that the rare but potentially atypical femoral shaft fractures now associated with bisphosphonate therapy tend to occur in individuals who for some reason did not have deficient vitamin D states corrected adequately and prior to initiation of bisphosphonate therapy. In my practice, I like to wait about 2 to 3 months after the correction is achieved in vitamin D levels before starting a bisphosphonate if it is used at all. These agents do show efficacy in some studies. Recent data indicate that vertebral fractures are reduced in men treated with zoledronic acid followed over 24 months compared to placebo groups (Bopomen et al., 2012). Besides oral and intravenous bisphosphonates, the anabolic agents tetrapeptide (Forteo) and the immune-modulating RANK ligand inhibitor Prolia, to shut down osteoclastic bone activity represent newer pharmacotherapies available to treat this condition. However, we don't know the long-term effects of this class of immunotherapy.

Although it is evident that there is a need to have more definitive data regarding fracture outcomes in men with respect to current available therapies (Ogrendk et al., 2011), maintaining an excellent exercise program for prevention is essential. Until more definitive guidelines for men have been established, prevention is key. Men should be encouraged to exercise for a multitude of reasons, including cardiovascular and cancer risk reduction and stress reduction. Resistive weight programs to build and maintain muscle tone also help build bone mass. High-intensity interval trainings decrease all-risk mortality in addition to burning fat. Yoga, Pilates, and tai chi are all great adjuncts to maintain balance and flexibility for fall reduction and fracture risk reduction. Men in particular need to be encouraged to stretch versus simply doing a quick free weight regimen, which is more of a habit entrenched from the "gym" mentality. These are great venues for stress reduction in addition to providing the benefit of bone health, and I highly recommend my patients to buddy up with other male friends to explore these other venues.

Finally, a last word about calcium. There is current debate if one should take it and how much. The calcium one ingests should be readily soluble. If you take the pill and place it in water, it should dissolve within 15 to 20 minutes. If it doesn't, get rid of it and try another brand. There are many designer calcium compounds available. I prefer hydroxyapatite microcrystalline compounds with vitamin K. The role of strontium was controversial but now it is available through compounding pharmacies nationally, and I recommend its use as an adjunct supplement. I believe 1,000 mg of elemental calcium is sufficient for the vast majority of people, and citrate absorbed on an empty stomach and gluconates with food is the rule of thumb. Overall, calcium is less critical than optimal levels of vitamin D and resistive exercise as factors to emphasize in a therapy or prevention program. Similarly, hormone replacement with testosterone for men has been virtually ignored as an additional therapeutic route for both therapy and prevention in andropausal males. It is certainly a therapy to consider, especially if intolerance or relative contraindications exist for tradition therapies to increase bone mass.

Finally, it should be noted that besides the *conventional anabolic agent tetrapeptide, or Forteo,* another anabolic exists for potential use as a bone mass enhancer: the *off-label use of growth hormone* (GH). This modality is FDA approved in children for clinical indications of severely delayed growth in the setting of low levels of growth hormone. In adults, the current indication would include Adult GH deficiency states as evidenced by the GH provocation test, a difficult and potentially dangerous testing protocol. Low serum levels of insulin-like growth factor 1 (IGF1) in the setting of clinical symptoms (fatigue, increasing adipose tissue, sarcopenia, hair loss, etc.) in a man over the age of 40 and low bone mass could be interpreted as a situation where GH could be utilized. It is quite effective in increasing bone mass and certainly an option for some, although it is not FDA approved for this purpose. The main drawback would be cost.

Diet recommendations for osteoporosis in men differs from those for women. Typically, women are advised to remain under 0.8 mg/kg of body weight with respect to protein intake (F, Chapter 36). For men, this could be very different. In the absence of renal disease, the healthy aging male wishing to build bone and muscle mass simultaneously requires a higher protein intake. Competitive athletes usually require a rule-of-thumb protein intake of 1 mg per pound body weight to maintain and build muscle mass (approximately 2 g/kg). For the vigorous man training 3 to 4 days per week with weights, this general guide also is applicable. Lean protein sources are best, including wild oily fish and grass-fed hormone-free red meat for occasional consumption. The anti-inflammatory Mediterranean/Paleolithic pattern is desirable with high-fiber, micronutrient-dense foods; grains; nuts; and healthy fats. Soy whole-food consumption (one to two servings per day) should be encouraged as a clean protein source assuming non-GMO sources in men as in for women.

Alcohol consumption should once again be moderate at most, as excessive consumption could reduce bone mass. Carbonated drinks may leach calcium, and attention to dietary beverage selection for the man with osteoporosis is important, as it is with women.

Fall prevention is another major area to address that may be more unique and a greater threat to men than women for reasons not commonly discussed. In this arena, cognitive function with balance and healthy brain aging are vital topics to address during a man's life span. Supplements that help the brain help not only cognition but also balance, vision, and reaction times. Exercises that enhance balance, coordination, and reaction time should be sought in addition to usual exercises men may choose out of simple familiarity. A *formal flexibility program* should be incorporated for minimizing injury if a fall were to occur. Men tend to work less on flexibility than women. Hence, they may be at higher risk for injury once they do fall. Men generally weigh more than women; hence, their impact of falling may do more harm than to women. Men have a higher mortality than women with falls, and fracture mortality data confirm this fact. Yoga, Pilates, tai qi, and other martial arts, along with daily stretching regimens and instruction, should be taught to and sought by men. Repeated falling episodes and osteoporosis morbidities should also be viewed as symptom continuum associated with the aging brain and decline of neuro-cognitive functions inclusive of balance, reaction time, and vision. Attention to both organ systems, not just their bones, is needed for men including brain cognitive stimulating activities such as crossword puzzles, foreign languages and strategy games such as chess.

In closing, the healthy aging man does have many options for prevention, detection, and treatment of potential skeletal disorders. These include strategic use of potent supplements coupled with a goal-oriented exercise regimen and detection of strategies stratified for risk. The therapies besides the standard forms have been discussed and hopefully have given the reader a broader view of possible options both inside and outside the box. The references cited are excellent sources for specific topics examined in more detail. The relative paucity of citations has more to do with this chapter being more of a 30-year summation of personal clinical observation, initially a traditional one and subsequently transforming into an *integrative approach*—one that addresses the mind, body, and spiritual aspects of health and healing of individuals and requires an expansion of the constraints of using evidence-based paradigms as the sole criterion for choosing therapies. Men deserve and should seek this approach too!

REFERENCES

Bopomen, S, et al. Fracture risk and zoledronic acid therapy in men with osteoporosis. New Engl J Med. 2012;367:1714–1723.

Center, JR, et al. Mortality after all types of osteoporotic fracture in men and women an observational study. Lancet. 1999;353:878–882.

Feldstein, AC. The near absence of osteoporosis in older men with fractures. Osteoporos Int. 2005;16:953–962.

Haentjens, P, et al. Meta-analysis: excess mortality after hip fracture among older women and men. Ann Intern Med. 2010;152:380–390.

Kolata, AL. "Quinoa". *Quinoa: Production, Consumption and Social Value in Historical Context.* 2009. Department of Anthropology, The University of Chicago.

Kremer, J, et al. Effects of high dose fish oil on rheumatoid arthritis after stopping nonsteroidal anti-inflammatory drugs. Amer Coll of Rheum. 1995;38(8):1107.

Lee, YK, et al. Has the microbiota played a critical role in the evolution of adaptive immune system? Science. 2010;330(6012):1768–1773.

Ogrendk, M, et al. Treatment of rheumatoid arthritis with roxithromycin: a randomized trial. Postgrad Med. 2011;123(5):220–227.

Tilley, BC, et al. Minocycline in rheumatoid arthritis. A 48 week, double blinded, placebo controlled trial. MIRA Trial Group. Ann Intern Med. 1995;122(2):81–89.

GENERAL REFERENCES

Integrative Rheumatology

A. Orwoll, Eric S. **Osteoporosis in Men**, Academic Press, 1999.

B. Horowitz, Randy; Muller, Daniel. **Integrative Rheumatology**, Weil Integrative Medicine Library, Oxford Press, 2011.

C. Rayman, Margaret; Callaghan, Alison. **Nutrition & Arthritis**, Blackwell Publishing, 2006.

Functional Medicine

D. Lord, Richard S.; Bralley, J Alexander. **Laboratory Evaluations for Integrative and Functional Medicine**, revised 2nd ed., Metemetrix Institute, 2012.

Integrative Medicine

E. Rakel, David. **Integrative Medicine**, 2nd ed., Saunders-Elsevier, 2007.

F. Maizes, Victoria; Low Dog, Tieraona. **Integrative Women's Health**, Oxford University Press, 2010.

15

Gastrointestinal Disease in Men

AJAY NAROLA, MYLES D. SPAR AND S. DEVI RAMPERTAB

The spectrum of gastrointestinal (GI) illness in men includes idiopathic disorders such as irritable bowel syndrome (IBS); inflammatory bowel disease (IBD), including ulcerative colitis and Crohn's disease; and various cancers.

Inflammatory Bowel Disease

IBD involves vigorous inflammation of the gut, causing damage and manifesting as pain, bleeding, and diarrhea. Both ulcerative colitis (UC) and Crohn's disease typically manifest from ages 15 to 30 years, with UC exhibiting a slightly higher prevalence among males and Crohn's being slightly more prevalent among females. UC is limited to the large intestine and affects the more superficial layers of the gut wall, causing bleeding, cramping, and loose stools. The inflammation can also affect other organ systems such as the skin and joints, and those with UC have a higher risk of colon cancer. Traditional Western therapy for UC includes the use of aminosalicylate medications, steroids, and immune-modifying medications including biologic agents like infliximab. Surgery may be indicated to remove the colon. Such surgery is curative.

Crohn's disease can affect any portion of the gastrointestinal (GI) tract, causing ulceration, pain, bleeding, and loose stools. The disease is often patchy and is associated with inflammation-related disease throughout the body, especially the skin, joints, and eyes. Traditional Western medicine treatment is similar to that for ulcerative colitis. Surgery is often required for sufferers of Crohn's disease. Crohn's disease, on the other hand, may recur in other parts of the gut.

An integrative medicine approach to IBD involves an aggressive anti-inflammatory plan including diet and lifestyle modification. The anti-inflammatory diet has been discussed in the nutrition chapter of this text. Supplements are important in further attenuating the inappropriately enhanced inflammation response in patients with IBD. Omega-3-fatty acids, turmeric, and high doses of probiotics can be especially helpful. Repletion of Vitamin D in Vitamin D deficient patients has been found to be helpful since Vitamin D is increasingly being recognized as a modulator of the immune system.

Other factors that contribute to chronic inflammation include undiagnosed infections, exposures to heavy metals or chemicals that cause constant stimulation of the immune system, and emotional stress. The 4-R approach is a broad approach to patients with IBD, as outlined to follow.

4-R APPROACH

An integrative approach to gastrointestinal disease such as IBD and IBS often involves the functional medicine approach called the 4-R approach. This approach provides a broad foundation for improved gut health and serves as an effective method for resolving complicated and undefined illness. The 4 Rs are removal, reinoculation, replacement, and repair. Removal refers to the eradication of the substances from the body or the diet that contribute to poor health. These can include foods, pesticides, food additives, unwanted bacteria, fungi, and parasites. Reinoculation refers to the use of probiotics, supplements containing *Lactobacillus acidophilus*, bifidobacteria, and other friendly flora that help to digest food, produce useful vitamins and keep away harmful microbes, and have antitumor effects. Prebiotics, such as fructooligosaccharides (FOSs) and inulin, may also be used to help healthy bacteria proliferate. Replacement refers to the addition of supplements to support digestive function and may include digestive enzymes, bile salts, and/or HCl. Repair refers to the nutritional support that helps quickly regenerate and heal the gut, such as with glutamine and mucinaligous substances including marshmallow or slippery elm.

Specifics on 4-R

In terms of the removal element of the 4-R approach, there are various methods of determining what needs to be removed from the diet. Often, foods are most likely the offending agents in a patient's symptoms. One effective way to determine which foods may be causing problems for a particular individual is the elimination diet. This involves removing all of the most common triggers of GI symptoms, usually including gluten, sugar, dairy, corn, soy, and any artificial additives, for a period of at least 3 weeks and then adding them back into the diet one at a time to help identify what dietary element may be contributing to symptoms.

Food sensitivity testing may also be used to help identify which foods trigger an immunoglobulin G (IgG)-mediated reaction in that individual patient. Gluten sensitivity testing is an important part of this. IgA tissue transglutaminase is the best test available with the highest sensitivity and specificity.

Besides food, other potential contributing factors to symptoms that need to be removed from the diet may be artificial flavorings or colorings, MSG, or meat raised with pesticide-treated grains, hormones, or antibiotics.

The reinoculation portion of the 4-R approach is becoming increasingly important, as the role of the human biome is becoming better understood in gut function as well as in neurologic and immunologic health.

Irritable Bowel Syndrome

IBS is not associated with such an elevated inflammatory response as IBD. Specific causes are unknown, but it is likely a disorder of the neurologic function of the gut causing abnormal motility, such as lack of coordination of the rhythm of relaxation and contraction along the gut that needs to happen to allow for normal transit of material down the GI tract. Some patients with IBS may have loose stools, some may have constipation, and most have alternating periods of both. IBS is more prevalent in women than men, so it will not be a focus in this book; however, the 4-R approach in combination with mind–body interventions such as mindfulness and meditation can be powerful treatment modalities for this condition.

Mind–body interventions, as discussed extensively in the chapter on mind–body medicine, work based on the principle that your mind is capable of affecting your body. In fact, there is a large neurologic component to the gut; thus, using the mind to alter neurotransmitter production and induce a relaxation response hormonally will affect the gut directly. Some examples of mind–body approaches include meditation, biofeedback, hypnosis, yoga, and guided imagery. Manipulative and body-based practice is another type of complementary and alternative medicine (CAM) approach, which includes massage, chiropractic care, reflexology, energy medicine, tai chi, Reiki, and therapeutic touch.

The rest of this chapter will focus on cancers of the GI tract given their increased prevalence in men. First, a general description of the common GI cancers among men will be presented. After all cancers are discussed, integrative approaches to GI cancers in general will be presented.

Esophageal Cancer

EPIDEMIOLOGY

The incidence of esophageal cancer is relatively low in the United States, whereas incidence worldwide is high. In the United States, an estimated 17,460 cases of esophageal cancer were diagnosed in 2012, and 15,070 deaths are expected from the disease.

The two major types of esophageal cancer are squamous cell carcinoma and adenocarcinoma.

In areas of the world where esophageal squamous cell carcinoma (SCC) is endemic, such as the Middle East and South East Asia, it is seen in greater than 100 per 100,000 people, with equal affliction of men and women. In the United States and other Western countries, the incidence is much lower and men are more frequently affected. African Americans have a threefold risk of development of this disease (Siegel et al., 2012).

The incidence of esophageal SCC is decreasing in the United States due to long-term reductions in tobacco use and alcohol consumption, which are felt to be the major risk factors, but the incidence of esophageal adenocarcinoma has been rising dramatically over the last three decades as a result of increases in known risk factors such as obesity and Barrett's esophagus.

ETIOLOGY

In areas of the world endemic for esophageal SCC, it is felt to arise from exposure to carcinogenic substances such as nitrosamines, fungal contaminants, and human papillovirus. The cases in the United States are felt to be a result of exposure to alcohol and/or tobacco. The magnitude of risk of cigar and pipe smoking appears to be less than with cigarettes. Tobacco and alcohol may synergistically increase risk, as they do in SCC of the head and neck. It has also been proposed that a diet low in fruits and vegetables accounts for an increased incidence of esophageal SCC in the United States. Esophageal diseases such as esophageal strictures, lye ingestion, celiac disease, achalasia, and scleroderma with esophageal involvement increase the risk as well.

The esophageal adenocarcinoma rate has increased substantially, particularly in White men (5:1 men vs. women), and mean age of onset is 65 years. It is not associated with alcohol (Siegel et al., 2012). Instead, it is seen in the setting of elevated body mass index (BMI) or in patients with a history of smoking. Chronic gastroesophageal reflux disease (GERD) with subsequent development of Barrett's metaplasia, which then progresses to esophageal adenocarcinoma, is the common pathway for development of this type of cancer. Among patients who have Barrett's esophagus, the risk of developing esophageal cancer is increased at least 30-fold above that of the general population. Once again, a diet low in fresh fruits and vegetables has also been implicated as a risk factor for this cancer.

CLINICAL FEATURES

Esophageal SCC arises from the midesophagus, whereas esophageal adenocarcinoma arises from the distal esophagus. Both types of cancer present in a similar fashion with progressive solid food dysphagia secondary to obstruction of the esophagus by the tumor associated with weight loss. Weight loss is multifactorial and is due to dysphagia, changes in diet, and loss of appetite.

Early clinical manifestations are nonspecific, including brief "sticking" of apples, meat, and such harder foods in the throat; retrosternal discomfort or a burning sensation; and regurgitation of saliva or food. Frank dysphagia to solid food and hoarseness of the voice secondary to recurrent laryngeal nerve involvement are manifestations of advanced disease. GI bleeding such as melena and hematemesis are unusual, but slow chronic GI bleeding in the form of iron deficiency anemia is frequently a feature of esophageal cancer. Tracheobronchial fistulas secondary to direct invasion through the esophageal wall into the mainstem bronchus are a late complication of esophageal cancer and may cause intractable coughing or frequent pneumonias.

DIAGNOSIS

Diagnostic workup can be initiated with barium studies, but the confirmatory diagnosis is always made with upper endoscopic biopsy. Early cancer can be visualized endoscopically as superficial plaques, nodules, or ulcers, whereas advanced disease appears as a stricture or an ulcerated or circumferential mass. Population-based studies show that the larger the number of biopsies taken (up to seven), the higher the diagnostic accuracy, up to 98%, which increases to 100% with added brush cytology.

Once biopsy confirms the diagnosis of esophageal cancer, the next step is staging to confirm the extent of disease in terms of both regional spread and distant organ metastasis. The tumor (T), node (N), and metastasis (M) staging system (TNM), which is beyond the scope of this book, is used universally and determines treatment options available to the patient depending on the level of involvement of the cancer.

Staging typically starts out with a noninvasive test such as computed tomography (CT) scan of the thorax and abdomen to assess for the presence of distant metastatic disease. Endoscopic ultrasonography (EUS) is useful to evaluate for local and regional disease. It is helpful to determine the depth of penetration of the esophageal mass and local lymph node involvement. Integrated positron emission tomography (PET)/CT scans are helpful to identify metastatic disease in patients who are otherwise thought to be surgical candidates after routine CT staging.

TRADITIONAL TREATMENT

Treatment options in esophageal cancer are based on the stage of the tumor. In early and locally advanced disease (stages I and II), radical surgery is the treatment of choice (Bosset et al., 1997). Endomucosal resection may be attempted endoscopically in patients with early disease who are poor surgical candidates. For stage II and III cancers, several trials and meta-analyses support chemoradiotherapy followed by surgery in terms of offering a survival benefit in contrast to surgery alone (Am Joint Com, 2010; Kelsen et al., 1998). Most patients, though, are not surgical candidates because the disease is too advanced and are therefore offered palliative measures. Esophageal strictures may be treated with a membrane-covered expandable metal stent or repeated esophageal dilation. Palliative chemoradiation with cisplatin and fluorouracil is currently the standard of care in patients with unresectable disease.

Gastric Cancer

EPIDEMIOLOGY

Rates of gastric cancer are greatest in Asia and parts of South America and are lowest in North America. In the United States, gastric cancer is currently the 14th most common cancer. The American Cancer Society estimates that more than 21,000 cases of gastric cancer occur annually, and that the male-to-female ratio is 1.5:1. Worldwide, however, gastric cancer rates are about twice as high in men as in women. Gastric cancer is the seventh leading cause of cancer deaths. Incidence rates are highest among Asian Americans, Blacks, and Latinos compared to Whites (Garcia et al., 2007).

Known risk factors of gastric cancer include Lynch syndrome (also known as hereditary nonpolyposis colorectal cancer [HNPCC]), familial adenomatous polyposis (FAP), Peutz-Jeghers syndrome, and a family history of a first-degree relative with gastric cancer. Other situations that put patients at increased risk include infection with *Helicobacter pylori*, intake of salted meats containing nitrites, pernicious anemia, and prior gastric surgery.

CLINICAL FEATURES

Most symptoms of gastric cancer reflect advanced disease because early disease is asymptomatic in the majority of patients. The most common symptoms include abdominal pain, weight loss, and early satiety or anorexia. Although frank blood loss in terms of hematemesis, melena, and hematochezia is less commonly seen, occult blood loss can frequently occur, resulting in iron deficiency anemia. The presence of a palpable abdominal mass is the most common physical finding and generally indicates long-standing, advanced disease. Difficulty swallowing (dysphagia) is not common except as a late manifestation of cancer of the proximal stomach, especially at or near the gastroesophageal junction. Late complications and signs of advanced disease include palpable abdominal mass, ascites (fluid collection in peritoneal cavity), pleural effusion (fluid collection in pleural cavity), gastric outlet obstruction, gastrointestinal bleeding, and intrahepatic and extrahepatic jaundice.

DIAGNOSIS

Gastric cancer workup can be initiated through laboratory studies including complete blood count to rule out anemia. Tumor biomarkers like carcinoembryonic antigen are elevated in 45% to 50% of cases, and cancer-associated antigen 19-9 (CA 19-9) is increased in 20% of cases.

Upper gastrointestinal endoscopy with biopsy of the suspicious lesion is the best diagnostic method. Upper endoscopy is highly specific and sensitive as compared to any other imaging studies such as barium studies. During endoscopy, any suspicious gastric lesion should be biopsied because 5% of gastric adenocarcinomas present as a gastric ulcer (Graham et al., 1982).

Once biopsy is positive for gastric carcinoma, staging of the cancer and preoperative evaluation is performed. The most commonly used staging system is based on TNM classification, which is beyond the scope of this book. Briefly, T1 to T4 staging suggests progressive invasion of tumor cells from the most inner layer of the stomach (called mucosa) toward the most outer layer of the stomach (called serosa) and its adjacent structures. N1 to N3 staging is directly proportional to involvement of the number of regional lymph nodes. M0 indicates no distant metastasis and M1 means involvement of distant organs like the liver, lungs, and brain.

Staging workup can be initiated with CT scan of the abdomen and pelvis to assess the presence of peritoneal and visceral metastasis. Peritoneal fluid cytoanalysis should be done in the presence of ascites. A preoperative chest x-ray or CT scan is also recommended for the detection of intrathoracic disease. Endoscopic ultrasound (EUS) with fine-needle aspiration is more specific than CT at assessing tumor depth (T stage) and lymph node involvement (N stage).

Surgical respectability should also be determined with a staging laparoscopy to rule out peritoneal involvement. Diagnostic laparoscopy is more invasive than CT or EUS but has the benefit of direct visualization of the liver surface, the peritoneum, and local lymph nodes. Between 20% and 30% of patients who have disease that is beyond the T1 stage on EUS will be found to have peritoneal metastases despite having a negative CT scan (Lowy et al., 1996). Integrated PET/CT is suggested as part of the preoperative staging assessment, primarily to screen for distant metastases. Serum tumor markers (including carcinoembryonic antigen [CEA] and CA-125) have more prognostic value but limited diagnostic utility.

TRADITIONAL TREATMENT

Modalities for early gastric cancer include endoscopic mucosal resection, surgery (gastrectomy), antibiotic treatment for eradication of *H. pylori*, and adjuvant therapies such as chemotherapy and radiation therapy. Surgical resection of the primary carcinoma with removal of affected lymph nodes is the treatment of choice. Palliative surgery can be performed in advanced stages to relieve abdominal pain and/or obstruction. In patients with metastatic disease, palliative therapy is warranted with the current standard regimen consisting of cisplatin, fluorouracil, and epirubicin (Agboola, 1994). Prognosis is poor in patients with gastric cancer. Those with extensive involvement/metastatic disease have 0% to 20% survival at the end of 5 years (Wanebo et al., 1993).

Hepatocellular Carcinoma

EPIDEMIOLOGY

Hepatocellular carcinoma (HCC) is a primary cancer of the liver and is a different entity from metastatic liver cancer. This type of cancer is more prevalent in men than women. In the United States, the incidence rates for men and women were 6.8 and 2.2 per 100,000 persons, respectively, in 2008. It is more commonly seen in sub-Saharan Africa and Asia. It is the fifth most frequently diagnosed cancer worldwide in men (Jemal et al., 2011).

ETIOLOGY

Outside of the United States, vertical transmission of hepatitis B is a common cause of HCC. Exposure to aflatoxin also serves as an important risk factor to the development of HCC. Aflatoxin is a mycotoxin that commonly contaminates corn, soybeans, and peanuts. Some case-control trials have suggested that Betel nut chewing, which is widespread in certain regions of Asia, may also be an independent risk factor for the development of cirrhosis and HCC (Tsai et al., 2001).

Most patients in the United States who develop HCC have underlying cirrhosis, which is secondary to either hepatitis C or alcohol. Cirrhosis alone, independent of its etiology, is a definite risk factor for the development of HCC. There is a 5% annual incidence of cirrhosis progressing to HCC. Other risk factors for liver cancer include cirrhosis due to autoimmune hepatitis, chronic long-term inflammation of the liver (chronic hepatitis), iron overload in the body (hemochromatosis), α_1-antitrypsin deficiency, Wilson's disease, and primary biliary cirrhosis.

Some observational studies have noted coffee consumption as a protective factor for liver cancer. A meta-analysis estimated that consumption of two or more cups per day was associated with a 43% reduction of liver cancer (95% confidence interval [CI] 0.49 to 0.67) (Larsson et al., 2007). Few epidemiologic studies suggest a possible link between diabetes mellitus and HCC (El-Serag et al., 2004), and other observational studies show consumption of red meat and saturated fat increases risk for HCC (Cross et al., 2007). However, these studies are small and limited, so results should be interpreted cautiously until large prospective randomized trials confirm the evidence.

CLINICAL FEATURES

Patients who develop HCC in the United States are many times asymptomatic and are incidentally found to be afflicted during their participation in screening programs for high-risk patients. Previously stable cirrhotic patients who start developing decompensating complications such as ascites, encephalopathy, jaundice, or variceal bleeding need to be screened for HCC because these complications indicate invasion of the tumor into the hepatic or portal veins.

Clinical features of advanced disease include upper abdominal pain, significant weight loss, early satiety, palpable mass in the upper abdomen, obstructive jaundice, and bone pain due to metastasis. There may be intraperitoneal bleeding due to tumor rupture. Fever may develop in association with central tumor necrosis.

Some people may develop paraneoplastic syndromes including hypoglycemia, hypercalcemia, erythrocytosis, watery diarrhea, and cutaneous manifestations like porphyria cutanea tarda.

The physical findings in most patients with HCC include enlarged spleen, ascites, jaundice, or other manifestations of chronic cirrhosis. Hepatomegaly or a bruit heard over the liver is rarely present.

DIAGNOSIS

Laboratory examination is usually nonspecific and depends on the type and stage of cirrhosis. The majority of patients who develop HCC have cirrhosis and may have thrombocytopenia, hypoalbuminemia, hyperbilirubinemia, hypoprothrombinemia, and mild anemia. Liver enzymes including serum aminotransferases (aspartate aminotransferase [AST] and alanine aminotransferase [ALT]), alkaline phosphatase, and γ-glutamyl transpeptidase are frequently abnormal (Lai et al., 1982).

The diagnosis of HCC is often suspected in a patient with underlying liver disease such as cirrhosis or chronic viral hepatitis who develops a rising serum α-fetoprotein (AFP) level.

Transabdominal ultrasound is a highly sensitive, specific, and cost-effective way to diagnose HCC. Triple-phase abdominal CT (three phases: phase 1 is prior to contrast injection, phase 2 is filling of hepatic arteries, and phase 3 is filling of the portal veins) and magnetic resonance imaging (MRI) are also very good studies to evaluate for HCC.

In cirrhotic patients, any dominant solid nodule that is not clearly a hemangioma should be considered an HCC unless proven otherwise. For noncirrhotic patients, the diagnosis of HCC should be considered for any hepatic mass that is not clearly a hemangioma or focal nodular hyperplasia, especially if it is hypervascular. Percutaneous biopsy should only be performed when diagnostic imaging is uncertain, because the risks of biopsy are bleeding, infection, and spread of the tumor cells along the line of the needle track. The most commonly used serum marker as aforementioned is the serum AFP concentration. Several other serologic markers such as des-γ-carboxy prothrombin are not as sensitive and specific but can be used in combination with the serum AFP to improve diagnostic precision.

Once the diagnosis has been made for primary HCC, the next step is to look for extrahepatic metastasis for staging. Detection of extrahepatic metastases can be done by multiple imaging modalities alone or in combination and include CT scan, bone scan, MRI, and PET scan.

TRADITIONAL TREATMENT

HCC is an aggressive tumor that is frequently diagnosed late in its course. The median survival following diagnosis ranges from 6 to 20 months, and mainstay of therapy is surgical resection. Surgical resection should be offered to all patients with a single lesion in an otherwise healthy liver. Liver transplantation is the treatment of choice in patients with more advanced cirrhosis as long as the tumor is less than 5 cm, there are no more than three tumors, and no lesion is greater than 3 cm.

Unfortunately, the majority of patients are not surgical candidates because of tumor extent or underlying liver dysfunction. In that setting, several other treatment modalities are available, including radiofrequency ablation (RFA), microwave ablation, percutaneous ethanol or acetic acid ablation, transarterial chemoembolization (TACE), radioembolization, cryoablation, radiation therapy, systemic chemotherapy, and molecularly targeted therapies, all of which are beyond the scope of this book (Bruix et al., 2005).

Pancreatic Cancer

EPIDEMIOLOGY

Cancer of the pancreas is the fourth most important cause of cancer-related death in the United States. The majority of these tumors (85%) are adenocarcinomas evolving from the ductal epithelium.

More than 44,000 cases are diagnosed per annum in the United States, and mortality rates are nearly similar to incidence rates because of poor prognosis. The incidence is greater in men than women (male-to-female ratio 1.3:1) and in Blacks (14.8 per 100,000 in Black males compared to 8.8 per 100,000 in the general population).

ETIOLOGY

Risk factors can be subdivided into hereditary and nonhereditary categories. A role for familial aggregation and/or genetic factors is suggested by the fact that 5% to 10% of patients with exocrine pancreatic cancer have a first-degree relative with the disease. Some conditions that predispose to pancreatic cancer include Peutz-Jeghers syndrome, FAP, BRCA2 mutation, Lynch syndrome, cystic fibrosis, and hereditary pancreatitis.

Nonhereditary risk factors include diabetes mellitus, insulin resistance, cigarette smoking, obesity, and physical inactivity. Diabetes mellitus and smoking are each related to pancreatic cancer development, with a twofold increased risk. A BMI of at least 30 kg/m^2 was associated with a significantly increased risk of pancreatic cancer compared with a BMI of less than 23 kg/m^2 (relative risk 1.72, 95% CI 1.19 to 2.48). Alcohol consumption also appears to play a role, especially in heavy drinkers. A multicenter study of more than 2,000 patients with chronic pancreatitis demonstrated a 26-fold increase in the risk of developing pancreatic cancer in heavy drinkers (Michaud et al., 2001).

The occurrence of pancreatic cancer is lower in persons with a diet rich in fresh fruits and vegetables (Nkondjock et al., 2005). On the other side, consumption of processed red meat is associated with a higher risk of pancreatic cancer. Poultry, dairy products, and coffee consumption do not augment the risk of this disease (Risch et al., 2003).

CLINICAL FEATURES

The initial presentation of pancreatic cancer varies according to tumor location. Tumors in the pancreatic body or tail usually present late in the course and common symptoms include abdominal pain and weight loss. Tumors originating in the head of the pancreas are usually discovered earlier because they present with jaundice secondary to obstruction of the common bile duct.

Most patients (80% to 85%) with locally advanced or advanced disease have upper abdominal dull vague pain, the pain usually radiates to the back and worsens with food intake, and there is associated profound weight loss, anorexia, early satiety, diarrhea, or steatorrhea.

In general, metastasis of pancreatic cancer starts from regional lymph nodes followed by involvement of distant organs like the liver and lungs. The cancer can also directly spread to adjacent visceral organs such as the duodenum, stomach, and colon, or to more distant organs in the abdominal cavity through peritoneal spread, which may result in ascites. Unfortunately, because of the late presentation of the disease, only 15% to 20% of patients are candidates for pancreatectomy.

An abdominal mass or ascites can be noted at presentation in patients with advanced pancreatic cancer. A nontender but palpable gallbladder is present in patients with jaundice.

DIAGNOSIS

Pancreatic cancer is notoriously difficult to diagnose in its early stage, and 52% of all patients already have distant disease during initial diagnosis. The initial diagnosis of pancreatic cancer is made by imaging studies most of the time, which include ultrasound, CT scan of the abdomen and pelvis, MRI, magnetic resonance cholangiopancreatography (MRCP), endoscopic ultrasound, and PET scan. EUS is highly sensitive and very useful in detecting small lesions and vascular involvement, both of which are key elements involved in staging. Endoscopic retrograde cholangiopancreatography (ERCP) was widely used as a diagnostic tool for pancreatic cancer in the past, but currently EUS is utilized more often for this purpose.

When a mass lesion of the pancreas is detected on CT or ultrasound, it is reasonable to proceed with helical CT angiography or EUS to assess resectability. Another purpose of imaging studies is to delineate tumor size, extent, and spread (whether metastatic or not) and decide on the management plan with regard to surgical resection and/or chemotherapy and radiation.

Several serum markers for pancreatic cancer have been evaluated, the most useful of which is CA 19-9. The reported sensitivity and specificity for pancreatic cancer are 80% and 90%, respectively. However, these values are closely related to tumor size. The accuracy of CA 19-9 to identify patients with small surgically resectable cancers is limited.

Radiographic criteria for unresectability include extrapancreatic involvement, including extensive peripancreatic lymphatic involvement, nodal involvement beyond the peripancreatic tissues, and/or distant metastases, and direct involvement of the superior mesenteric artery (SMA), inferior vena cava, aorta, celiac axis, or hepatic artery.

TRADITIONAL TREATMENT

The treatment plan depends on the location of the primary tumor. The standard treatment for tumors of the head of the pancreas that meet resectability criteria is a Whipple procedure or pancreaticoduodenectomy, which is resection of the pancreatic head, the duodenum, part of the jejunum, the common bile duct, the gallbladder, and part of the stomach. A modified Whipple procedure has been developed that preserves the pylorus, which is important for stomach emptying.

Management for tumors in the body or tail of the pancreas is different because tumors in the body or tail of the pancreas do not cause the same symptoms as those in the head of the pancreas, and therefore these cancers tend to be diagnosed in an advanced stage. If the tumor can be removed with surgery, a laparoscopy is usually done first to make sure the cancer has not spread. If surgery is an option, part of the pancreas is removed, usually along with the spleen.

Adjuvant therapy after surgery includes chemotherapy, radiation, or a combination of both, which is helpful to prolong survival by eliminating the tiny cancer cells before they have a chance to grow. In people with locally advanced pancreatic cancer, there are two ways to give adjuvant therapy after surgery for pancreatic cancer: chemotherapy alone versus combination of chemotherapy and radiation therapy, which is called chemoradiotherapy. In the United States, chemoradiotherapy is recommended for most patients.

For patients who are initially diagnosed with metastatic pancreatic cancer, prognosis is very poor and chemotherapy might be recommended to slow the spread of the cancer, alleviate symptoms, and prolong life. The 1-year survival rate for pancreatic cancer is barely 24%, and the overall 5-year survival is less than 5% (Ries et al., 2000).

Colorectal Cancer

Colorectal cancer has the highest incidence among gastrointestinal cancers in the United States, and according to the American Cancer Society, colorectal cancer is the third leading cause of cancer-related deaths in the United States in both men and women. Nevertheless, early diagnosis frequently leads to a complete cure.

Nearly all colon cancers begin as noncancerous (benign) polyps, which gradually develop into cancer. The most important risk factors for colon cancer are age older than 50 years and family history. Male sex; African American ethnicity; high-fat, low-fiber diet with red or processed meats; inflammatory bowel disease (Crohn's disease or ulcerative colitis); and hereditary syndromes also increase risk (Rex et al., 2009).

SYMPTOMS

Patients with benign polyps called adenomas and early cancer are often asymptomatic. Symptoms associated with colorectal cancer include blood in the stool, diarrhea, constipation, or other change in bowel habits; narrow-caliber stools; unintentional weight loss; pain and tenderness in the abdomen; and tenesmus. Chronic blood loss in the form of iron deficiency anemia may be the only symptom in 10% to 20% of people with colorectal cancer.

DIAGNOSIS

Colonoscopy is the gold standard method to diagnose colorectal cancer because it allows for visualization of the entire colon and will allow for biopsies/removal of suspicious lesions. Barium enema is useful only for large advanced lesions, and therefore has fallen out of favor. Abdominal/pelvic CT is essential to help delineate whether there has been spread of the primary tumor to other areas such as the liver.

STAGES OF COLON CANCER

The stages of colon cancer are as follows:
- Stage 0: Very early cancer on the innermost layer of the intestine
- Stage I: Cancer is in the inner layers of the colon
- Stage II: Cancer has spread through the muscle wall of the colon
- Stage III: Cancer has spread to the lymph nodes
- Stage IV: Cancer has spread to other organs, called metastasis

TRADITIONAL TREATMENT

Treatment depends primarily on the stage of the cancer. Treatments may include surgery (mostly colon resection), chemotherapy, and/or radiation therapy. Most studies show that stages 0, I, and II require surgery, which is partial or complete colonic resection depending on stage and degree of spread. There are some cases where patients with stage II colon cancer are given chemotherapy after surgery.

Almost all patients with stage III colon cancer should be given chemotherapy after surgery for about 6 to 8 months. Chemotherapy agents include irinotecan, oxaliplatin, capecitabine, and 5-fluorouracil. In patients with stage IV disease, surgery is often palliative to prevent bowel obstruction. Chemotherapy is offered but may not improve survival. Radiation therapy can be localized or generalized depending on extent, staging of disease, and type of organ involved.

PROGNOSIS

Prognosis mainly depends on staging of the disease at initial presentation. Five-year survival is 85% to 95% in stage I cancer, but plummets to less than 5% for stage IV cancers (Cunningham et al., 2010).

PREVENTION

The death rate for colon cancer has declined in the last 15 years. This may be due to increased consciousness and screening by colonoscopy. Almost all men and women age 50 and older should have a colon cancer screening. Patients at risk may require earlier screening as discussed previously (Levin et al., 2008; Whitlock et al., 2008).

Change in diet and lifestyle is also essential. Some data propose that low-fat and high-fiber diets may decrease the risk of colon cancer.

Some studies have reported that nonsteroidal anti-inflammatory drugs (aspirin, ibuprofen, etc.) may diminish the risk of colorectal cancer. On the flip side, these medicines can augment the risk for gastrointestinal bleeding as well, and most professionals do not suggest these medicines to prevent colon cancer.

Integrative Medicine Approaches to Gastrointestinal Cancers

Dietary supplements may improve gastrointestinal health and can help prevent GI cancers. Calcium and omega-3 fatty acids may decrease the risk of getting colon cancer, and coenzyme Q10 may relieve cancer symptoms and increase energy. Omega-3 fatty acids work as an anti-inflammatory and antioxidant that may prevent or treat cancer (Velicer et al., 2008). Selenium may protect colonic cells from external and internal stressors. Folic acid, vitamin B complex, and vitamins C, D, and E can help prevent cancer (Greenwald et al., 2007) and rebuild the body after chemotherapy (Lippman et al., 2009; Verhoef et al., 2005). One herb in the news is turmeric, a yellow plant in the ginger family. Research in several countries indicates that this anti-inflammatory herb can slow the spread of cancer, slow down the growth of new tumor blood vessels, and cause cancer cells to die. According to Bharat B. Aggarwal, MD, professor of cancer medicine, Department of Experimental Therapeutics, University of Texas, the active component of turmeric is an excellent blocker of tumor necrosis factor, which contributes to cancer treatment (Miller et al., 2008).

Other natural herbs that can help with side effects from chemotherapy such as nausea, depression, and insomnia include but are not limited to blackberry, fenugreek, ginger, cinnamon, peppermint, St John's wort, saw palmetto, valerian, and kava (Miller et al., 2008).

Ayurvedic medicine, traditional Chinese medicine, and homeopathy can be used for GI cancers and other gastrointestinal conditions. These are discussed in their respective chapters.

To date, comparatively little is known about the safety and efficiency of complementary health practices that people may use for cancer (Dy et al., 2004). However, some of these practices have undergone careful evaluation, and many more studies are being carried out every year. In 2009, the Society for Integrative Oncology issued evidence-based clinical practice guidelines for health care providers to evaluate when incorporating complementary health practices in the care of cancer patients.

Here we tried to provide an overview of results from a few reviews and studies in the areas of cancer prevention, treatment, and management of symptoms and side effects.

COMPLEMENTARY AND ALTERNATIVE MEDICINE FOR CANCER PREVENTION

Although researchers continue to investigate the possible role of vitamin and mineral supplements in preventing cancer, available evidence is limited and does not support taking these supplements for this purpose. A 2003 Agency for Healthcare Research and Quality (AHRQ) review found little evidence of cancer prevention benefits from three antioxidants (vitamins C and E and coenzyme Q10) (Coulter et al., 2003). A 2008 review of 20 clinical trials found no convincing evidence that antioxidant supplements prevent gastrointestinal cancer (Bjelakovic et al., 2008). Higher intake of calcium may be associated with reduced risk of colorectal cancer, but the National Cancer Institute has concluded that the available evidence does not support taking calcium supplements to prevent colorectal cancer (NCI, 2010).

COMPLEMENTARY AND ALTERNATIVE MEDICINE
FOR CANCER TREATMENT

A 2008 review of the research literature concluded that some botanical supplements used in Ayurvedic medicine and traditional Chinese medicine may have some role in cancer treatment, but scientific evidence is limited because most of the research on botanicals and cancer treatment is in the early stages (Barnes et al., 2008; Boehm et al., 2010). There is also concern about side effects and interaction with cancer drugs (Lawenda et al., 2008).

Because of lack of solid evidence, it is unclear so far whether use of vitamin and mineral supplements and antioxidants in cancer treatment is beneficial or harmful because taking a daily multivitamin might improve the overall nutritional status of patients, but there is concern that some supplements might interfere with cancer treatment or increase the risk of a recurrence.

COMPLEMENTARY AND ALTERNATIVE MEDICINE
FOR CANCER SYMPTOMS AND SIDE EFFECTS

Studies have found acupuncture to be useful in managing chemotherapy-associated vomiting in some cancer patients. Although some early studies have shown beneficial effects, research on acupuncture for cancer pain control and for management of other cancer symptoms is limited because of inconsistent and inconclusive studies (Ezzo et al., 2010).

Various studies also propose probable benefits of hypnosis, massage, meditation, and yoga in helping cancer patients manage side effects and symptoms of the disease. For example, a study of 380 patients with advanced cancer concluded that massage therapy may offer some immediate help for these patients (Kutner et al., 2008).

A 2008 review of the research literature on botanicals and cancer concluded that although several botanicals have shown promise for managing side effects and symptoms such as nausea and vomiting, pain, fatigue, and insomnia, the scientific evidence is inconclusive (Deng et al., 2009). More information on botanicals for such symptoms can be found in the chapter on integrative oncology.

Overall, the data on integrative medicine and CAM with regard to the prevention and treatment of cancer are scarce and not compelling. More research in the form of clinical trials is needed to further investigate this.

Conclusion

In general, the most important integrative medicine approaches to gastrointestinal disease include specific dietary recommendations, supplement use, and mind–body techniques. Such approaches can be important adjuncts to conventional treatment for inflammatory bowel disease, irritable bowel syndrome, and cancers of the GI tract.

REFERENCES

Agboola O. Adjuvant treatment in gastric cancer. Cancer Treat Rev. 1994;20:217.

Barnes PM, Bloom B, Nahin RL. Complementary and alternative medicine use among adults and children: United States, 2007. CDC National Health Statistics Report #12, 2008.

Bjelakovic G, Nikolova D, Simonetti RG, et al. Antioxidant supplements for preventing gastrointestinal cancers. Cochrane Database Syst Rev. 2008;(3):CD004183. Accessed at http://www.thecochranelibrary.com on April 7, 2010.

Boehm K, Borrelli F, Ernst E, et al. Green tea (Camellia sinensis) for the prevention of cancer. Cochrane Database Syst Rev. 2009;(3):CD005004. Accessed at http://www.thecochranelibrary.com on April 10, 2010.

Bosset JF, Gignoux M, Triboulet JP, et al. Chemoradiotherapy followed by surgery compared with surgery alone in squamous-cell cancer of the esophagus. N Engl J Med. 1997;337:161.

Bruix J, Sherman M, Practice Guidelines Committee, American Association for the Study of Liver Diseases. Management of hepatocellular carcinoma. Hepatology. 2005;42:1208.

Colon cancer. A.D.A.M. Medical Encyclopedia. November 2007. http://www.ncbi.nlm.nih.gov/pubmedhealth/PMH0001308

Coulter I, Hardy M, Shekelle P, et al. *Effect of the Supplemental Use of Antioxidants Vitamin C, Vitamin E, and Coenzyme Q10 for the Prevention and Treatment of Cancer. Evidence Report/Technology Assessment No. 75. AHRQ Publication No. 04-E003.* Rockville, MD: Agency for Healthcare Research and Quality, 2003.

Cross AJ, Leitzmann MF, Gail MH, et al. A prospective study of red and processed meat intake in relation to cancer risk. PLoS Med. 2007;4:e325.

Cunningham D, Atkin W, Lenz HJ, et al. Colorectal cancer. Lancet. 2010;375:1030–1047.

Deng GE, Frenkel M, Cohen L, et al. Evidence-based clinical practice guidelines for integrative oncology: complementary therapies and botanicals. J Soc Integrat Oncol. 2009;7(3):85–120.

Dy G, Bekele L, Hanson L, et al. Complementary and alternative medicine use by patients enrolled onto phase I clinical trials. J Clin Oncol. 2004;22(23):4810–4815.

Edge SB, Byrd DR, Compton CC, et al. (Eds.). *American Joint Committee on Cancer Staging Manual*, 7th ed. New York: Springer, 2010, pp. 10, 241.

El-Serag HB, Tran T, Everhart JE. Diabetes increases the risk of chronic liver disease and hepatocellular carcinoma. Gastroenterology. 2004;126(2):460.

Ezzo J, Richardson MA, Vickers A, et al. Acupuncture-point stimulation for chemotherapy-induced nausea or vomiting. Cochrane Database Syst Rev. 2006;(2):CD002285. Accessed at http://www.thecochranelibrary.com on April 7, 2010.

Garcia M, Jemal A, Ward EM, et al. Global cancer facts & figures 2007. American Cancer Society. Accessed at http://www.cancer.org/downloads/STT/Global_Facts_and_Figures_2007_rev2.pdf on October 19, 2009.

Graham DY, Schwartz JT, Cain GD, et al. Prospective evaluation of biopsy number in the diagnosis of esophageal and gastric carcinoma. Gastroenterology. 1982;82:228.

Greenwald P, Anderson D, Nelson SA, et al. Clinical trials of vitamin and mineral supplements for cancer prevention. Am J Clin Nutr. 2007;85(1):314S–317S.

Jemal A, Bray F, Center MM, et al. Global cancer statistics. CA Cancer J Clin. 2011;61:69.

Kelsen DP, Ginsberg R, Pajak TF, et al. Chemotherapy followed by surgery compared with surgery alone for localized esophageal cancer. N Engl J Med. 1998;339:1979.

Kutner J, Smith M, Corbin S, et al. Massage therapy versus simple touch to improve pain and mood in patients with advanced cancer: a randomized trial. Ann Intern Med. 2008;149(6):369–379.

Lai CL, Ng RP, Lok AS. The diagnostic value of the ratio of serum gamma-glutamyl transpeptidase to alkaline phosphatase in alcoholic liver disease. Scand J Gastroenterol. 1982;17:41.

Larsson SC, Wolk A. Coffee consumption and risk of liver cancer: a meta-analysis. Gastroenterology. 2007;132:1740.

Lawenda BD, Kelly KM, Ladas EJ, et al. Should supplemental antioxidant administration be avoided during chemotherapy and radiation therapy? J Natl Cancer Inst. 2008;100(11):773–783.

Levin B, Lieberman DA, McFarland B, et al. Screening and surveillance for the early detection of colorectal cancer and adenomatous polyps, 2008: a joint guideline from the American Cancer Society, the U.S. Multi-Society Task Force on Colorectal Cancer, and the American College of Radiology. CA Cancer J Clin. 2008;58:130–160.

Lippman SM, Klein EA, Goodman PJ, et al. Effect of selenium and vitamin E on risk of prostate cancer and other cancers: the Selenium and Vitamin E Cancer Prevention Trial (SELECT). JAMA. 2009;301(1):39–51.

Lowy AM, Mansfield PF, Leach SD, et al. Laparoscopic staging for gastric cancer. Surgery. 1996;119:611.

Michaud DS, Giovannucci E, Willett WC, et al. Physical activity, obesity, height, and the risk of pancreatic cancer. CSSOJAMA. 2001;286(8):921.

Miller S, Stagl J, Wallerstedt DB, et al. Botanicals used in complementary and alternative medicine treatment of cancer: clinical science and future perspectives. Expert Opin Invest Drugs. 2008;17(9):1353–1364.

National Cancer Institute. Calcium and cancer prevention: strengths and limits of the evidence. Accessed at http://www.cancer.gov/cancertopics/factsheet/prevention/calcium#9 on April 9, 2010.

National Cancer Institute. Complementary and alternative medicine in cancer treatment (PDQ), patient version. Accessed at http://www.cancer.gov/cancertopics/pdq/cam/cam-cancer-treatment/patient/allpages on April 13, 2010.

National Cancer Institute, National Center for Complementary and Alternative Medicine. Thinking about complementary and alternative medicine: a guide for people with cancer. Accessed at http://nccam.nih.gov/health/cancer/camcancer.htm.

National Comprehensive Cancer Network (NCCN) guidelines. http://www.nccn.org

Nkondjock A, Ghadirian P, Johnson KC, et al. Dietary intake of lycopene is associated with reduced pancreatic cancer risk. J Nutr. 2005;135(3):592–597.

Rex DK, Johnson DA, Anderson JC, et al. American College of Gastroenterology. American College of Gastroenterology guidelines for colorectal cancer screening 2009 [corrected]. Am J Gastroenterol. 2009;104:739–750.

Ries LA, Eisner MP, Kosary CL, et al. SEER Cancer Statistics Review, 1973–1996. Bethesda, MD: National Cancer Institute, 2000.

Risch HA. Etiology of pancreatic cancer, with a hypothesis concerning the role of N-nitroso compounds and excess gastric acidity. J Natl Cancer Inst. 2003;95(13):948–960.

Siegel R, Naishadham D, Jemal A. Cancer statistics, 2012. CA Cancer J Clin. 2012;62:10.

Smith RA, Cokkinides V, Brooks D, et al. Cancer screening in the United States, 2010: a review of current American Cancer Society guidelines and issues in cancer screening. CA Cancer J Clin. 2010;60:99–119.

Tsai JF, Chuang LY, Jeng JE, et al. Betel quid chewing as a risk factor for hepatocellular carcinoma: a case-control study. Br J Cancer. 2001;84:709.

Velicer CM, Ulrich CM. Vitamin and mineral supplement use among U.S. adults after cancer diagnosis: a systematic review. J Clin Oncol. 2008;26(4):665–673.

Verhoef MJ, Balneaves LG, Boon HS, et al. Reasons for and characteristics associated with complementary and alternative medicine use among adult cancer patients: a systematic review. Integrat Cancer Ther. 2005;4(4):274–286.

Wanebo HJ, Kennedy BJ, Chmiel J, et al. Cancer of the stomach. A patient care study by the American College of Surgeons. Ann Surg. 1993;218:583.

Whitlock EP, Lin JS, Liles E, et al. Screening for colorectal cancer: a targeted, updated systematic review for the U.S. Preventive Services Task Force. Ann Intern Med. 2008;149:638–658.

16

Integrative Treatment of Common Cancers in Men

MARY L. HARDY

Introduction

PREVALENCE AND COSTS

Cancer remains a major public health challenge and is expected to be the cause of 25% of all deaths in the United States this year (Siegel et al., 2011). Although death rates for men's cancers are declining, male deaths from cancer still exceed that of women. The three most common cancers in men, prostate, lung, and colon cancers, account for 427,800 cases yearly or over half of all cancers in men. In men, 300,430 cancer deaths are expected this year, with over 85,000 from lung cancer alone. (See Table 16.1 for details.)

Prostate cancer, the most common cancer in men, is much less lethal than lung cancer. The lifetime risk for men of developing prostate cancer is one in six, and the majority of new patients are expected to survive their initial diagnosis for years. Even though African American men have shown the steepest decline in cancer incidence of any racial/ethnic group in the last 10 years, they still have higher incidence rates of prostate cancer than White men. Racial differences in prostate cancer risk are not easily explainable and seem unrelated to many of the obvious, modifiable risk factors. Factors such as health disparities and differences in vitamin D levels are among the factors that have been postulated to account for these differences (Mordukhovich et al., 2011; Siegel et al., 2011).

Costs for cancer care are expected to exceed $124 billion in 2010 and increase an additional 28% by 2020 (Mariotto et al., 2011), with the greatest increase in costs occurring in prostate cancer survivors due to the long period of ongoing care needed after diagnosis.

UTILIZATION OF COMPLEMENTARY AND ALTERNATIVE MEDICINE THERAPIES AND LIFESTYLE CHANGE IN CANCER

Utilization of complementary and alternative medicine (CAM) by men with cancer is common; however, men were two to five times less likely to

Table 16.1: Male Cancer: New Cases and
Deaths 2011 (Estimated)

	New Cases	*Deaths*
Total cases	822,300	300,430
Prostate	240,890	33,720
Lung	115,060	85,600
Colon	71,850	25,250

From Siegel R, Ward E, Brawley O, Jemal A. The impact
of eliminating socioeconomic and racial disparities on premature cancer deaths. CA Cancer J Clin. 2011;61(4):212–236.

use alternative medicine than women in a recent population-based survey
(Patterson et al., 2002). The average cost for CAM use per year in this survey
was not high ($68), but costs varied widely and at the highest end were very
significant ($4 to $14,659) (Patterson et al., 2002).

A systematic review of 42 studies showed that an average of 30% (range 8%
to 50%) of men with prostate cancer used CAM therapies. Higher socioeconomic status, higher education, younger age, and more advanced disease were
associated with higher use (Bishop et al., 2011). Although more complicated
therapeutic regimens predicted double the use of CAM therapies (Patterson
et al., 2002), there were no differences in the rates of use of CAM in a group of
prostate cancer patients based on type of initial conventional therapy (Lippert
et al., 1999). Overall, vitamins, herbs, and mind–body therapies were the most
commonly used modalities (Patterson et al., 2002).

The most often reported reasons for use included boosting the immune
system and preventing cancer recurrence (Eng et al., 2003). A strong desire
for personal control was also significantly associated with higher intake of
dietary supplements (Patterson et al., 2003). Utilization remained high even
when a majority of users thought that CAM was only "somewhat helpful" for
their condition (McDermott & Blough, 2012). Although CAM use was often
directed at cancer treatment, over 80% of respondents reported using CAM
for other medical conditions or to increase well-being (Patterson et al., 2002).

Less than half of CAM users disclosed use to any health care professional,
and only 30% told the physician involved in their prostate cancer care in one
study, although these results are not uniformly reported (Eng et al., 2003;
McDermott & Bloush, 2010).

Receiving a cancer diagnosis can be a very motivating circumstance for
patients. Following a diagnosis of prostate or colon cancer, 30% of men made
specific dietary changes. Fifteen percent began a new physical activity, and 36%
took one or more new dietary supplements. A third of men made two changes,
but less than 10% made all three changes (diet, exercise, and supplements). After

three or more treatment episodes, men more than doubled their rate of all lifestyle changes. Rates of change were substantially the same whether the diagnosis was made recently (<1 year) or up to 2 years previously (Patterson et al., 2003).

Most patients rely on anecdotal information from friends and family (39%) to make decisions regarding CAM use, especially after a cancer diagnosis. They are more likely to consult the Internet (19%) than either their primary care provider (15%) or their oncologist for guidance (Eng et al., 2003). CAM therapies were generally considered more safe or less toxic than conventional treatments, and scientific evidence played a relatively small part in choosing CAM therapies (Evans et al., 2007). Most users combined CAM use with conventional therapy. CAM users were more likely to delay or decline conventional treatment, but the numbers are small (5% and 4%, respectively, in one survey; Eng et al., 2003).

Diet and Lifestyle Modification of Cancer Risk

It has been suggested that only 5% to 10% of all cancers are the direct result of genetic abnormalities. Therefore, the vast majority (90% to 95%) of cancer development is the result of dietary and other potentially modifiable lifestyle factors such as obesity, exercise, smoking, and so forth. Thirty-five percent of all cancer deaths in men are estimated to be the result of diet alone. Obesity, a consequence at least in part of the same choices, accounts for 14% of cancers in men (Anand, Kunnumakkara, et al., 2008). The percentage of risk attributable to poor dietary choices is even higher in higher income countries (34% vs. 37%), presumptively reflecting the higher intake of meat, fat, and processed foods in the typical Western diet (TWD). For certain cancers, the risk associated with these lifestyle factors is much higher. Seventy-five percent of cancer deaths in both prostate and colon cancer can be attributed directly to diet. For lung cancer, the dietary risk is low (20%), but the tobacco-related risk is high (84% in men; Anand, Kunnumakkara, et al., 2008). Worldwide, men were twice as likely as women to die from cancer deaths due to potentially preventable lifestyle factors (1.6 million vs. 830,000, respectively) according to the World Health Organization (WHO). Thus, men could be considered an at-risk population in need of lifestyle intervention.

Not only do dietary choices affect the development of cancer, but also they influence the stage at which cancers present, if they progress or recur, and how lethal they are. In light of this evidence, many organizations, including the American Cancer Society (ACS), have made recommendations regarding diet and lifestyle choices to optimize cancer risk prevention (Box 16.1).

Box 16.1 American Cancer Society (ACS) Guidelines on Nutrition and
Physical Activity for Cancer Prevention

ACS Recommendations for Individual Choices
- Achieve and maintain a healthy weight throughout life.
- Be as lean as possible throughout life without being underweight.
- Avoid excess weight gain at all ages. For those who are currently over-weight or obese, losing even a small amount of weight has health benefits and is a good place to start.
- Engage in regular physical activity and limit consumption of high-calorie foods and beverages as key strategies for maintaining a healthy weight.
- Adopt a physically active lifestyle.
- Adults should engage in at least 150 minutes of moderate-intensity or 75 minutes of vigorous-intensity activity each week, or an equivalent combination, preferably spread throughout the week.
- Children and adolescents should engage in at least 1 hour of moderate- or vigorous-intensity activity each day, with vigorous-intensity activity occurring at least 3 days each week.
- Limit sedentary behavior such as sitting, lying down watching television, or other forms of screen-based entertainment.
- Doing some physical activity above usual activities, no matter what one's level of activity, can have many health benefits.
- Consume a healthy diet, with an emphasis on plant foods.
- Choose foods and beverages in amounts that help achieve and maintain a healthy weight.
- Limit consumption of processed meat and red meat.
- Eat at least 2.5 cups of vegetables and fruits each day.
- Choose whole-grain instead of refined-grain products.
- If you drink alcoholic beverages, limit consumption.
- Drink no more than one drink per day for women or two per day for men.

ACS Recommendations for Community Action
Public, private, and community organizations should work collaboratively at national, state, and local levels to implement policy and environmental changes that:
- Increase access to affordable, healthy foods in communities, worksites, and schools and decrease access to and marketing of foods and beverages of low nutritional value, particularly to youth.
- Provide safe, enjoyable, and accessible environments for physical activity in schools and worksites and for transportation and recreation in communities.

From Kushi LH, Doyle C, McCullough M, Rock CL, Demark-Wahnefried W, Bandera EV, Gapstur S, Patel AV, Andrews K, Gansler T; American Cancer Society 2010 Nutrition and Physical Activity Guidelines Advisory Committee. American Cancer Society Guidelines on nutrition and physical activity for cancer prevention: reducing the risk of cancer with healthy food choices and physical activity. CA Cancer J Clin. 2012;62(1):30–67. doi:10.3322/caac.20140

Men following the ACS guidelines reduced their risk of death. Increased compliance with a "healthy diet" reduced all-cause and cancer-related mortality by around 11% (p = 0.001). Moderate alcohol use, defined as less than two but more than zero drinks per day, decreased overall (14%) and cancer-related (25%) mortality as well (p < 0.0001 and p = 0.0008, respectively). Maintenance of a normal weight significantly reduced all-cause (30%) and cancer-related (23%) mortality (p for both <0.0001). Moderate physical activity did decrease all-cause but not cancer-related mortality. However, newly emergent data to be discussed later suggest a more protective role for exercise.

Obesity, often the result of injudicious dietary choices, is also an independent risk factor for a number of cancers. Higher body mass index (BMI), increased abdominal obesity, and lower lean body mass are all associated with increased risk of developing colorectal cancer (CRC), as is higher adult height (Gonzalez & Riboli, 2010). Counterintuitively, lung cancer risk decreases with increasing body weight and fat (AICR). This observation is probably related to confounders such as smoking's effect on weight or of weight loss associated with an undiagnosed malignancy.

Moderate levels of physical activity can affect cancer risk directly and through aiding in controlling weight gain and obesity (AICR). The data for the protective effect of physical activity is strongest with respect to the risk of CR. Various individual dietary components have been associated with risk modification for the most common cancers in men: lung cancer (LC), CRC, and prostate cancer (PC; AICR). The following sections contain a review of the epidemiologic evidence of cancer risk and diet.

PROTEIN (RED MEAT, PLANT-BASED PROTEINS, DAIRY)

The source and amount of dietary protein have been consistently implicated in cancer risk. Increased red meat consumption, especially of processed meat, increases risk of all three cancers (LC, CRC, PC), but the effect is strongest for CRC (Hu et al., 2011). The Health Professionals Follow Up Study (HPFS), a prospective cohort study of 37,698 men, quantified the mortality risk from eating red meat (Pan et al., 2012). A one-serving-per-day increase in red meat increased all-cause mortality by 13% for unprocessed meat and 20% for processed meat such as bacon and cold cuts. Increases in cancer mortality were similar (13% and 17%, respectively).

Happily, substituting a healthier source of protein (poultry, fish, legumes, or nuts) for the red meat led to a 7% to 19% reduction in all-cause mortality (Pan et al., 2012). More specifically, increased consumption of plant-based proteins is associated with a decreased risk of development of PC. Increased fish consumption decreases the risk of LC and CRC (AICR).

High red meat consumption may also be a marker for a more generally unfavorable diet and lifestyle. In the HPFS, participants who ate more meat also ate more total calories and fewer whole grains, fruits, and vegetables. Further, meat eaters were more likely to be less physically active, to drink alcohol, and to have a higher BMI (Pan et al., 2012). Given these observations, although it has not been tested, asking patients how many servings of red meat per week they eat may represent an appropriate proxy for overall dietary quality and perhaps even lifestyle risk. At the least, high red meat consumption should be a cue to examine other risk factors more closely.

Milk is a major dietary source of protein but also calcium; thus, assessment of the relationship between consumption of milk and milk products and cancer risk is more complicated. Diets rich in milk products and calcium have opposite effects on PC (increased risk, especially of more aggressive forms) and CRC (decreased risk; AICR). Calcium contained in milk likely accounts for the decreased CRC. Conversely, calcium has been associated with a decrease in the differentiation of prostate cancer (i.e., return to a less malignant cell type), thus explaining the higher risk of advanced or fatal prostate cancers associated with higher milk intake (Giovannuci et al., 2006). This effect is less significant once cancer is established.

FAT

Risk modification by dietary fat depends on the amount, type, and source of fat. Diets high in total fat, regardless of the source, increase the risk of CRC and LC. When the diet is high in animal fat, the rate of CRC is increased, and increasing amounts of butter predict higher rates of LC. For early-onset PC (in patients younger than 60 years), the type and the amount of fat determined the effect. Increased total fat and saturated fat (SF) increased the risk of PC development 2.5 times (Lophatananon et al., 2010), suggesting that a diet high in fat regardless of the source increases the risk of early-onset PC.

CARBOHYDRATES

Most cancer patients have heard the assertion that "sugar feeds cancer," and it is true that glucose utilization by tumors increases. However, despite this belief, very little direct evidence for increased risk of cancer with increased sugar consumption exists, especially when separated from insulin effects. Only for CRC have diets high in sugar and other simple carbohydrates been consistently suggestive of an increased risk. These associations were stronger for fructose than for sucrose and more pronounced in men than women (AICR).

On the other hand, fiber and other complex carbohydrates have long been considered a significant component of a healthy diet, in part because of their favorable effects on glycemic index. The 2010 Dietary Guidelines for Americans recommends consuming three servings of whole-grain foods per day. Whole grains are rich in fiber, defined as the edible carbohydrate part of plants that is resistant to digestion and absorption in the small intestine. They also contain many other phytonutrients that have been implicated in reduced carcinogenesis, such as lignans, oligosaccharides, carotenoids, flavonoids, and phenolic acids (Lattimer & Haub, 2010). Increases in whole-grain and dietary fiber consumption has been associated with decreased polyp formation and decreased risk of colon cancer (Aune et al., 2011). Reduction of the colon cancer rate has also been seen in a largely vegetarian population with increasing amounts of lentils in the diet. In the Adventist Health Study, a dose-response effect was seen for cooked green vegetables, dried fruit, legumes, and brown rice with colon polyp formation. Consumption of legumes three times per week decreased the risk of CRC development by 33% (Tantamango et al., 2011). There does not appear to be any consistent association of increasing fiber consumption with rates of LC or PC (AICR).

In summary, insulin resistance and/or a high glycemic index may be more significant factors in tumorigenesis than sugar alone. Diabetic patients generally have higher cancer rates, and metformin has recently been added to cancer prevention and treatment regimens with beneficial effects. Of course, both insulin resistance and diabetes are complex metabolic conditions that can increase cancer risk through a variety of mechanisms, such as increased levels of insulin-like growth factor 1 (IGF-1), changes in sex hormone–binding globulins, and inflammation (Arcidiacono et al., 2012).

FRUITS AND VEGETABLES

Diets rich in fruits and vegetables are generally considered to be "anticancer," so it is recommended for the general population to eat a minimum of five servings per day. For those at higher risk, intake should increase to 9 to 12 servings per day (Table 16.2; AICR). Risk reduction may vary for particular cancers in relationship to individual foods. Decreased risk is associated with diets rich in fiber (CRC), nonstarchy vegetables (CRC, LC), garlic (CRC, maybe PC), and fruits (LC, CRC). A great deal of attention has been paid to certain vegetable types, for example, cruciferous vegetables such as broccoli, cauliflower, cabbage, and so forth. High consumption of these vegetables is inversely associated with lung cancer risk (Kim & Park, 2009). High fruit and vegetable consumption can also decrease the risk of lung cancer for current smokers (Gonzalez & Riboli, 2010). Diets rich in lycopene, a carotenoid present in high

Table 16.2: What Is One Serving?

Fruits	Vegetables
• One medium fruit (size of a baseball) • ½ cup chopped, cooked, or frozen fruit (like applesauce) • ¼ cup dried fruit • 6 oz of juice: limit to 0–1/day	• 1 cup leafy vegetables (like salad) • ½ cup cooked or chopped vegetables • 6 oz of juice without extra sugar or salt

levels in concentrated tomato products, have shown decreased rates of pros-tate cancer. More than two servings of tomato sauce per week in the Health Professionals Follow Up Study resulted in a highly significant 23% reduction in prostate cancer risk (Van Poppel & Tombal, 2011).

BEVERAGES (ALCOHOL, TEA, AND COFFEE)

For beverages, evaluable evidence exists for milk (discussed earlier), alcohol, tea, and coffee. Convincing evidence exists that alcohol consumption in excess of 25 to 30 grams/day (about two standard drinks) increases risk of colon can-cer development in men (AICR). As with the mortality data discussed earlier, a J-shaped dose-response curve exists. Risk is higher with high consump-tion but reduces with consumption of two or fewer drinks per day until it rises again at zero drinks per day (AICR), suggesting that nondrinkers have a slightly increased risk while men who have between one and two standard drinks per day have a decreased risk. Over this level, risk of developing cancer increases. There does not appear to be an increased risk of LC in drinkers that is not associated first with smoking (Fedirko and Tramacere, 2011).

Tea, the second most widely consumed beverage worldwide after water, has received a great deal of attention as a possible chemopreventative agent. In gen-eral, benefit for cancer reduction has largely been shown in association with green tea, not black tea (Yuan et al., 2011). These beverages, although made from the same plant, are handled differently, which affects their phytochemical composition and presumptively their health effects. Green tea, when picked, is immediately steamed to destroy enzymes in the leaf and thus prevents the oxidation of the polyphenols, the active ingredient. Black tea, once picked, is allowed to ferment and the polyphenols are changed into a related but different set of compounds called theaflavones. It is assumed that the different effects of these two beverages are largely related to their phytochemical composition.

Green tea polyphenols known as catechins have proved extremely active in preclinical models. Green tea polyphenols are unique in their ability to affect car-cinogenesis at multiple stages of tumor development and at a large number of different cancer sites. Dozens of different molecular activities of green tea have been identified and involve targets affecting proliferation, angiogenesis, apoptosis, inhibition of key cancer-promoting enzymes, and inhibition of molecular receptors such as the epidermal growth factor receptor (C. S. Yang & Wang, 2010).

Despite strong mechanistic and preclinical studies, human epidemiologic evidence has not been as clear-cut. A large number of confounders likely account for these differences. For example, there is significant heterogeneity in the populations studied, the quality and quantity of the tea consumed, and the presence of other risk factors such as smoking and alcohol consumption. When these factors are absent or adjustments are made in the analysis to remove their effects, the action of green tea is more clearly beneficial (C. S. Yang & Wang, 2010). For LC and CRC, despite promising preclinical data, meta-analyses of the existing human epidemiologic data have not shown evidence of consistent benefit in decreasing the risk of cancer development (Tang & Wu, 2009).

The strongest epidemiologic data supports a significant inverse relationship between increasing green tea production and decreasing prostate cancer results. The most direct evidence of benefit for green tea polyphenols and PC progression has come from three human clinical trials involving treatment with a green tea extract (GTE). These trials will be discussed in the dietary supplement section later.

Coffee, a beverage enjoyed by millions, is not only a significant dietary caffeine source but also a complex mixture of active phytochemicals including caffeic acid hydrocyhydroquinone and chlorogenic acid (Butt & Sultan, 2011). The effects of coffee depend on the target tissue and the type of coffee in a series of recent meta-analyses. For lung cancer, decaffeinated coffee drinking was associated with a reduced risk, whereas high rates of caffeinated coffee drinking or an increase of two cups of coffee per day was associated with an increase in lung cancer rates (Tang & Wu, 2010). A modest but consistent benefit was seen for coffee drinkers and colon cancer risk. For the highest quartile of coffee intake, risk reductions of up to 30% were seen (Galeone et al., 2010). Data were mixed for prostate cancer. A small but statistical increase in risk was seen (relative risk [RR], 1.16; confidence interval [CI] 1.01–1.33) when all studies were pooled. However, all of the adverse effects were seen in the case-control studies, whereas the cohort studies (a better research design) showed no risk; the conclusion of this research group was that no evidence existed of an increased risk of prostate cancer with caffeine consumption (Park et al., 2010).

PUTTING IT ALL TOGETHER: EATING WELL

The Dietary Guidelines for Americans 2010 reflects the growing evidence that dietary choices affect health and risk of chronic disease. The best presentation

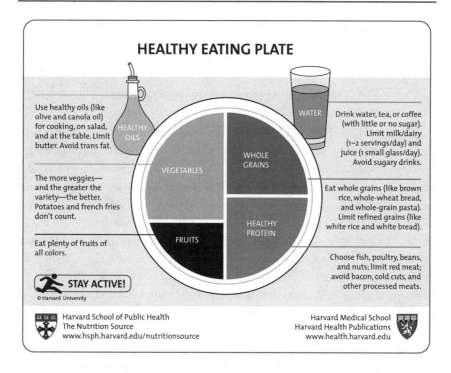

FIGURE 16.1. An Anti-Inflammatory Healthy Eating Plate.

Copyright © 2011, Harvard University. For more information about The Healthy Eating Plate, please see The Nutrition Source, Department of Nutrition, Harvard School of Public Health, http://www.thenutrition-source.org, and Harvard Health Publications, http://www.health.harvard.edu.

of these guidelines is found on the nutrition website of the Harvard School of Public Health (Figure 16.1).

Dietary Patterns: Vegetarian and Vegan

Vegetarian diets are associated with a generally decreased risk of cancer based on multiple dietary factors. Vegetarians replace higher risk meat with plant-based proteins such as nuts, whole grains, and soy but also have diets higher in fruits and vegetables. Therefore, vegetarian diets are higher in fiber and phytonutrients while being lower in cholesterol and harmful fats. Vegetarians also, in part as a result of diet, maintain a lower BMI and total body fat. People who make healthier dietary choices also tend to have healthier overall health habits, thus making it difficult to isolate the effect of diet alone. Finally, to derive benefit from this dietary pattern, it isn't necessary to be completely vegetarian or vegan. Inclusion of fish has been shown to be healthy in its own right, and moderate use of poultry shows little increase in risk for PC, LC, or CRC.

Dietary Patterns: Mediterranean

A good model for an overall healthy eating pattern exists in the Mediterranean diet, and a growing body of evidence supports its positive effect on cancer risk reduction. Men adherent to a Mediterranean diet (MD) showed a 21% reduction in cancer risk (Verberne et al., 2010). This traditional pattern includes large amounts of nuts, fruits, vegetables, legumes, whole-wheat bread, fish, and olive oil and moderate amounts of red wine, largely drunk with meals (Pauwels, 2011). This diet is a rich source of constituents that decrease inflammation and interfere with carcinogenesis. For CRC, an inverse relationship exists with oleic acid and even more clearly with omega-3 fatty acids. Seventy-six percent of the variation in CRC rates throughout Europe can be accounted for by three foods: increased meat intake with increased rates and increased olive oil and fish intake with decreased rates. For PC, there is no association with olive oil consumption per se, but omega-6 fatty acid intake is associated with increased risk whereas omega-3 intake is associated with inhibition of progression of PC. Increasing risk of PC is seen with increased meat intake, whereas a decrease is seen with increasing fish consumption (Pauwels, 2011).

Dietary Pattern and Recurrence or Progression

Evidence of dietary effect on disease progression following diagnosis does exist. Despite the observation that continued consumption of red meat, both processed and unprocessed, negatively affects PC progression, neither fish nor skinless poultry showed any adverse effect in a prospective trial (Richman et al., 2010). A low-fat vegan diet (LFVD) did increase prostate-specific antigen (PSA) doubling time in cohorts of early prostate cancer patients during a period of watchful waiting. Patients were assigned to a lifestyle intervention created initially for heart disease, which included a 10% fat vegan diet, yoga, and stress management, as well as group support. PSA doubling times increased significantly in the treatment group while decreasing in the controls. Also, serum from the treated men was shown to reduce the growth of prostate cancer cell lines in an ex vivo study. Decreased PSA and/or increased PSA doubling time was also seen in additional trials of LFVD, use of a soy beverage, or consumption of 8 ounces of pomegranate juice concentrate (Van Patten et al., 2008).

Higher intake of the typical Western diet (high intake of meat, fat, refined grains, and dessert) versus the prudent diet (high intake of fruit, vegetables, poultry, and fish) was associated with a greater risk of recurrence and cancer-related mortality in previously treated stage III colon cancer survivors (Meyerhardt et al., 2007).

Exercise

Increased physical activity is recommended as a means to decrease cancer risk (see ACS recommendations earlier in the chapter). Adequate exercise is defined as 2.5 or more hours of moderate or intense exercise per week (Table 16.3). Overall cancer risk is decreased with increases in both leisure and occupational activity, but this association is not strong (Thune & Furberg, 2001). For men, increased physical activity is directly associated with decreased risk of colon cancer. Colon cancer risk is reduced modestly with increased leisure time exercise but substantially reduced with higher rates of occupational physical activity. There does not seem, however, to be a correlation between physical activity and the development of rectal cancer (AICR).

The beneficial effects of exercise can also be seen after CRC diagnosis. Following conventional treatment of colorectal carcinoma, patients with

Table 16.3: Examples of Moderate- and Vigorous-Intensity Physical Activities

	Moderate Intensity	*Vigorous Intensity*
Exercise and leisure	Walking, dancing, leisurely bicycling, ice and roller skating, horseback riding, canoeing, yoga	Jogging or running, fast bicycling, circuit weight training, swimming, jumping rope, aerobic dance, martial arts
Sports	Downhill skiing, golfing, volleyball, softball, baseball, badminton, doubles tennis	Cross-country skiing, soccer, field or ice hockey, lacrosse, singles tennis, racquetball, basketball
Home activities	Mowing the lawn, general yard and garden maintenance	Digging, carrying, and hauling, masonry, carpentry
Occupational activity	Walking and lifting as part of the job (custodial work, farming, auto or machine repair)	Heavy manual labor (forestry, construction, firefighting)

From Kushi LH, Doyle C, McCullough M, Rock CL, Demark-Wahnefried W, Bandera EV, Gapstur S, Patel AV, Andrews K, Gansler T; American Cancer Society 2010 Nutrition and Physical Activity Guidelines Advisory Committee. American Cancer Society Guidelines on nutrition and physical activity for cancer prevention: reducing the risk of cancer with healthy food choices and physical activity. CA Cancer J Clin. 2012;62(1):30–67. doi:10.3322/caac.20140

increased physical activity (30 to 45 minutes daily) reduced significantly their risk of cancer recurrence and cancer mortality (Meyerhardt et al., 2006). In this study, patients with stage III colon cancer who performed 18 to 27 MET hours per week of exercise had a 50% reduction in risk of recurrence and a significant increase in disease-free survival and overall survival. Increasing exercise intensity or endurance led to only small, nonsignificant increases in response.

Suggestive but less strong evidence exists for reduction of lung cancer with increased exercise as well. Sedentary lifestyle is associated with an increased risk of lung cancer, and increased leisure activity was frequently associated with decreased risk (Box 16.2). No mechanism for this interaction has been proposed, but this effect is observed in both former and current smokers (AICR).

In general, effects of leisure activity/exercise on prostate cancer risk have not been shown to be protective. However, a recent evaluation of a large European cohort demonstrated an inverse relationship between occupational activity and PC risk (Johnsen et al., 2009). To the contrary, several studies show a correlation between intense leisure physical activity and increased risk

---

Box 16.2 Suggested Ways to Reduce Sedentary Behavior

Limit time spent watching TV and using other forms of screen-based entertainment.

Use a stationary bicycle or treadmill when you do watch TV.

Use the stairs rather than an elevator.

If you can, walk or bike to your destination.

Exercise at lunch with your coworkers, family, or friends.

Take an exercise break at work to stretch or take a quick walk.

Walk to visit coworkers instead of sending an e-mail.

Go dancing with your spouse or friends.

Plan active vacations rather than only driving trips.

Wear a pedometer every day and increase your number of daily steps.

Join a sports team

From Kushi LH, Doyle C, McCullough M, Rock CL, Demark-Wahnefried W, Bandera EV, Gapstur S, Patel AV, Andrews K, Gansler T; American Cancer Society 2010 Nutrition and Physical Activity Guidelines Advisory Committee. American Cancer Society Guidelines on nutrition and physical activity for cancer prevention: reducing the risk of cancer with healthy food choices and physical activity. CA Cancer J Clin. 2012;62(1):30–67. doi:10.3322/caac.20140

of aggressive prostate cancer. Thus, it seems prudent to recommend to those who are at risk of developing or who are surviving prostate cancer and who do not engage in physically demanding work to exercise moderately in their leisure time (AICR).

Indirectly, exercise contributes to risk reduction for a number of cancers by helping maintain a normal BMI (AICR).

Obesity

Obesity is an independent risk factor for a number of cancers, and risk increases with rising BMI. The cancer death rate at a BMI of 27 to 30 is 1.5 times higher than in the normal-weight cohort. At a BMI of 40, it is almost four times higher [AICR]. Increased body fat, especially abdominal fat, is thought to increase cancer risk through the release of inflammatory cytokines, stimulation of higher insulin levels, and increased insulin resistance, all of which favor increased cancer carcinogenesis. Recent studies have shown that for every increase in BMI by 5 kg/m^2, cancer mortality increases by 10% (Basen-Engquist & Chang, 2011). Higher rates of obesity were seen with sedentary behaviors and increased consumption of sugary drinks, "fast food," animal fats, starchy vegetables, and other energy-dense foods. Higher consumption of nonstarchy vegetables, high-fiber foods, whole grains, and low-energy dense foods was correlated with lower weight. Increased TV watching and screen time in general were independently associated with increased weight (AICR).

For colon cancer, increased body fat and abdominal body fat are strongly associated with increased CRC risk. For each 0.1 increment in the waist-to-hip ratio, there is a 30% increase in colon cancer rate. Another way to look at the same risk is that each inch increase in waist circumference was associated with a 5% increase in colon cancer rate (AICR). Further, patients with a BMI greater than 35 at diagnosis have an increased risk of recurrence of colon cancer as well. Unfortunately, weight reduction after diagnosis does not seem to affect recurrence rates (Meyerhardt, 2011).

Conversely for lung cancer, risk decreases with increasing body weight, but this may not be directly due to total body weight or body fat. Rather, increased smoking is associated with lower body weight, and the relationship of risk to weight may represent confounding by smoking (AICR). A recent analysis did confirm this association but did not support the hypothesis of attributing the apparently protective effect of high BMI to a confounding effect of smoking decreasing weight (Smith & Brinton, 2012).

Although intuitively it seems likely that obesity would adversely affect prostate cancer risk, the data are far from clear on this point. Obesity may be a risk factor for PC, but the association barely reached statistical significance (p = 0.03). Results were somewhat stronger for waist circumference (p = 0.02). This suggests that abdominal fat may have more influence on prostate cancer carcinogenesis than body weight in general. Supporting this hypothesis, obesity associated with central adiposity (BMI >35 or waist circumference >102 cm) was more strongly associated with prostate cancer risk (odds ratio [OR] 1.66, p = 0.03). All measures of obesity were most strongly associated with more aggressive, high-grade disease (De Nunzio et al., 2011).

Smoking

The causal relationship between smoking and LC has been well established, and 85% of all LC is smoking related. Second-hand smoke is also considered a significant risk factor for LC carcinogenesis. The latest trend in smoking for young adults, a water pipe or hookah smoking, is also associated with a two times increased risk of developing LC (Akl et al., 2010). The harmful effects of smoking are partially mitigated if smokers engage in vigorous physical activity and eat five or more servings of vegetables and fruits per day (ACS). Fortunately, smoking cessation after early-stage lung cancer does improve prognosis regarding recurrence (Parsons et al., 2010). Nonsmoking status is strongly (almost five times higher; p = 0.001) associated with the favorable epidermal growth factor receptor gene mutation.

Cigarette smoking also significantly elevates CRC risk, although not to the degree that it does for LC (Botteri et al., 2008). The RR of CRC is 1.18 with an absolute increase of approximately 11 cases for each 100,000 person-years. However, this risk only became statistically significant after 30 years of smoking. Unfortunately, smoking cessation after the diagnosis of colon cancer does not favorably affect recurrence rates (Meyerhardt, 2011).

There is also a negative, albeit weaker, association between smoking and prostate cancer, especially as smoking exposure increased (Huncharek et al., 2010). Current smokers were at increased risk for fatal PC, with the heaviest smokers showing a 24% to 30% increased risk of death compared to nonsmokers.

Smoking cessation should be an active component of cancer therapy for any current smoker diagnosed with cancer, especially lung cancer. Unassisted attempts to quit are usually only successful 2% to 3% of the time. Simple advice by the physician to stop smoking doubles this rate. The U.S. Department of Public Health (USDPH) provides an excellent document that reviews the 5 A's approach: ask, assess, advise, assist, and arrange (http://www.surgeongeneral. gov/tobacco/tobaqrg.html). The majority of long-term smokers will require pharmacotherapy for sustained abstinence. Therapeutic options are reviewed in the USDPH document. Hospitalization provides an excellent opportunity for smoking cessation, and strategies for abstinence should be included in discharge planning (Rigotti et al., 2007). Smoking cessation provides benefit and improves prognosis even after an LC diagnosis is made (Parsons et al., 2010).

Helping Patients Make Lifestyle Changes

The diagnosis of cancer has been identified as a teaching moment, a time in which patients are more likely to be ready to make lifestyle changes (Demark-Wahnefried et al., 2005). Despite this observation, only 5% of cancer survivors meet all three basic cancer prevention recommendations: eat five fruits and vegetables per day, get physically active, and don't smoke.

Health care providers can successfully influence patients by sending effective health behavior messages. Primary care providers, nurses, pharmacists, and so forth have multiple opportunities during routine contact with cancer survivors and should use these opportunities because oncologists generally don't have this routine contact. While almost three quarters of oncologists surveyed agree that they should be providing ongoing preventative care to cancer patients, 20% rarely or never provide this service and almost 50% do only sometimes (Demark-Wahnefried et al., 2005).

Effectively motivating and guiding patients through behavior change can be a tricky business, but the basic steps are fairly straightforward. Begin by assessing patient adherence to the ACS recommendations using open-ended questions. If adherence is good, reinforce this behavior and encourage the patient to continue. If adherence is poor, assess the patient's readiness to change using Prochaska's States of Change model (Figure 16.2; Prochaska et al., 1994). Different strategies are needed for different states of readiness. It is not helpful to engage a patient who is still in the precontemplation or contemplation state of change in a discussion of action-oriented strategies.

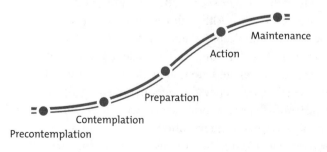

FIGURE 16.2. Prochaska States of Change Model.
http://www.prochange.com/ttm

For those not ready to act, raising awareness of the need to change and the possibility of change are the appropriate actions. The most appropriate question to ask may be: How about letting me help you reduce your risk of getting cancer or of the cancer coming back? If you meet resistance, probe gently using motivational interviewing techniques or open-ended questions to understand what is keeping the patient from moving forward (Rollnick & Miller, 2007). Agree with the patient to revisit the topic (stopping smoking, eating more vegetables) and schedule another visit. Provide appropriate tools or materials at the end of the visit.

Active planning, the determination of concrete steps to take in the near future, is reserved for those ready to engage in behavioral change (preparation, action, or maintenance). For these patients, collaborative planning is crucial. Aid the patient (not tell the patient) in finding concrete manageable steps to achieve the targeted change. It is usually best to work on one change at a time, but some patients prefer to make a more global intervention. Write down the agreed-upon change on a prescription pad or letterhead (this is official business!). Then ask the patient how confident he or she feels about executing the plan you have made, with 0 being no confidence and 10 being perfectly confident. If the patient's rating is not a 7 or higher, there is less chance of him or her being successful. Return to probing questions to find out where there is resistance, an unacknowledged barrier, and so forth. Redo the plan and check again. Once an appropriate plan is made, give the patient appropriate tools (website, books, handouts, community resources, classes) and schedule a return visit to check on progress (Rollnick et al., 1999).

Cancer Screening and Detection

Cancer screening and early detection have been prominent components of the ACS guidelines since their inception. It was felt that appropriate screening would lead to earlier diagnosis, resulting in more effective treatment and better outcomes for patients. Although this goal has been more successful with some cancers, for example, breast and cervical cancer, for the three most common cancers in men, colon, lung, and prostate cancer, screening guidelines are complicated and recommendations are not always uniform (Table 16.4; Smith et al., 2012). Further, frequency and rigor of screening may vary depending on personal or family history of prior cancer as well presence of risk factors. As with all population-based interventions, cost/benefit analyses sometimes do not favor screening. In addition, the cost and risk of any false-positive screening test should be considered in applying these guidelines as well. Effective and early detection of precancerous lesions or even frank cancer provides an

Table 16.4: ACS Recommendations for the Early Detection of Cancer in Average-Risk, Asymptomatic Individuals

Cancer Site	Population	Test or Procedure	Frequency
Colorectal	Men and women, ages ≥50 years	FOBT with at least 50% test sensitivity for cancer, or FIT with at least 50% test sensitivity for cancer, or	Annual, starting at age 50. Testing at home with adherence to manufacturer's recommendation for collection techniques and number of samples is recommended. FOBT with the single stool sample collected on the clinician's fingertip during a DRE in the health care setting is not recommended. gFOBT tests also are not recommended. In comparison with guaiac-based tests these are more patient friendly and are likely to be equal or better with regard to sensitivity and specificity. There is no justification for repeating FOBT in response to an initial positive finding.
		Stool DNA tests, or	Internal uncertain, starting at age 50.
		FSIG, or	Every 5 years, starting at age 50. FSIG can be performed alone, or consideration can be given to combining FSIG performed every 5 years with a highly sensitive gFOBT or FIT performed annually.
		DCBE, or	Every 5 years, starting at age 50.
		Colonoscopy, or	Every 10 years, starting at age 50.
		CT Colonoscopy	Every 5 years, starting at age 50.
Prostate	Men, ages ≥50 years	DRE and PSA	Men who have at least a 10-years life expectancy should have an opportunity to make an informed decision with their health care provider about whether to be screened for prostate cancer after receiving information about the potential benefits, risks, and uncertainties associated with prostate cancer screening. Prostate cancer screening should not occur without an informed decision-making process.
Cancer-related checkup	Men and women age ≥20 years		On the occasion of a periodic health examination, the cancer-related checkup should include examination for cancers of the thyroid, testicles, ovaries, lymph nodes, oral cavity, and skin, as well as health counseling about tobacco use, sun exposure, diet and nutrition, risk factors, sexual practices, and environmental and occupational exposures.

ACS, American Cancer Society; FOBT, fecal occult blood test; FIT, fecal immunochemical test; DRE, digital rectal examination; gFOBT, guaiac-based toilet bowl FOBT test; FSIG, flexible sigmoidoscopy; DCBE, double-contrast barium enema; CT, computed tomography; PSA, prostate-specific antigen.

Beginning at age 40 years, annual clinical breast examination should be performed prior to mammography.

Adapted from Smith RA, Cokkinides V, Brawley OW. Cancer screening in the United States, 2012: a review of current American Cancer Society guidelines and current issues in cancer screening. CA Cancer J Clin. 2012.

opportunity to use the lifestyle modifications discussed earlier to interrupt carcinogenesis and perhaps restore the patient to health.

For lung cancer, no screening routine, even in high-risk smokers, had been demonstrated to decrease mortality; therefore, no recommendation for lung cancer screening is included in the current ACS guidelines. However, a recent 3-year clinical trial comparing annual computerized tomography (CT) screening to annual chest x-ray screening has reported a 20% reduction in mortality in the CT group. Colon cancer screening is recommended for the general population to begin at age 50, but many options are listed for the method of screening, ranging from the least invasive but potentially the most inaccurate method, fecal occult blood (FOB) sample, to the most accurate but most invasive, colonoscopy. Screening is especially important in this cancer because of the presence of a precancerous condition (polyps) and the long latency period for colorectal cancer carcinogenesis (perhaps up to 10 years). Choice of screening technique depends on patient compliance, access to care, and perceived degree of risk. Less invasive methods (positive stool FOB, for example) are often used to select patients to advance to more accurate techniques (colonoscopy, for example) that can be both diagnostic and therapeutic (polypectomy). However, some experts recommend that around age 50 all patients should have a screening colonoscopy. Follow-up interval is determined by the findings at endoscopy.

Prostate cancer screening by means of digital rectal exam (DRE) or PSA is controversial and the "best" pathway in not always clear-cut. This uncertainty is the result of some unique features of the natural history of prostate cancer and the concern that too much potentially unnecessary treatment is being used to treat low-risk lesions. The development of PC is very common as men age, but some, perhaps most, incidentally diagnosed PCs are not aggressive and therefore would most appropriately be treated with lifestyle management or watchful waiting. Our current technology does not allow for us to discern with any degree of reliability which PCs do not require treatment. Therefore, the ACS recommends that patients be informed of the information contained in Box 16.3 before screening tests are done. Further, it is also recommended that patients should be counseled in a manner that allows them to become effective participants in all decision making (Smith et al., 2012). Tests such as free PSA percent and urinary prostate cancer gene 3 (PCA3) testing may help to refine screening, but their usefulness is for subpopulations of men at risk.

Conventional Treatment and Toxicity of Treatment

A detailed discussion of the current state of the art of conventional treatment for CRC, PC, and LC is far beyond the scope of this chapter. Surgical treatment

Box 16.3 Core Elements of the Information to Be Provided to Men to Assist With Their Decision About Prostate Cancer Screening

Prostate cancer is an important health concern for men:

- Screening with the PSA blood test alone or with the DRE is more likely to detect cancer at the earliest stage than if no screening is performed.
- Prostate cancer screening may be associated with a reduction in the risk of dying from prostate cancer. However, evidence is conflicting and experts disagree about the value of screening.
- For men whose prostate cancer is detected by screening, it is currently not possible to predict which men are likely to benefit from treatment. Some men who are treated may avoid death and disability from prostate cancer. Others who are treated would have died of unrelated causes before their cancer became serious enough to affect their health and shorten their lives.
- Depending on the treatment selected, treatment of prostate cancer can lead to urinary, bowel, sexual, and other health problems. These problems may be significant or minimal, permanent or temporary.
- The PSA and DRE may have false-positive or false-negative results, meaning men without cancer may have abnormal results and undergo unnecessary additional testing and clinically significant cancers may have been missed. False-positive results can lead to sustained anxiety about prostate cancer risk.
- Abnormal results from screening with the PSA or DRE require prostate biopsies to determine whether the abnormal findings are cancer. Biopsies can be painful, may lead to complications such as infection or bleeding, and can miss clinically significant cancer.
- Not all men whose prostate cancer is discovered through screening require treatment, but they may require periodic blood tests and prostate biopsies to determine the need for future treatment.
- In helping men reach the screening decision based on their personal values, once they understand the uncertainties, risks, and potential benefits, it can be helpful to provide reasons why some men decide for or against undergoing screening. For example:
  - A man who chooses to be screened might place a higher value on finding cancer early and might be willing to risk injury to urinary, sexual, and/or bowel function.
  - A man who chooses not to be screened might place a higher value on avoiding the potential harms of screening and treatment such as anxiety or risk of injury to urinary, sexual, and/or bowel function.

PSA, prostate-specific antigen; DRE, digital rectal examination.

From Smith RA, Cokkinides V, Brawley OW. Cancer screening in the United States, 2012: a review of current American Cancer Society guidelines and current issues in cancer screening. CA Cancer J Clin. 2012.

is often considered first-line care, especially if complete resection is possible. However, considerable toxicity may attend that choice—for example, impotence and loss of bladder control in prostate cancer or the need to use a colostomy, temporarily or permanently, in some colorectal carcinomas. Classical chemotoxic chemotherapy, while providing benefit, is often accompanied by significant side effects, some of which (e.g., neuropathy) may be permanent. Additionally, radiation therapy itself may harm tissues around or underneath the target site. Finally, hormone sensitivity of many early prostate cancers permits the use of androgen blockade as an effective therapy, but there are side effects such as erectile dysfunction, loss of bone and muscle, feminization, and hot flashes, making this a difficult therapy for most patients.

Although there are strategies that should be used to reduce the toxicity of conventional treatments (see later), the quest for more precise and less harsh interventions has led to a new area of treatment that involves the use of therapies targeted to molecular mechanisms or gene mutations in individual patients. This represents the transformation of oncology from the uniform treatment of large groups of patients to the targeted therapy of individual subjects. Most experts consider this the future of conventional oncology. By and large, the therapies are less toxic than the therapies they seek to replace and many are oral, thereby improving the disruptions of parenteral cancer treatment. Significant toxicity still accompanies a number of these therapies as well.

MITIGATING TOXICITY OF COMMON CHEMOTHERAPEUTIC AGENTS

Cytoxic chemotherapy, newer targeted therapy, and radiation all have significant side effect profiles. The majority of these symptoms (e.g., nausea) resolve with the completion of treatment. Others, such as neuropathy, can be permanent and if severe enough will necessitate modification of the chemotherapy regimen either by delaying treatment or decreasing the dose given. Although there are many effective pharmaceutical medications for side effects, dietary supplements and other CAM therapies can do an excellent job in blunting some of these symptoms as well, often with fewer side effects of their own. There is a growing body of literature in this area, so a limited review will have to suffice here.

Conventional oncologists have raised concerns regarding the risk of antioxidant (AO) dietary supplement use during chemotherapy and radiation. It is known that antioxidant status decreases during conventional chemotherapy, so the idea of antioxidant repletion has at least the benefit of biologic plausibility (Ladas et al., 2004). A systematic review analyzed 19 randomized clinical trials that involved the concurrent use of AO vitamins and conventional chemotherapy and reported on treatment efficacy. There was no evidence reported of significant decreases in the efficacy of conventional chemotherapy (Block et al., 2007). Further analysis demonstrated that a number of supplemental AOs actually decreased symptom toxicity. The agents tested, including glutathione, melatonin, vitamin A, AO mixtures, N-acetylcysteine, vitamin E (VE), selenium, L-carnitine, coenzyme Q10, and ellagic acid, showed reduction in a variety of dose-limiting toxicities (Block et al., 2008). A meta-analysis showed that selenium supplementation decreased the nephrotoxicity of cis-platinum and the side effects of radiation during active treatment (Fritz et al., 2011).

Stomatitis and mucositis are predictable side effects of a number of therapies including cytotoxic chemotherapy (taxanes, platinum-based agents, 5-FU, methotrexate, etoposide, etc.), radiation, and certain targeted therapies. These symptoms are particularly difficult because it interferes with proper nutrition. Further, the condition seen in the mouth is continued throughout the mucosa of the rest of the digestive tract and can result in increased intestinal permeability or malabsorption. Good oral hygiene using agents formulated for dry mouth and simple saline mouthwash constitute the first line of treatment. Oral glutamine, an amino acid, has been used effectively as a preventative agent. Doses tested in clinical trials ranged from 8 to 24 g/day given during the first 4 to 7 days of the chemotherapy cycle. Topical VE in a dose of 100 mg applied directly to the mouth tissues and an oral mouthwash consisting of 400 mg/ml have decreased mucositis. Oral zinc decreased the development of mucositis in head and neck radiation patients when 25 to 50 mg was given three times a day. Mild improvements that were not always statistically significant were seen with two herbal mouthwashes containing either aloe vera or a German chamomile extract. Even something as simple as sucking on ice during the intravenous administration of chemotherapy or using honey in a sore mouth provided at least some relief. Benefit for all therapies was much more limited with 5-FU chemotherapy (Hardy, 2008).

Peripheral neuropathy can be a permanent, debilitating side effect of taxanes, 5-FU, and platinum-based drugs, among others. Once again, glutamine is an effective preventative agent for neuropathy in similar doses to those used for mucositis. Improvements were seen in dysesthesias, pain, and weakness. There was less interference with walking and activities of daily living. Overall, less modification of the chemotherapy routines was needed in glutamine-treated patients. Using a 300- to 600-mg dose of VE per day decreased neuropathy associated with taxane and platinum-based chemotherapy significantly without any evidence of adverse effects (Hardy, 2008). α-Lipoic acid, often used for diabetic neuropathy, has shown some success in small trials using doses of

1,800 mg/day (Pachman et al., 2011). Melatonin in high doses of 10 to 20 mg has improved neuropathy symptoms in lung cancer patients. In addition, these doses have shown increased survival for LC and CRC patients in clinical trials. All of these trials but two have been conducted by one group, indicating the need for caution in interpreting these data until they are replicated by more trials. No significant side effects were seen, even with high doses of melatonin (Seeley et al., 2012). More recent preclinical work suggests that melatonin may be as effective at substantially lower doses.

Nausea

Ginger, very popular in herbal traditions around the world, both as a food and as a medicine, decreases nausea from a wide variety of causes (including chemotherapy-induced nausea and vomiting [CINV]). Ginger in doses as low as 1 g of powdered encapsulated herb daily has been shown to decrease nausea following gynecologic oncology surgery. This dose of ginger also performed as well as metoclopramide for patients receiving cis-platinum-based chemotherapy (Hardy, 2008). However, a study testing oral ginger (1 or 2 g daily) used adjunctively with the newer 5-HT3 receptor agonists did not show that ginger provided any additional benefit for acute or delayed CINV (Zick et al., 2009). A second trial in children and adolescents taking a highly emetogenic chemotherapy for sarcoma found different results. Children taking 1 or 2 g of powdered ginger a day, depending on their weight, had one-third the incidence of moderate to severe nausea as the nonginger group (15% vs. 47%; $p = 0.022$; Pillai et al., 2011). The addition of high-protein foods to a ginger regimen can augment the antiemetic effects as well (Levine et al., 2008).

RADIATION DERMATITIS

Radiation frequently causes skin changes that induce significant morbidity in patients undergoing this type of treatment. Risk factors for radiation-induced dermatitis include fairer skin and higher dose of ionizing radiation. Conventional care recommendations include advice to use mild soaps without perfumes or other potentially irritating ingredients. Any skin that will be sun exposed after treatment should also be protected with high-SPF sunblock. Additional benefit can be gained by topical application of certain herbal remedies. Aloe vera is the plant most patients identify for this use, and many will advocate splitting a fresh leaf and then putting the extruded gel directly on the skin. This strategy probably should be discouraged given the risk of contaminating the skin with inadequately prepared plant material. Results for commercially prepared aloe products were mixed likely due to the great variation in this category of goods. Thus, a firm conclusion regarding the effectiveness of aloe generally cannot be drawn. The largest controlled clinical trial of nonconventional treatment of radiation dermatitis ($n = 254$) was conducted using a homeopathic calendula cream applied twice a day starting at the beginning of a course of radiation therapy. The incidence of grade II or higher dermatitis was significantly less in the calendula-treated group (41% vs. 61%; $p < 0.001$; Hardy, 2008).

Advising patients appropriately on the use of dietary supplements during cancer care leads to safe and effective use of supplements and improvements in outcomes if a few simple guidelines are followed (see Box 16.4). Patients are often reluctant to disclose use to the oncologist, leaving the primary care provider often in a better position to have a clearer idea of what the patient is taking. Questioning about use should be done in an open-ended nonjudgmental manner, and the patient should be encouraged to disclose use to the oncologic team as well. The safety margin of the products discussed in this section is quite high as long as the products are well made and without any adulterants or other unexpected additions (Hardy, 2008).

Acupuncture has been shown to be helpful in the management of a variety of difficult cancer treatment–related side effects. Three separate articles have demonstrated benefit for the use of acupuncture for the relief of pain

---

Box 16.4 Recommendations to Maximize Gain and Minimize Risk in Use of Dietary Supplements During Cancer Care

Encourage full disclosure from patients.
  Assist patients to establish reasonable goals.
  Develop a nuanced message about dietary supplement use.
  Develop knowledge base regarding dietary supplement.
  Favor dietary supplements from well-known, reputable companies.
  Favor simpler over more complex dietary supplements.
  Favor products that have been tested in human clinical trials.
  Ask to see the actual products the patients are using.
  Ask to see the resources patients use to guide decisions.
  Collaborate with the patients to form a treatment plan.
  Monitor patients during use of dietary supplements.

From Hardy M. Dietary supplement use in cancer care: help or harm. Hematol Oncol Clin N Am. 2008;22:581–617.

postoperatively after thoracotomy and following surgery for a variety of other solid tumors including tumors of the prostate. One study also showed modest improvement in chemotherapy-induced neuropathy. A large study in China ($n = 682$) demonstrated that the white blood cell (WBC) counts were higher in lung cancer patients treated with acupuncture than the untreated control group when both groups were given equivalent conventional therapy. Another large trial ($n = 739$) showed that acupuncture treatment decreased chemotherapy-related nausea, and a smaller trial using conventional antiemetics and electropoint acupuncture induced a complete remission of nausea in two thirds of postoperative cancer patients. For radiation-induced xerostomia, small studies have shown benefit even after completion of head and neck cancer therapy. Modest improvements in postchemotherapy fatigue were shown in a small, uncontrolled study (Lu & Dean-Clower, 2008). Acupuncture has been suggested to be helpful for hot flashes associated with androgen deprivation therapy. Despite positive reports in uncontrolled studies, few randomized controlled trials have been conducted.

Massage therapy has been evaluated in a number of different cancer patient populations. Benefit in terms of decrease of symptoms such as pain, anxiety, depression, fatigue, and nausea has been reported in a number of clinical trials. A variety of different touch therapies were used and involved everything from limited massage (foot, neck, back, and shoulders) to full-body massage. These interventions were often combined with other relaxing therapies such as meditation or aromatherapy (Meyers et al., 2008).

Mindfulness-based stress reduction (MBSR), relaxation training, meditation, guided imagery, hypnosis, art and music therapy, and biofeedback are mind–body therapies that have proven useful for cancer patients. Exercise, yoga, and other physical movement therapies benefit the patient beyond the benefit derived from the physical activity alone. One of the most closely studied therapies, MBSR, has shown highly significant effects in a pooled analysis of global improvement in quality of life of cancer patients ($p < 0.00005$). Highly statistical results were also seen for improved mood and reduced distress ($p < 0.0001$; Musial et al., 2011).

Individualization of mind–body therapies based on patient preferences is essential, and patients may be more comfortable in nonmedical settings. These therapies are often delivered at cancer treatment centers but more often in community support settings. Although many men are reluctant to participate in group activities, strong psychosocial networks and active support help mitigate some of the stress engendered by cancer diagnosis and treatment. Involvement of the family and other care providers as well as the patient improves the efficacy of these treatments. It has been the experience at our center that mind–body therapies not only relieve physical symptoms but also help relieve the suffering (as opposed to the pain) experienced following a cancer diagnosis.

Dietary Supplement Use

Epidemiologic data has provided convincing evidence of cancer risk reduction based on dietary components and other lifestyle factors. Paradoxically, chemoprevention studies using the same nutrients as isolated chemoprevention agents have, with several exceptions, not shown positive results. It is assumed that artificial versions of these nutrients do not have the same effects as complex mixtures in foods. For other nutrients, associations with lower risk of disease occurrence and mortality are firm, but prospective studies of prevention have not been done.

Nutraceutical prevention studies are difficult to perform and are fraught with confounders. Endpoints of cancer occurrence or death are hard endpoints but take years to develop, making these trials difficult and expensive. Finally, it is also possible that there are subpopulations at increased risk or with inadequate diets that will benefit more from supplementation than the general population, but trials have not generally been designed to identify these subjects. Despite the fact that dietary supplements do not achieve the same results as dietary components, because many men take dietary supplements on a regular basis, it is important to be familiar with the literature in this area to facilitate effective counseling for patients.

MULTIVITAMINS AND SUPPLEMENTS

Supplement use is common in men. Male members of the VITamins and Lifestyle Cohort (VITAL) were questioned about their dietary supplement use and then observed prospectively. Over 1,600 prostate cancers were reported during this trial. No association with risk or benefit was seen for chondroitin, fish oil, ginkgo, coenzyme Q10, ginseng, glucosamine, or saw palmetto. A 42% reduction in risk of developing prostate cancer was seen in association with grapeseed extract, but no additional studies have been performed to validate this association (Brasky et al., 2011). A meta-analysis of 14 randomized controlled trials or case cohort studies testing a variety of supplements, including multivitamin (MVI) vitamin E, vitamin C (VC), Zn, Se, and β-carotene, did not show any effect of these supplements on prostate cancer rate or severity (Stratton & Godwin, 2011).

Further, long-term use of MVI, VC, VE, and folic acid did not decrease the risk of lung cancer in the VITAL cohort. In fact, it is possible that VE supplementation may have represented a small increased risk, which was confined to current smokers (Slatore et al., 2008).

Vitamin D and Calcium

A review of 63 observational trials using surrogates of ultraviolet (UV) exposure such as latitude, season, ambient sunlight, and the risk of cancer shows a strong inverse association between higher sun exposure and lower cancer rates, with the exception of skin cancers. This difference is attributable to lower vitamin D (VD) levels in populations with lower sun exposure, leading to lower serum VD levels. This relationship was strongest for colon and prostate cancers (Garland & Garland, 2006).

An epidemic of VD deficiency has been identified because a majority of the Western populations, particularly African Americans, have very low levels. Ninety percent of the adult population of Great Britain is considered to be VD deficient, and cases of rickets are now being diagnosed with greater frequency. Serum VD levels are considered sufficient for osteoporosis prevention if they are above 30 to 35 ng/ml and toxic if they are over 150 ng/ml. However, for cancer prevention low levels may not be high enough. In a cohort of newly diagnosed cancer patients, 19% of men presented with VD levels of less than 12 ng/ml, and only 27% were VD sufficient with a serum VD level of greater than 32 ng/ml. The mean VD at presentation was 19 ng/ml (Vashi et al., 2010). Supplementation with 8,000 IU VD_3/day raised the mean serum VD level to 36 ng/ml after 14 weeks of supplementation. Very deficient patients were still unlikely to raise their VD to the sufficient range by the end of this period of supplementation.

Compelling evidence exists to support VD supplementation as a strategy to decrease the incidence and severity of cancer. VD levels less than 16 ng/ml were associated with a 70% increase in the incidence of PC and a sixfold increase in the incidence of invasive cancer (Garland & Garland, 2006). Low VD levels have been correlated with a worse prognosis in colon and prostate cancer. Unfortunately, supplementation with VD in men with advanced prostate cancer did not always improve prognosis (Buttigliero et al., 2011). The proposed ideal range for serum VD to mitigate cancer risk is between 40 and 60 ng/ml. At that level, it is postulated that almost 50,000 new cases of colon cancer would be prevented each year in the United States and Canada and deaths from colon cancer would be reduced by three quarters Further, it has been estimated that ensuring a serum VD of 34 ng/ml in the general population would decrease the rate of colon cancer by 50% (Garland & Gorham, 2009). Estimates of epidemiologic studies suggest that supplementing every

American with 1,000 IU of VD$_3$ would decrease the rate of cancer mortality in men by 7%, and in higher latitude countries that rate would be doubled. In this era of cost constraints, cost estimates for this intervention, $1 billion, must also be balanced against an expected savings in reduced treatment costs of $16 billion to $25 billion (Grant et al., 2007).

Calcium supplementation alone was not associated with risk reduction for CRC in a general population of average risk according to a recent meta-analysis (C. Carroll et al., 2010). However, further analysis showed that calcium supplementation in the range of 1,200 to 2,000 mg/day statistically significantly reduced the risk of recurrence of adenomas (RR. 80; p = 0.006). There is some evidence that nondairy calcium intake may be associated with an increased risk of prostate cancer. Data from the European Prospective Investigation into Cancer and Nutrition (EPIC) study found that high intake of calcium from dairy products was positively associated with risk of prostate cancer (RR 1.2) in 142,000 men over nearly a 9-year period (Allen et al., 2008).

The Institute of Medicine's (IOM's) most recent recommendation for the general population for intake of VD is 600 IU for adults and 800 IU for those over 70 years of age. The recommendation for calcium was 1,000 mg for males and 1,200 mg for females and males over 50 years of age (IOM Report on Vitamin D, 2010). Many experts concerned with cancer risk do not agree with the IOM recommendations and would recommend a daily dose of at least 1,000 IU and preferably 2,000 IU. Following blood levels and supplementing with as much VD as needed to achieve a serum VD of 40 to 60 ng/ml allows the most individualized and precise control of VD dosage (Garland & Gorhan, 2009).

Selenium

Early data from randomized controlled trials (RCTs) indicated a protective role for selenium supplementation as well as VE. For example, in a meta-analysis of nine large RCTs, selenium was the only nutritional supplement that was found to reduce by 25% the overall risk of all types of cancer tested including lung, colon, and prostate cancer (Lee et al., 2011). A second meta-analysis, looking only at lung cancer and including a wider range of evidence, suggested that selenium may protect patients with an initially low serum selenium.

Vitamin E

Although a 10-year history of supplemental VE use in the VITAL study was not associated with an overall decrease in PC rate, it was associated with a significant decrease in risk of advanced prostate cancer (hazard ratio [HR]

0.43; p for trend <0.03) (Peters et al., 2008). A report from the Prostate, Lung, Colorectal and Ovarian Cancer Screening (PLCOS) prospective cohort trial showed a decreasing risk of advanced PC with increasing dose and duration of VE supplementation in current or recent smokers (within the last 10 years; Kirsh et al., 2006).

To test the hypothesis that VE and selenium would decrease the risk of developing PC, the Selenium and Vitamin E Cancer Prevention trial (SELECT) was started. Selenium (200 mcg) and vitamin E (400 IU of all-rac-α-tocopheryl acetate) were tested in a multifactorial randomized controlled trial. The study was stopped because it appeared that the VE supplementation in this form increased the risk of PC (Klein & Thompson, 2001). More information on this trial can be found in Chapter 3 on nutritional supplements.

Folic Acid

In the United States fortification of grains with folic acid (FA) to prevent birth defects provides a baseline supplementation for the general population. In numerous epidemiologic studies folate-rich foods have shown an inverse dose-response relationship with the incidence of colon cancer, but the results from clinical studies have been mixed (AICR). A large prospective observational trial (Cancer Prevention Study II) following more than 43,000 men showed a significantly decreased risk of CRC development with high dietary or supplemental folic acid (Stevens & McCullough, 2011). Two additional large clinical trials, one cohort trial and one randomized controlled trial, using a lower dose of FA (1 mg/day) did not show any benefit in reducing recurrence of colorectal adenomas (Cole et al., 2007; Wu et al., 2009). In fact, in the RCT, FA supplementation was significantly associated with a higher risk of developing multiple lesions and more advanced adenomas (Cole et al., 2007). High-dose supplementation (5 mg/day) decreased the recurrence of polyps in a Veterans Administration population (n = 95) over 3 years in a randomized double-blind placebo-controlled trial. Response was better in younger patients (under 70 years of age) and those with left-sided lesions or with more advanced adenomas (Jaszewski et al., 2008). A meta-analysis of 27 recent cohort and case-control studies found a small beneficial effect on CRC incidence rather than any harm (Kennedy et al., 2011). This variability of response may be explained by the observation that FA and folate have a U-shaped response curve, suggesting a dual action in carcinogenesis. Early in the process increased levels suppress growth, but once the process is established, growth promotion occurs.

Limited data on FA supplementation and prostate cancer risk exists. In a single randomized controlled trial, the Aspirin/Folate Polyp Prevention Study,

FA supplementation decreased the risk of PC threefold (3.3% incidence vs. 9.7%; p = 0.01; Figueiredo et al., 2009). However, a meta-analysis of six RCTs showed a light increase in risk of prostate cancer (RR = 1.24 with 95% CI 1.03–1.49) for men receiving folic acid (Wien et al., 2012).

Many confounders could modify the effect of FA on cancer risk. The timing in the carcinogenic process and dose of FA as well as the form (natural or artificial) likely contribute to the effect. Significant genetic mutations play a role, as does alcohol intake, which depletes B vitamins and other key nutrients. For now, it seems prudent in general populations to avoid high chronic doses of FA (>800 mcg), and in high-risk populations or those with low serum folate levels, higher supplementation still could be beneficial but close observation is recommended.

Carotene and Other Carotenoids

In a meta-analysis of six RCTs involving more than 40,000 participants, no evidence of a risk reduction was seen for cancer in general or for cancer mortality. The lack of effect was similar for both primary and secondary prevention trials (Jeon et al., 2011). There may be subpopulations that would benefit from supplementation. For example, β-carotene supplementation at a rate of at least 2,000 mcg/day decreased the risk of PC in men with low dietary β-carotene intake (Kirsch et al., 2006).

An increased risk of lung cancer development was seen in two large randomized trials conducted on current male smokers using β-carotene and vitamin E. Unexpectedly, lung cancer risk was increased with the use of β-carotene alone. These trials very famously highlighted the risk of single-agent antioxidants in patients with high oxidative load (i.e., smokers) and highlighted risks of supplementation not predicted by dietary studies. In confirmation of these findings, the VITAL study looked at associated risk for a broader range of carotenoids: β-carotene, retinol, lycopene, and lutein. Longer use of β-carotene, retinol, and lutein was associated with increased risk of lung cancer (all histological types). Neither gender nor smoking status significantly changed these risks (Satia & Littman, 2009). In a meta-analysis of large RCTs, a small 7% increase in the rate of cancer among current smokers was reported (Jeon et al., 2011). Long-term use of isolated carotenoids in patients at risk for lung cancer should be discouraged.

Soy Isoflavones

Because the incidence of prostate cancer is lower in Asian than in Western countries, there has been much interest in unique aspects of the Asian diet, especially soy. A large prospective study (n = 45,509) of soy product consumption in Japanese men showed that increased consumption of miso soup, soy food, and their isoflavones genistein and daidzein was correlated with an overall decreased rate of localized cancer (Kurahashi et al., 2007). For men over 60 years of age, increased soy food consumption was associated in a dose-dependent fashion with a decreased rate of advanced PC. In American Adventists (vegetarians), high consumption of soy milk predicted a 70% decreased risk of prostate cancer (p = 0.03; Jacobsen et al., 1998).

Soy foods have been associated with decreased PC rates in observational trials, and isolated isoflavones have in clinical trials as well. A phase II trial of 54 men with early prostate cancer awaiting prostatectomy who took 30 mg of genistein for 3 to 6 weeks demonstrated a decrease in the PSA of 7.8% without any effect on either thyroid or sex hormones (Lazarevic et al., 2011). Another study in prostate cancer patients with rising PSAs evaluated the effect of 50 mg of mixed isoflavones taken twice a day. Patients were either in a period of watchful waiting, were on antiandrogen therapy, or had just completed local therapy. Although this study did not show a significant decline in PSA, PSA stabilized in 83% of the patients in the hormone-treated group and 35% of the hormone-refractory group. Overall, the total group showed a significant slowing in the rate of rise of PSA (Hussain et al., 2003). A 66% response rate was reported in another small case series of androgen-naïve patients who failed prostatectomy and salvage radiation therapy. In castration-resistant patients, a 33% response rate was seen using commercially available soy isoflavone products, suggesting a role for isolated isoflavones even after conventional treatments have failed (Joshi et al., 2011).

Soy isoflavones have also been shown to mitigate the side effects of radiation therapy in PC patients. Patients treated with 200 mg of isoflavones for 6 months beginning at the onset of radiation therapy had significantly less leakage or dribbling of urine, less painful bowel movements, less rectal cramping and diarrhea, and a greater ability to have erections (Ahmad et al., 2010).

A recent meta-analysis was performed to explore the relationship between lung cancer and soy intake (W. S. Yang et al., 2011). Eleven epidemiologic studies and eight case-control studies were analyzed and revealed a significant inverse relationship between increasing soy intake and lung cancer risk (RR 0.7795 CI 0.65, 0.92). Effects were higher in women than men, for never smokers, and for Asians.

Although increased soy intake was associated with an overall reduction in colon cancer risk of approximately 10% in a recent meta-analysis, this result was not statistically significant. Furthermore, when analyzed on the basis of gender, significant benefit accrued to women but not to men (Yan & Spitznagel,

2010). However, a subsequent large observational study in a Japanese population found a small benefit. For men in the highest quintile versus the lowest of use, the RR was 0.65 (p for trend = 0.03) soy foods and 0.68 (p for trend = 0.051; Budhathoki et al., 2011). These two studies, taken together, suggest that a small benefit would accrue to men eating soy to reduce colon cancer risk, but the greatest value of these foods would be to replace red meat in the diet, allowing for less red meat consumption.

Green Tea Extract

Epidemiologic data suggest a protective effect from CRC for patients who consume ten 6-ounce cups of green tea per day (AICR). Further, a pilot study (n = 136) followed patients after removal of colorectal adenoma for 1 year, during which time they were randomized to either take 1.5 g of green tea extract or placebo. All members of this group did drink green tea but at a dose lower than the protective level. Follow-up colonoscopy demonstrated half the rate of new polyp formation in the supplemented group than the control group (15% vs. 31%; p < 0.05). The polyps formed in the treated group were smaller as well (p < 0.001; Shimizu et al., 2008).

Curcumin

Extensive preclinical investigation into the molecular activity of curcumin, the active ingredient in the Indian spice tumeric, has generated great interest in this molecule and initiated early human clinical trials. Curcumin adversely affects multiple cell signaling pathways including those regulating cell cycle arrest, apoptosis, proliferation, cell survival, invasiveness, angiogenesis, and metastasis. Underlying these observed effects are the profoundly anti-inflammatory actions of curcumin on the molecular regulators of inflammation such as cyclooxygenase-2 (COX-2) and lipoxygenase-5 (LOX-5) enzymes; the inflammatory mediators tumor necrosis factor (TNF), interleukin-6 (IL-6), and IL-1; and the cellular mediator nuclear factor-κB (NF-κB). In cell lines, animal models, and/or early human trials, benefit has been seen for colon cancer principally but also for prostate cancer (Anand, Sundaram, et al., 2008).

Human clinical trials have mainly focused on high-risk conditions (ulcerative colitis [UC] and familial adenomatous polyposis) as well as colon cancer. Curcumin has been able to reduce inflammation and presumptively the progress of disease in UC, a high-risk condition for colon cancer. Curcumin supplementation was also shown to be a promising adjunctive therapy to maintain remission in UC patients undergoing medical treatment in a randomized double-blind placebo-controlled trial (Hanai et al., 2006). For familial ade-nomatous polyposis patients, the combination of curcumin and quercetin decreased polyp number and size (Cruz-Correa et al., 2006). In a phase IIa clinical trial, 4 g/day of curcumin decreased by 40% the number of aberrant crypt foci (ACF) in 44 smokers with prior ACFs ($p < 0.005$; R. E. Carroll et al., 2011). In a phase I study in refractory colorectal cancer patients, doses of a proprietary tumeric extract demonstrated safety and tolerability up to a dose of 2.2 g of extract containing 180 mg of curcumin. In addition, radiologi-cally stable disease was demonstrated in 5 of 15 patients included in this trial (Sharma et al., 2001). Curcumin has also been reported in preclinical studies to protect normal tissue while sensitizing cancer cells for chemotherapy and radiotherapy. Due to the very poor solubility of curcumin, novel drug delivery methods are under active investigation, although for colon cancer prevention, this may be of lesser importance because topical effects in the colonic mucosa would presumptively provide benefit (Bansal et al., 2011).

Summary

Integrative medicine approaches can be very important in cancer prevention and treatment. Dietary constituents including macronutrient composition and supplement use have been shown to have an impact on cancer incidence, especially with regard to the cancers most common in men. Lung, prostate, and colorectal cancer are the three most common cancers in men, and their incidence and treatment and the tolerance of treatment for these cancers are all especially amenable to lifestyle changes that form the basis for the integra-tive medicine approach.

REFERENCES

Ahmad IU, Forman JD, Sarkar FH, Hillman GG, Heath E, Vaishampayan U, Cher ML, Andic F, Rossi PJ, Kucuk O. Soy isoflavones in conjunc-tion with radiation therapy in patients with prostate cancer. Nutr Cancer. 2010;62(7):996–1000. doi:10.1080/01635581.2010.509839

Akl EA, Gaddam S, Gunukula SK, Honeine R, Jaoude PA, Irani J. The effects of waterpipe tobacco smoking on health outcomes: a systematic review. Int J Epidemiol. 2010;39(3):834–857. doi:10.1093/ije/dyq002

Allen NE, Key TJ et al. EPIC Trial Br J Cancer 2008 May 6;98(9):1574-1581.

Anand P, Kunnumakkara AB, Sundaram C, Harikumar KB, Tharakan ST, Lai OS, Sung B, Aggarwal BB. Cancer is a preventable disease that requires major lifestyle changes. Pharm Res. 2008;25(9):2097–2116. doi:10.1007/s11095-008-9661-9

Anand P, Sundaram C, Jhurani S, Kunnumakkara AB, Aggarwal BB. Curcumin and cancer: an "old-age" disease with an "age-old" solution. Cancer Lett. 2008; 267(1): 133–164. doi:10.1016/j.canlet.2008.03.025

Arcidiacono B, Iiritano S, Nocera A, Possidente K, Nevolo MT, Ventura V, Foti D, Chiefari E, Brunetti A. Insulin resistance and cancer risk: an overview of the pathogenetic mechanisms. Exp Diabetes Res. 2012;2012:789174. doi:10.1155/2012/789174

Aune D, Chan D, et al. Dietary fibre, whole grains and risk of colorectal cancer: a systematic review and dose-response meta-analysis of prospective studies. BMJ. 2011;343:d6617.

Bansal SS, Goel M, Aqil F, Vadhanam MV, Gupta RC. Advanced drug delivery systems of curcumin for cancer chemoprevention. Cancer Prev Res (Phila). 2011;4(8):1158–1171. doi:10.1158/1940-6207.CAPR-10-0006

Basen-Engquist K, Chang M. Obesity and cancer risk: recent review and evidence. Curr Oncol Rep. 2011;13(1):71–76. doi:10.1007/s11912-010-0139-7

Bishop FL, Rea A, Lewith H, Chan YK, Saville J, Prescott P, von Elm E, Lewith GT. Complementary medicine use by men with prostate cancer: a systematic review of prevalence studies. Prostate Cancer Prostatic Dis. 2011;14(1):1–13. doi:10.1038/pcan.2010.38

Block KI, Koch AC, Mead MN, Tothy PK, Newman RA, Gyllenhaal C. Impact of antioxidant supplementation on chemotherapeutic efficacy: a systematic review of the evidence from randomized controlled trials. Cancer Treat Rev. 2007;33(5):407–418.

Botteri E, Iodice S, Bagnardi V, Raimondi S, Lowenfels AB, Maisonneuve P. Smoking and colorectal cancer: a meta-analysis. JAMA. 2008;300(23):2765–2778. doi:10.1001/jama.2008.839

Brasky TM, Kristal AR, Navarro SL, Lampe JW, Peters U, Patterson RE, White E. Specialty supplements and prostate cancer risk in the VITamins and Lifestyle (VITAL) cohort. Nutr Cancer. 2011;63(4):573–582. doi:10.1080/01 635581.2011.553022

Budhathoki S, Joshi AM, Ohnaka K, Yin G, Toyomura K, Kono S, Mibu R, Tanaka M, Kakeji Y, Maehara Y, Okamura T, Ikejiri K, Futami K, Maekawa T, Yasunami Y, Takenaka K, Ichimiya H, Terasaka R. Soy food and isoflavone intake and colorectal cancer risk: the Fukuoka Colorectal Cancer Study. Scand J Gastroenterol. 2011;46(2):165–172. doi:10.3109/00365521.2010.522720

Butt MS, Sultan MT. Coffee and its consumption: benefits and risks. Crit Rev Food Sci Nutr. 2011;51(4):363–373. doi:10.1080/10408390903586412

Buttigliero C, Monagheddu C, Petroni P, Saini A, Dogliotti L, Ciccone G, Berruti A. Prognostic role of vitamin d status and efficacy of vitamin D supplementation in cancer patients: a systematic review. Oncologist. 2011;16(9):1215–1227. doi:10.1634/theoncologist.2011-0098

Carroll C, et al. Supplemental calcium in the chemo-prevention of colorectal cancer: a systematic review and meta-analysis. Clin Ther. 2010;32(5):789–803.

Carroll RE, Benya RV, Turgeon DK, Vareed S, Neuman M, Rodriguez L, Kakarala M, Carpenter PM, McLaren C, Meyskens FL Jr, Brenner DE. Phase IIa clinical trial of curcumin for the prevention of colorectal neoplasia. Cancer Prev Res (Phila). 2011;4(3):354–364. doi:10.1158/1940-6207. CAPR-10-0098

Cole BF, Baron JA, Sandler RS, Haile RW, Ahnen DJ, Bresalier RS, McKeown-Eyssen G, Summers RW, Rothstein RI, Burke CA, Snover DC, Church TR, Allen JI, Robertson DJ, Beck GJ, Bond JH, Byers T, Mandel JS, Mott LA, Pearson LH, Barry EL, Rees JR, Marcon N, Saibil F, Ueland PM, Greenberg ER; Polyp Prevention Study Group. Folic acid for the prevention of colorectal adenomas: a randomized clinical trial. JAMA. 2007;297(21):2351–2359.

Cruz-Correa M, Shoskes DA, Sanchez P, Zhao R, Hylind LM, Wexner SD, Giardiello FM. Combination treatment with curcumin and quercetin of adenomas in familial adenomatous polyposis. Clin Gastroenterol Hepatol. 2006;4(8):1035–1038.

De Nunzio C, Albisinni S, Freedland SJ, Miano L, Cindolo L, Finazzi Agrò E, Autorino R, De Sio M, Schips L, Tubaro A. Abdominal obesity as risk factor for prostate cancer diagnosis and high grade disease: a prospective multicenter Italian cohort study. Urol Oncol. 2011; Sep 16. [Epub ahead of print]

Demark-Wahnefried W, Aziz NM, Rowland JH, Pinto BM. Riding the crest of the teachable moment: promoting long-term health after the diagnosis of cancer. J Clin Oncol. 2005;23(24):5814–5830.

Eng J, Ramsum D, Verhoef M, Guns E, Davison J, Gallagher R. A population-based survey of complementary and alternative medicine use in men recently diagnosed with prostate cancer. Integr Cancer Ther. 2003;2(3):212–216.

Evans M, Shaw A, et al. Decisions to use complementary and alternative medicine by male cancer patients: information-seeking roles and types of evidence used. BMC Complement Altern Med 2007;7:25.

Fedirko V, Tramacere I, Bagnardi V, Rota M, Scotti L, Islami F, Negri E, Straif K, Romieu I, La Vecchia C, Boffetta P, Jenab M. Alcohol drinking and colorectal cancer risk: an overall and dose-response meta-analysis of published studies. Ann Oncol. 2011;22(9):1958–1972. doi:10.1093/annonc/mdq653

Figueiredo JC, Grau MV, Haile RW, Sandler RS, Summers RW, Bresalier RS, Burke CA, McKeown-Eyssen GE, Baron JA. Folic acid and risk of prostate cancer: results from a randomized clinical trial. Natl Cancer Inst. 2009;101(6):432–435. doi:10.1093/jnci/djp019

Fritz H, Kennedy D, Fergusson D, Fernandes R, Cooley K, et al. Selenium and lung cancer: a systematic review and meta analysis. PLoS ONE 2011;6(11): e26259. doi:10.1371/journal.pone.0026259

Galeone C, Turati F, La Vecchia C, Tavani A. Coffee consumption and risk of colorectal cancer: a meta-analysis of case-control studies. Cancer Causes Control. 2010;21(11):1949–1959. doi:10.1007/s10552-010-9623-5

Garland CF, Garland FC. Do sunlight and vitamin D reduce the likelihood of colon cancer? Int J Epidemiol. 2006;35(2):217–220.

Garland CF, Gorham ED, et al. Vitamin D for cancer prevention: global perspective. Ann Epidemiol 2009 Jul;19(7):468-483.

Giovannucci E, Liu Y, Stampfer MJ, Willett WC. A prospective study of calcium intake and incident and fatal prostate cancer. Cancer Epidemiol Biomarkers Prev. 2006;15(2):203–210.

Gonzalez CA, Riboli E. Diet and cancer prevention: contributions from the European Prospective Investigation into Cancer and Nutrition (EPIC) study. Eur J Cancer. 2010;46(14):2555–2562. doi:10.1016/j.ejca.2010.07.025

Grant WB, Garland CF, Gorham ED. An estimate of cancer mortality rate reductions in Europe and the US with 1,000 IU of oral vitamin D per day. Recent Results Cancer Res. 2007;174:225–234.

Hanai, H et al. Curcumin maintenance therapy for ulcerative colitis: randomized, multicenter, double-blind, placebo-controlled trial. Clin Gastroenterol Hepatol. 2006;4(12):1502–1506.

Hardy M. Dietary supplement use in cancer care: help or harm. Hematol Oncol Clin N Am. 2008;22:581–617.

Huncharek M, Haddock KS, Reid R, Kupelnick B. Smoking as a risk factor for prostate cancer: a meta-analysis of 24 prospective cohort studies. Am J Public Health. 2010;100(4):693–701. doi:10.2105/AJPH.2008.150508

Hussain M, Banerjee M, Sarkar FH, Djuric Z, Pollak MN, Doerge D, Fontana J, Chinni S, Davis J, Forman J, Wood DP, Kucuk O. Soy isoflavones in the treatment of prostate cancer. Nutr Cancer. 2003;47(2):111–117.

Jacobsen BK, Knutsen SF, Fraser GE. Does high soy milk intake reduce prostate cancer incidence? The Adventist Health Study (United States). Cancer Causes Control. 1998;9(6):553–557.

Jaszewski R, Misra S, Tobi M, Ullah N, Naumoff JA, Kucuk O, Levi E, Axelrod BN, Patel BB, Majumdar AP. Folic acid supplementation inhibits recurrence of colorectal adenomas: a randomized chemoprevention trial. World J Gastroenterol. 2008;14(28):4492–4498.

Jeon YJ, Myung SK, Lee EH, Kim Y, Chang YJ, Ju W, Cho HJ, Seo HG, Huh BY. Effects of beta-carotene supplements on cancer prevention: meta-analysis of randomized controlled trials. Nutr Cancer. 2011;63(8):1196–1207. doi:10.1080/01635581.2011.607541

Johnsen NF, Tjønneland A, et al. Physical activity and risk of prostate cancer in the European Prospective Investigation into Cancer and Nutrition (EPIC) cohort. Int J Cancer. 2009;125(4):902–908. doi:10.1002/ijc.24326

Joshi M, et al. Effects of commercially available soy products on PSA in androgenic-deprivation – naïve and castration-resistant prostate cancer. South Med J. 2011;104(11):736–740.

Kennedy DA, et al. Folate intake and the risk of colorectal cancer: a systematic review and meta-analysis. Cancer Epidemiol. 2011;35(1):2–10.

Kim MK, Park JH. Conference on "Multidisciplinary approaches to nutritional problems". Symposium on "Nutrition and health". Cruciferous vegetable intake and the risk of human cancer: epidemiological evidence. Proc Nutr Soc. 2009;68(1):103–110. doi:10.1017/S0029665108008884

Kirsch VA, et al. Supplemental and dietary vitamin E, beta carotene and vitamin C intakes and prostate cancer risk. JNCI J Natl Cancer Inst. 2006;98(4):221. doi:10.1093/jnci/djj108

Klein EA, Thompson IM jr et al. Vitamin E and the risk of prostate cancer: the Seenium and Vitamin E cancer prevention trial (SELECT). JAMA. 2011;306(14):1549-1556.

Kurahashi N, et al. Soy product and isoflavone consumption in relation to prostate caner in Japanese men. Cancer Epidemiol Biomarkers Prev. 2007;16:538.

Kushi LH, Doyle C, McCullough M, Rock CL, Demark-Wahnefried W, Bandera EV, Gapstur S, Patel AV, Andrews K, Gansler T; American Cancer Society 2010 Nutrition and Physical Activity Guidelines Advisory Committee. American Cancer Society Guidelines on nutrition and physical activity for cancer prevention: reducing the risk of cancer with healthy food choices and physical activity. CA Cancer J Clin. 2012;62(1):30–67. doi:10.3322/caac.20140

Ladas EJ, Jacobson JS, Kennedy DD, Teel K, Fleischauer A, Kelly KM. Antioxidants and cancer therapy: a systematic review. J Clin Oncol. 2004;22(3):517–528.

Lattimer J, Haub M. Effects of dietary fiber and its components on metabolic health. Nutrients. 2010;2:1266–1289. doi:10.3390/nu2121266

Lazarevic B, Boezelijn G, Diep LM, Kvernrod K, Ogren O, Ramberg H, Moen A, Wessel N, Berg RE, Egge-Jacobsen W, Hammarstrom C, Svindland A, Kucuk O, Saatcioglu F, Taskèn KA, Karlsen SJ. Efficacy and safety of short-term genistein intervention in patients with localized prostate cancer prior to radical prostatectomy: a randomized, placebo-controlled, double-blind Phase 2 clinical trial. Nutr Cancer. 2011;63(6):889–898. doi:10.1080/01635581.2011.582221

Lee EH, Myung SK, Jeon YJ, Kim Y, Chang YJ, Ju W, Seo HG, Huh BY. Effects of selenium supplements on cancer prevention: meta-analysis of randomized controlled trials. Nutr Cancer. 2011;63(8):1185–1195. doi:10.1080/016355 81.2011.607544

Levine ME, Gillis MG, Koch SY, Voss AC, Stern RM, Koch KL. Protein and ginger for the treatment of chemotherapy-induced delayed nausea. J Altern Complement Med. 2008;14(5):545–551. doi:10.1089/acm.2007.0817

Lippert MC, McClain R, Boyd JC, Theodorescu D. Alternative medicine use in patients with localized prostate carcinoma treated with curative intent. Cancer. 1999;86(12):2642–248.

Lophatananon A, Archer J, Easton D, Pocock R, Dearnaley D, Guy M, Kote-Jarai Z, O'Brien L, Wilkinson RA, Hall AL, Sawyer E, Page E, Liu JF, Barratt S, Rahman AA; UK Genetic Prostate Cancer Study Collaborators; British Association of Urological Surgeons' Section of Oncology, Eeles R, Muir K. Dietary fat and early-onset prostate cancer risk. Br J Nutr. 2010;103(9):1375–1380. doi:10.1017/S0007114509993291

Lu W, Dean-CLower, E et al. The value of acupuncture in cancer care. Hematol Oncol Clin N Am. 2008 Aug;22(4):631-648.

Mariotto AB, Yabroff KR, Shao Y, Feuer EJ, Brown ML. Projections of the cost of cancer care in the United States: 2010–2020. J Natl Cancer Inst. 2011;103(2):117–128. doi:10.1093/jnci/djq495

McDermott CL, Blough DK, et al. Complementary and alternative medicine use among newly diagnosed prostate cancer patients. Support Care Cancer. 2012 Jan;20(1):65–73.

Meyerhardt JA, Heseltine D, Niedzwiecki D, Hollis D, Saltz LB, Mayer RJ, Thomas J, Nelson H, Whittom R, Hantel A, Schilsky RL, Fuchs CS. Impact of physical activity on cancer recurrence and survival in patients with stage III colon cancer: findings from CALGB 89803. J Clin Oncol. 2006;24(22):3535–3541.

Meyerhardt JA, Niedzwiecki D, Hollis D, Saltz LB, Hu FB, Mayer RJ, Nelson H, Whittom R, Hantel A, Thomas J, Fuchs CS. Association of dietary patterns with cancer recurrence and survival in patients with stage III colon cancer. JAMA. 2007;298(7):754–764.

Mordukhovich I, Reiter PL, Backes DM, Family L, McCullough LE, O'Brien KM, Razzaghi H, Olshan AF. A review of African American-white differences in risk factors for cancer: prostate cancer. Cancer Causes Control. 2011;22(3):341–357. doi:10.1007/s10552-010-9712-5

Musial F, Büssing A, Heusser P, Choi KE, Ostermann T. Mindfulness-based stress reduction for integrative cancer care: a summary of evidence. Forsch Komplementmed. 2011;18(4):192–202. doi:10.1159/000330714

Myers CD, Walton T, Bratsman L, Wilson J, Small B. Massage modalities and symptoms reported by cancer patients: narrative review. J Soc Integr Oncol. 2008;6(1):19–28.

Pachman DR, Barton DL, Watson JC, Loprinzi CL. Chemotherapy-induced peripheral neuropathy: prevention and treatment. Clin Pharmacol Ther. 2011;90(3):377–387. doi:10.1038/clpt.2011.115

Pan A, Sun Q, Bernstein AM, Schulze MB, Manson JE, Stampfer MJ, Willett WC, Hu FB. Red meat consumption and mortality: results from 2 prospective cohort studies. Arch Intern Med. 2012;172(7):555–563. doi:10.1001/archinternmed.2011.2287

Park CH, Myung SK, Kim TY, Seo HG, Jeon YJ, Kim Y; Korean Meta-Analysis (KORMA) Study Group. Coffee consumption and risk of prostate cancer: a meta-analysis of epidemiological studies. BJU Int. 2010;106(6):762–769. doi:10.1111/j.1464-410X.2010.09493.x

Parsons A, Daley A, et al. Influence of smoking cessation after diagnosis of early stage lung cancer on prognosis: a systematic review of observational studies with meta-analysis. BMJ. 2010;340:b5569.

Patterson RE, Neuhouser ML, Hedderson MM, Schwartz SM, Standish LJ, Bowen DJ, Marshall LM. Types of alternative medicine used by patients with breast, colon, or prostate cancer: predictors, motives, and costs. J Altern Complement Med. 2002;8(4):477–485.

Pauwels EK. The protective effect of the Mediterranean diet: focus on cancer and cardiovascular risk. Med Princ Pract. 2011;20(2):103–111. doi: 10.1159/000321197

Peters U, et al. Vitamin E and selenium supplementation and risk of prostate cancer in the vitamins and lifestyle (VITAL) study cohort. Cancer Causes Control. 2008;19:75–87.

Pillai AK, Sharma KK, Gupta YK, Bakhshi S. Anti-emetic effect of ginger powder versus placebo as an add-on therapy in children and young adults receiving high emetogenic chemotherapy. Pediatr Blood Cancer. 2011;56(2):234–238.

Prochaska JO, Norcross JC, DiClemente CC. *Changing for Good.* New York: Morrow, 1994. Released in paperback by Avon, 1995.

Richman EL, Stampfer MJ, Paciorek A, Broering JM, Carroll PR, Chan JM. Intakes of meat, fish, poultry, and eggs and risk of prostate cancer progression. Am J Clin Nutr. 2010;91(3):712–721. doi:10.3945/ajcn.2009.28474

Rigotti NA, Munafo MR, Stead LF. Interventions for smoking cessation in hospitalised patients. Cochrane Database Syst Rev. 2007;(3):CD001837.

Rollnick S, Mason P, Butler C. *Health Behavior Change: A Guide for Practitioners.* New York: Churchill Livingstone, 1999.

Rollnick ST, Miller W. *Motivational Interviewing in Health Care: Helping Patients Change Behavior.* Guilford Press, 2007.

Satia JA, Littman A, et al. Associations of herbal and specialty supplements with lung and colorectal cancer risk in the VITamins and Lifestyle study. Cancer Epidemiol Biomarkers Prev. 2009 May;18(5):1419-1428.

Seely D, Wu P, Fritz H, Kennedy DA, Tsui T, Seely AJ, Mills E. Melatonin as adjuvant cancer care with and without chemotherapy: a systematic review and meta-analysis of randomized trials. Integr Cancer Ther. 2012;11(4):293–303. doi:10.1177/1534735411425484

Sharma RA, McLelland HR, Hill KA, Ireson CR, Euden SA, Manson MM, Pirmohamed M, Marnett LJ, Gescher AJ, Steward WP. Pharmacodynamic and pharmacokinetic study of oral Curcuma extract in patients with colorectal cancer. Clin Cancer Res. 2001;7(7):1894–1900.

Shimizu M, Fukutomi Y, Ninomiya M, Nagura K, Kato T, Araki H, Suganuma M, Fujiki H, Moriwaki H. Green tea extracts for the prevention of metachronous colorectal adenomas: a pilot study. Cancer Epidemiol Biomarkers Prev. 2008;17(11):3020–3025. doi:10.1158/1055-9965.EPI-08-0528

Siegel R, Ward E, Brawley O, Jemal A. The impact of eliminating socioeconomic and racial disparities on premature cancer deaths. CA Cancer J Clin. 2011;61(4):212–236.

Slatore CG, Littman AJ, Au DH, Satia JA, White E. Long-term use of supplemental multivitamins, vitamin C, vitamin E, and folate does not reduce the risk of lung cancer. Am J Respir Crit Care Med. 2008;177(5):524–530.

Smith L, Brinton LA et al. Body mass Index and risk of lung cancer among never, former and current smokers. JNCI 2012 May 16;104(10):778-789.

Smith RA, Cokkinides V, Brawley OW. Cancer screening in the United States, 2012: a review of current American Cancer Society guidelines and current issues in cancer screening. CA Cancer J Clin. 2012.

Stevens VL, McCullough ML, et al. High levels of folate from supplements and fortification are not associated with increased risk of colorectal cancer. Gastroenterology. 2011 Jul;141(1):98–105.

Stratton J, Godwin M. The effect of supplemental vitamins and minerals on the development of prostate cancer: a systematic review and meta analysis. Fam Pract 2011 Jun;28(3):243-252.

Tang N, Wu Y, Zhou B, Wang B, Yu R. Green tea, black tea consumption and risk of lung cancer: a meta-analysis. Lung Cancer. 2009;65(3):274–283. doi:10.1016/j.lungcan.2008.12.002

Tantamango YM, Knutsen SF, Beeson WL, Fraser G, Sabate J. Foods and food groups associated with the incidence of colorectal polyps: the Adventist Health Study. Nutr Cancer. 2011;63(4):565–572.

Thune I, Furberg AS. Physical activity and cancer risk: dose-response and cancer, all sites and site-specific. Med Sci Sports Exerc. 2001;33(6 Suppl):S530–550; discussion S609–610.

Van Patten CL, de Boer JG, Tomlinson Guns ES. Diet and dietary supplement intervention trials for the prevention of prostate cancer recurrence: a review of the randomized controlled trial evidence. J Urol. 2008;180(6):2314–2321; discussion 2721–2722. doi:10.1016/j.juro.2008.08.078

Van Poppel H, Tombal B. Chemoprevention of prostate cancer with nutrients and supplements. Cancer Manag Res. 2011;3:91–100. doi:10.2147/CMR. S18503

Vashi PG, et al. Impact of oral vitamin D supplementation on serum 25-hydroxyvutamin D levels in oncology. Nutr J. 2010;9:60.

Verberne L, Bach-Faig A, Buckland G, Serra-Majem L. Association between the Mediterranean diet and cancer risk: a review of observational studies. Nutr Cancer. 2010;62(7):860–870. doi:10.1080/01635581.2010.509834

Wien TN, Pike E et al. Cancer risk with folic acid supplements: a systematic review and meta-analysis. BMJ Open 2012 Jan;2(1):e000653.

World Health Organization. Global Health Observatory, Cancer Mortality and morbidity. http://www.who.int/gho/ncd/mortality_morbidity/cancer_text/en/. Accessed 12/1/13.

Wu K, Platz EA, Willett WC, Fuchs CS, Selhub J, Rosner BA, Hunter DJ, Giovannucci E. A randomized trial on folic acid supplementation and risk of recurrent colorectal adenoma. Am J Clin Nutr. 2009;90(6):1623–1631. doi:10.3945/ajcn.2009.28319

Yan L, Spitznagel EL. Soy consumption and colorectal cancer risk in humans: a meta-analysis. Cancer Epidemiol Biomarkers Prev. 2010 Jan;19(1):148-158.

Yang CS, Wang X. Green tea and cancer prevention. Nutr Cancer. 2010;62(7): 931–937. doi:10.1080/01635581.2010.509536

Yang WS, Va P, Wong MY, Zhang HL, Xiang YB. Soy intake is associated with lower lung cancer risk: results from a meta-analysis of epidemiologic studies. Am J Clin Nutr. 2011;94(6):1575–1583. doi:10.3945/ajcn.111.020966

Yuan JM, Sun C, Butler LM. Tea and cancer prevention: epidemiological studies. Pharmacol Res. 2011;64(2):123–135. doi:10.1016/j.phrs.2011.03.002

Zick SM, Ruffin MT, Lee J, Normolle DP, Siden R, Alrawi S, Brenner DE. Phase II trial of encapsulated ginger as a treatment for chemotherapy-induced nausea and vomiting. Support Care Cancer. 2009;s17(5):563–572. doi:10.1007/s00520-008-0528-8

17

Dermatologic Conditions

PHILIP D. SHENEFELT AND ROBERT A. NORMAN

Introduction

KEY TO ASSESSING COMMON SKIN CONDITIONS

D ermatologic diagnoses are largely pattern recognition processes. A brief focused history is quickly followed by physical examination of the skin. Based on the physical findings, a further focused history may be appropriate, or laboratory tests or skin biopsy may be indicated. Table 17.1 lists physical findings and differential diagnoses of common skin disorders. This does not replace the need for consultation with a dermatologist if there is any question about the diagnosis or appropriate treatment. Further descriptions of the common skin disorders can be found in alphabetical order in the text.

Therapeutic choices include observation, conventional medical treatments, doing nothing, homeopathy, placebo, aromatherapy, dietary measures, nutritional supplements, herbal treatments, hypnosis, biofeedback, acupressure, and other physical and energy methods. The common dermatological conditions and their integrative treatments are listed in alphabetical order.

Dietary measures and nutritional supplements can correct deficiencies and can provide anti-inflammatory actions to help reduce inflammatory skin disorders. In this sense food can be considered a form of medicine. On the other hand, inflammatory foods can increase the inflammation (Cannon & Vierck, 2006).

Placebo, homeopathy, and aromatherapy can produce positive results based on positive expectations and conditioning. Conditioning of paired stimulus and response can occur not only in the nervous system but also in the immune system, as experiments in psychoneuroimmunology have revealed (Tausk, Elenkov, & Moynihan, 2008). On the other side of the coin, nocebo can produce negative results based on negative expectations and conditioning. Biofeedback training can help to alter negative conditioning. Heart rate

Table 17.1: Physical Findings and Differential Diagnosis of Common Skin Disorders

Physical Findings	Differential Diagnosis
Macule or patch (flat spot)—white	Vitiligo, pityriasis alba, scar
Macule or patch (flat spot)—brown	Solar lentigo, melasma, postinflammatory hyperpigmentation, nevus (mole), melanoma
Macule or patch (flat spot)—purple	Purpura, bruise, venous lake
Papules (small bumps)	Acne, rosacea, folliculitis, nevus (mole), precancer (actinic keratosis), skin cancer (basal cell, squamous cell, melanoma), cherry angioma, seborrheic keratosis, lichen planus, wart, molluscum contagiosum, callus, corn (clavus), scabies, insect bites, skin tags
Nodules (large bumps)	Abscess, skin cancer, boil, cyst, prurigo nodularis, keloids, erythema nodosum
Plaques (large flat-topped bumps)	Psoriasis, lichen simplex chronicus, mycosis fungoides
Wheals (hives)	Hives (urticaria), drug allergy
Comedones (blackheads)	Acne, steroid-induced acne
Pustules	Acne, folliculitis, hidradenitis suppurativa
Rash—linear	Contact dermatitis, shingles (herpes zoster), warts, scratch marks (excoriations), neurodermatitis (psychogenic excoriations)
Rash—patchy	Contact dermatitis, atopic dermatitis, drug eruption, ringworm (tinea corporis), yeast (Candida), seborrheic dermatitis, stasis dermatitis, nummular dermatitis, mycosis fungoides, erythema multiforme, lupus erythematosus, cellulitis
Rash—confluent red	Sunburn, viral exanthem, drug eruption, erythroderma
Rash—scaly	Psoriasis, seborrheic dermatitis, pityriasis rosea, dry skin (asteatotic dermatitis), ichthyosis,
Vesicles (small blisters)	Athlete's foot (tinea pedis), cold sores (herpes simplex), shingles (herpes zoster), contact dermatitis, dyshidrosis
Bullae (large blisters)	Burn, contact dermatitis, friction, drug reaction, insect bite, autoimmune blistering disorders (pemphigus, pemphigoid, others), impetigo
Ulcer—mouth	Aphthous stomatitis (canker sores), autoimmune blistering disorders (pemphigus, lupus, oral pemphigoid), Stevens-Johnson syndrome, erythema multiforme, drug reaction, oral skin cancer

(continued)

Table 17.1: (continued)

Physical Findings	Differential Diagnosis
Ulcer—skin	Bedsore (decubitus ulcer), leg ulcer, deep fungal ulcer, other infectious ulcer, trauma, pyoderma gangrenosum
Hair loss	Androgenetic alopecia, alopecia areata, trichotillomania, telogen effluvium
Hair gain	Hypertrichosis, hirsutism
Nail abnormalities	Fungal nail (tinea unguium), traumatic, psoriasis, lichen planus
Excess sweating	Hyperhidrosis
Dilated leg veins	Varicose veins

variability biofeedback can calm and relax. Fingertip temperature biofeedback via a color-changing card or thermometer can produce warming and relaxation. Galvanic skin resistance biofeedback can help reduce sweating. Psychodermatology plays a significant role in many inflammatory skin conditions (Shenefelt, 2011). Hypnosis can benefit many of these inflammatory skin disorders (Shenefelt, 2000).

Herbal therapies for skin diseases (Bedi & Shenefelt, 2002) vary from ancient and modern traditional Chinese medicine (Yihou, 2004) and ayurvedic ("knowledge for long life") medicine of India (Khan & Khanum, 2009), to European and Native American and other ethnic herbal remedies, to well-researched scientific study monographs on herbs (Blumenthal, 1998).

Acupuncture is part of traditional Chinese medicine and requires specialized training, but acupressure is available to all. The commonly used acupressure sites are listed in Table 17.2, and specific acupressure points are listed under the corresponding diseases they can be used to treat. Acupuncture charts and books are also available to identify the acupressure sites more precisely. Most acupressure sites are in small hollows with fascia between bones, muscles, and tendons. With pressure, often slight tenderness can be felt at the correct site. The pressure should be firm enough to produce some discomfort and should be done three times a day for about 3 minutes at each indicated point on each side of the body. Acupressure can be used synergistically with hypnosis to modify expectations, emotions, and attention and increase self-regulation (Muenke & Draeger-Muenke, 2011).

For all skin disorders, consultation with an appropriate health care provider is recommended and self-diagnosis and self-treatment are risky. The information contained in this chapter is not warranted to be safe, correct, and efficacious for everyone.

Abscesses and Boils

Abscesses in the skin are tender, red, hot, tense, raised areas most commonly due to bacterial infection with *Staphylococcus aureus*. An abscess usually develops a central suppuration from which pus can be drained when it ruptures spontaneously or is lanced. The contents are contagious. A boil or furuncle is an abscess that starts at a hair follicle. Conventional treatment in the early stages consists of warm compresses and an appropriate oral antibiotic such as amoxicillin/clavulanate or broad-spectrum cephalothin while awaiting culture and sensitivity results. Cleaning the area with a topical antimicrobial such as chlorhexidine can help reduce spread to other areas. If fluctuance develops later, incision and drainage with culture and possibly packing of the cavity may be done along with continued appropriate oral antibiotic.

Dietary recommendations include yellow-orange fruits and vegetables, minimizing food with sugar and other carbohydrates, and increasing fluid intake. Supplements that may be of benefit include vitamin A, B-complex vitamins, vitamin C, and zinc. Herbal treatments include topical tea tree oil, oral garlic, calendula ointment, and a topical paste of goldenseal root powder.

Acne

Acne is a common disorder of the pilosebaceous apparatus associated with the hair follicles of the oily areas of skin on the face, chest, and back. It most commonly starts postpuberty and may resolve in the 20s in many people but may extend into the 30s, 40s, or 50s in others. Factors associated with acne include obstruction of hair follicle openings with skin that does not flake away properly, oil production in the hair follicles under hormonal influence, bacteria that digest the oil, and the body's inflammatory response to the bacteria and breakdown products of the oil. Acne often flares with stress. Conventional treatments are topical and oral. Topical treatments include benzoyl peroxide, topical antibiotics such as clindamycin or erythromycin, topical retinoids, and topical azelaic acid. Oral treatments include oral antibiotics such as doxycycline, tetracycline, minocycline, erythromycin, sulfa-trimethoprim, and, for severe acne, isotretinoin (Savage & Layton, 2010). Intralesional therapy may include intralesional corticosteroids for resistant acne cysts. Physical therapies include blue light therapy and cryotherapy. Repair of acne scars can be done with chemical peels, dermabrasion, laser ablation, surgical excision, or dermal fillers (Choudhary et al., 2011).

Diet can play a significant role in acne in some individuals (Logan & Treloar, 2007). Dietary measures include avoiding proinflammatory foods such as sugar, processed foods, french fries, fast foods, white bread, pasta,

Table 17.2: Acupressure Point and Locations

Acupressure Point	Location
Gallbladder 20	Occipital base of skull at muscular groove lateral to trapezius
Gallbladder 34	Lateral proximal lower leg anterior and inferior to head of fibula
Kidney 3	Posterior top of ankle medial malleolus at groove anterior to Achilles
Kidney 8	Medial two thumb widths above top of ankle medial malleolus
Large intestine 4	Dorsal midweb between thumb and index finger
Large intestine 11	End of outer crease of antecubital fossa of elbow
Liver 3	Dorsal midweb between big and second toe
Small intestine 10	Posterior between lateral scapula and humeral head
Small intestine 18	Two finger widths below lateral canthus of eye
Spleen 7	Medial midcalf
Spleen 9	Midlower border of tibial medial condyle
Spleen 10	Medial distal thigh two finger widths above top of patella
Stomach 2	On cheek one finger width below center of lower eyelid
Stomach 3	On cheek two finger widths below center of lower eyelid at ala nasi
Stomach 4	On cheek below center of lower eyelid at corner of mouth
Stomach 36	One hand width below bottom of patella and one thumb width lateral
Urinary bladder 10	Posterior paraspinal just below atlas
Urinary bladder 18	Paraspinal two finger widths lateral to midline at T9 midback
Urinary bladder 23	Paraspinal just above top of gluteal cleft
Urinary bladder 47	Four finger widths lateral to midline at T9 midback
Urinary bladder 64	On lateral hollow at proximal base of fifth toe metatarsal
Urinary bladder 65	On lateral fifth toe metatarsal-phalangeal joint
Urinary bladder 66	On lateral second phalanx of fifth toe

whole milk, ice cream, cheddar cheese, snack foods, corn oil, soda, caffeine, and alcohol while including anti-inflammatory foods such as wild salmon, fresh whole fruits and bright multicolored vegetables, green tea, water, olive oil, lean poultry, nuts, legumes and seeds, dark green leafy vegetables, and old-fashioned oatmeal (Cannon & Vierck, 2006). Nutritional supplements include β-carotene 25,000 IU, vitamin C 1,000 mg with bioflavonoids, vitamin E 400 IU, zinc 25 mg, and selenium 200 mcg per day, and flaxseed or evening primrose oil 2 teaspoons per day. Herbal treatments topically include calendula soap and tea tree oil. Herbal treatments orally include burdock root 500 mg and grapeseed or pine bark extract 250 mcg three times daily. Acupressure may be used to reduce stress, with pressing for about 3 minutes each three times daily on large intestine 4, large intestine 11, liver 3, and stomach 36 on each side of the body (Jacknin, 2001). Adequate sleep, adequate exercise, and daily use of relaxation or meditation techniques are also important.

Age Spots

Mottled skin with darker and lighter spots occurs as a result of sun damage. The darker brown flat spots are known as solar lentigines and are harmless but a sign of excess sun exposure over time. Conventional treatments include daily use of sunscreen, cover-up makeup, topical hydroxyquinone lightening creams, topical glycolic or lactic acid creams or peels, topical trichloroacetic acid peels, and topical tretinoin. Cryosurgery with liquid nitrogen selectively destroys melanocytes and is effective. Laser ablation with 532-nm light from diode or frequency-doubled Q-switched Nd:YAG lasers are effective, as is the alexandrite laser (Ho et al., 2011).

Nutritional supplement options are antioxidant vitamins C 500 to 1,000 mg and E 400 to 800 IU orally and selenium 50 to 200 mcg orally daily. Vitamins C and E can also be used topically. Herbal treatments include aloe vera gel topically, kojic acid from mushroom topically, fresh lemon juice topically, and oral grapeseed extract.

Autoimmune Blistering Disorders

Autoimmune blistering disorders occur when the body makes autoantibodies against specific target normal structures in the skin. The ensuing inflammatory response produces separation of the skin at that point and the separated areas fill with blister fluid. Relatively common autoimmune blistering disorders include pemphigus, bullous pemphigoid, and dermatitis herpetiformis. Conventional treatments with various immunosuppressive drugs should be managed by an experienced dermatologist. Dietary, nutritional, and herbal treatments are similar to that for blistered second-degree burns (see later).

Dietary measures include a balanced diet with plenty of fluids. Nutritional supplements include a multivitamin, vitamin B complex, vitamin C 1,000 to 3,000 mg/day, vitamin E 400 IU/day, selenium 50 mcg/day, zinc 50 mg/day, and flaxseed oil, evening primrose oil, or fish oil 1 tablespoon or equivalent daily. Immune stimulatory herbs such as echinacea should be avoided as they may worsen the autoimmune condition. Herbal anti-inflammatory measures include pine bark extract, grapeseed extract, and turmeric extract.

Bites and Stings: Insect, Tick, Scorpion, and Spider

Most bug bites are merely annoying, but some can become secondarily infected with bacteria, especially if scratched. Bee and wasp stings can be quite painful. If the honeybee leaves its stinger, scrape it off with a knife rather than pulling on it, as the squeezing may inject more venom. Some individuals can have potentially life-threatening anaphylactic reactions from bee or wasp stings and should carry an epinephrine kit and go to the emergency room if stung. To minimize bee stings, don't look like a flower (don't wear floral print clothes) or smell like a flower (cologne). Fire ants also sting and can produce white pustules. Mosquitoes may carry arthropod-borne viruses and in some parts of the world malaria and other diseases. Ticks may carry the organisms for Lyme disease, Rocky Mountain spotted fever, and other diseases. Tick removal is best done with forceps grasping the head and pulling back slowly and firmly. Prevention involves avoiding known habitats, wearing protective clothing, using insect repellants, and inspecting skin for ticks after possible exposure. Small scorpions can produce painful stings, but larger desert scorpions can produce highly toxic stings. Most spider bites are harmless, but the black widow has a neurotoxin and the brown recluse has a necrotoxin. Conventional treatments for bite sites include cleansing with soap and water or with rubbing alcohol and applying a topical antibiotic. Itching or swelling can be treated with oral antihistamines such as diphenhydramine, chlorpheniramine, or cetirizine and with topical pramoxine and hydrocortisone. For severe reactions or for scorpion stings or black widow spider bites, seek emergency medical care. Nutritional supplements include vitamin B complex twice daily as a repellant. Herbal topical citronella oil can be used as a repellant. Oral garlic 500 mg twice a day can also repel insects. Topical aloe vera gel or calendula cream can be applied to bite sites. For stings, ice packs, cold packs, or pastes of meat tenderizer, baking soda, mud, comfrey, or tobacco may offer relief. Topical or oral echinacea extract may also help to neutralize the hyaluronidase in the sting venom. Acupressure over liver 3 or bladder 65 for 3 minutes can help to ease the discomfort from stings (Jacknin, 2001).

Body Odor and Hyperhidrosis

Most repulsive body odors come from bacterial overgrowth in apocrine sweat in the axillae or in eccrine sweat on the feet. Garlic and spices such as curry can also add odor to sweat. Emotional sweating occurs mainly in the axillae, hands, feet, and forehead, whereas thermal sweating occurs over the whole body. Conventional treatment to reduce odor and sweating is to wash the area once or twice a day with deodorant or antibacterial soap, use deodorants, and use drying powders. Prescription drying agents with aluminum chloride are the next step. Iontophoresis is another prescriptive choice for hyperhidrosis. Paralyzing the nerves associated with sweating with local injections of dilute botulinum toxin can also be effective (Walling & Swick, 2011).

Dietary measures include avoiding garlic and odorous spices. Nutritional supplements include vitamin A 25,000 IU daily for 2 weeks, vitamin B complex, vitamin C 1,000 to 3,000 mg daily, and zinc 50 mg daily. Biofeedback with galvanic skin resistance can be used to help retrain autonomic sweating patterns. Herbal treatments with oral chlorophyll include alfalfa tablets, chlorophyll capsules, or parsley. Acupressure to reduce excessive sweating may be performed on bladder 64 and 66 and kidney 3 and 8 for 3 minutes three times daily (Jacknin, 2001).

Bruises

Blunt trauma can produce pain, swelling, and blood pigment discoloration, initially red, then black and blue, then yellowish brown as the blood pigment is resorbed. Skin that has had chronic sun exposure, especially on the forearms, and skin that has been affected by topical or internal corticosteroids can be thin and fragile, bruising and tearing readily. Medical conditions, drugs, and herbs that inhibit platelet function or clotting can enhance bruising. Conventional treatment consists of initial application of a cold pack for about 15 minutes that can be repeated several times in the first 24 hours. Avoid taking aspirin and other nonsteroidal anti-inflammatory drugs. If bruising seems excessive, investigate possible medical conditions or antiplatelet drugs or herbs such as ginkgo, garlic, or ginger that could account for it. Dietary measures include dark green leafy vegetables for vitamin K and citrus fruits for vitamin C. Supplement options include vitamin C, vitamin D, vitamin K orally and in topical cream form, and oral zinc. Herbal treatments include topical arnica gel and oral bromelain.

Burns

Burns damage the skin by heat, ultraviolet exposure, chemicals, or electricity. First-degree burns involve only the top layer of skin, the epidermis, with redness. Second-degree burns cause blister formation. Third-degree burns char or damage the leathery dermis. Fourth-degree burns penetrate to destroy underlying muscle or other internal structures. Third- and fourth-degree burns are medical emergencies, as are extensive second-degree burns. Conventional treatment is to remove the burning agent if still present, and in the case of a chemical burn rinse the area thoroughly with cool running water. Extensive second-degree burns, electrical burns, and third- and fourth-degree burns should be evaluated as soon as possible in the emergency room. A mild burn can be cooled with tap water. Blisters should be left intact.

Dietary measures include lean high-protein foods, green and yellow vegetables, and drinking sufficient water to replace fluids lost through the burn. Nutritional supplements include vitamin C, vitamin E, calcium, zinc, and protein powders. Herbal treatments include aloe vera gel, calendula cream, comfrey cream, and, for oozing areas, cool tea compresses. Acupressure pain relief may be done for 3 minutes three times daily at bladder 65 (Jacknin, 2001).

Canker Sores (Aphthous Stomatitis)

Canker sores, or aphthous stomatitis, are painful small oral mucosa ulcers with a gray base and red rim. Most are smaller than 1 cm and are called minor and usually heal spontaneously in a week or two. Those larger than 3 cm are called major and may take 6 weeks to heal, often with scarring. Both minor and major tend to recur, singly or in crops. Triggers include stress, minor injury to the oral mucosa, and smoking. There may be a burning or tingling sensation prior to onset, and early treatment can be productive in minimizing their occurrences. Conventional treatments include topical lidocaine for pain relief, topical corticosteroids, and oral anti-inflammatory antibiotic suspensions. In severe cases immune suppressants such as azathioprine, dapsone, or colchicine may be considered. Oral thalidomide may also be considered for extreme cases in males (Preeti et al., 2011).

Dietary considerations include trials of eliminating wheat and milk and keeping a food diary. Avoid acid foods, chewing gum, spicy foods, crunchy foods, and anything else that seems to irritate the mouth. Nutritional supplements include vitamin B complex, vitamin C with bioflavonoids 1,000 to 3,000 mg/day, zinc 50 mg/day, iron 15 mg/day, acidophilus powder, and topical vitamin E. Herbal treatments include aloe vera juice, chlorophyll tablets, licorice, powdered myrrh, and tannin from tea bag contact. Acupressure points include liver 3 and small intestine 4 and 10, stomach 4, and bladder 10 (Jacknin, 2001).

Cold Sores (Herpes Simplex)

Cold sores or fever blisters are herpes simplex virus infection. Most commonly they occur on the lips or genitals, but may also occur on other skin areas depending on where the contact with the virus occurred. They are infectious to others by direct contact. They can be new onset, sometimes accompanied by fever and malaise, or they can be recurrent, usually without systemic symptoms. Recurrence generally occurs in the same area as the original infection because the virus lies dormant in the dorsal root ganglia of the associated nerve. The recurrence is often preceded by tingling, itching, burning, or pain at the site before the blisters develop. Recurrences may be triggered by stress, fatigue, colds, fever, sun exposure, or other factors. Conventional treatment includes oral episodic acyclovir, valacyclovir, or famciclovir, and topical lidocaine (Nguyen et al., 2010). If recurrence is frequent, suppressive therapy may be considered.

Dietary measures when lesions are active include eating foods high in lysine such as dairy, seafood, chicken, turkey, eggs, beans, and potatoes and avoidance of foods high in arginine such as grains, seeds, nuts, peanuts, chocolate, coconut, beer, and raisins. For lip or mouth lesions, avoid acidic citrus fruits and juices. Nutritional supplements include L-lysine 1,500 mg/day for 2 weeks, multivitamin, vitamin B complex, vitamin C 3,000 mg/day, vitamin E 400 IU/ day, zinc 50 mg/day, flaxseed oil 1 tablespoon daily, and selenium 100 mcg/day. Herbal treatments include echinacea, garlic, and lemon balm tea. Acupressure point is spleen 7 (Jacknin, 2001).

Cuts and Scrapes

Cuts and scrapes can lead to bleeding, infections, and scarring. Conventional treatment for a cut that does not stop bleeding or is deep or long or on the lip is prompt medical evaluation and it may need suturing. Usually suturing can only be done within the first 12 hours after the injury. A tetanus shot may also be indicated if it has been more than 5 years since the last booster. For more minor cuts and scrapes, cleansing the area with soap and water, using pressure to control bleeding, and applying an antibiotic ointment and bandage are often all that is necessary. Diet requires adequate protein intake for healing. Nutritional supplements include vitamin C 3,000 mg/day, vitamin E 400 IU/ day, and zinc 50 mg/day. Herbal treatments include calendula gel, powdered cloves, comfrey cream, powdered yarrow, and tea tree oil. Honey may also be used as a dressing. See information later on scars if scarring occurs.

Dandruff (Seborrheic Dermatitis)

Dandruff or scaly scalp with or without itching and redness generally occurs with seborrheic dermatitis. The itching, scaling, and redness can occur on the nasolabial folds, eyebrows, eyelashes, and central chest and back in addition to the scalp. It occurs on oily areas where a yeast, *Pityrosporum ovale,* grows and digests the oil, creating products that the body reacts to with inflammation. Scratching the skin produces damage and further itching. Conventional treatment is with medicated shampoos containing ketoconazole, selenium sulfide, or zinc pyrithione to inhibit the yeast; coal tar shampoo to reduce itching and inflammation; and salicylic acid shampoo to remove scales. Cortisone solutions or foams or creams can also help to reduce inflammation in severe cases. Dietary measures include avoiding proinflammatory foods and eating anti-inflammatory foods as discussed under acne. Nutritional supplements include biotin 2 to 5 mg/day, flaxseed oil 1 tablespoon/day, and zinc 50 mg/day. Herbal rinses include thyme or rosemary 2 tablespoonfuls boiled in 1 cup water, strained, and allowed to cool before use. Apple cider vinegar diluted in half with water may be applied to the scalp as a compress for 30 minutes, then washed out.

Dermatitis and Eczema

Dermatitis is superficial inflammation of the skin. Eczema is another name for dermatitis. The acute phase is red and itchy with or without blisters and oozing. The subacute phase is less red but still itchy. The chronic phase is dry and itchy and sometimes thickened. The most common kinds of dermatitis are atopic dermatitis, irritant contact dermatitis, allergic contact dermatitis, dyshidrotic dermatitis, nummular dermatitis, and stasis dermatitis. Atopic dermatitis results from a minor genetic defect that produces a less effective skin barrier (Boguniewicz & Leung, 2011). The skin is drier and itchier than normal, and the rash is produced by scratching. Interleukin (IL)-31 appears to play a significant role in atopic dermatitis and correlates with scratching (Nobbe et al., 2012). Often a psychological component helps determine the atopic dermatitis flares through psychoneuroimmunologic mechanisms (Suarez et al., 2012). Irritant contact dermatitis is produced by repetitive skin exposure to mildly or moderately irritating chemicals such as washing the hands too frequently with soap and water. Allergic contact dermatitis is due to a delayed hypersensitivity reaction to one or more chemicals that are allergens. Which specific chemicals are causing the problem is determined by patch testing. Dyshidrotic dermatitis is tiny blistering and peeling usually along the sides of the fingers. Nummular dermatitis is coin-shaped patches on the legs and sometimes flank. Stasis dermatitis is on the lower legs and is usually associated with varicose veins. Conventional treatment consists of removing any inciting factors such as allergens or irritants, using topical corticosteroid or other anti-inflammatory creams such as tacrolimus or pimecrolimus, drying oozing areas, moisturizing dry areas, and checking for any secondary bacterial infection or overgrowth.

Dietary measures include avoiding proinflammatory foods and eating anti-inflammatory foods as discussed under acne. Nutritional supplements include a multivitamin, vitamin B complex, vitamin C 1,000 to 3,000 mg/day, vitamin E 400 IU/day, zinc 50 mg/day, and flaxseed oil, evening primrose oil, or fish oil 1 tablespoon or equivalent daily. Herbal treatments include aloe vera gel, calendula cream, chamomile cream, and comfrey ointment. Menthol 0.25% and/or camphor 0.5% may be added to creams for their anti-itch effects. Acupressure points include spleen 7 and 10; liver 3; bladder 18, 23, and 47; and large intestine 4 and 11 (Jacknin, 2001).

Drug Eruptions

Drug eruptions most commonly are morbilliform (measles-like) or urticarial (hives) but can mimic many inflammatory skin diseases from acne to xerosis (Al-Niaimi, 2011). They may have a pharmacologic or an allergic basis. Most drug eruptions are symmetrical, but photodrug eruptions are in photodistributed areas, and fixed drug eruptions often are solitary lesions. Conventional treatment consists of discontinuing the drug and giving appropriate supportive care.

Dietary measures include avoiding proinflammatory foods and eating anti-inflammatory foods as discussed under acne. Nutritional supplements include a multivitamin, vitamin B complex, vitamin C 1,000 to 3,000 mg/day, vitamin E 400 IU/day, zinc 50 mg/day, and flaxseed oil, evening primrose oil, or fish oil 1 tablespoon or equivalent daily. Herbal treatments include aloe vera gel, calendula cream, chamomile cream, and comfrey ointment.

Dry Skin (Xerosis)

Dry skin occurs when there is not enough water to keep the keratin supple in the stratum corneum, the top dead layer of skin that serves as a barrier. Water does not stay in the skin without some oil on top to hold it there. Drying occurs more readily when the relative humidity is low, promoting easier evaporation of water from the skin. When the skin dries excessively it cracks easily and has a less effective barrier function. This occurs more intensely in persons with atopic dermatitis, where there is already a barrier defect. Excess sweating washes away some of the natural oils, causing the skin to be susceptible to later drying. Soaps and water and solvents also remove natural oils. Conventional treatments consist of using less drying and less irritating fragrance-free soaps or cleansers, blotting the skin dry after a bath or shower, then coating the dry areas with a fragrance-free moisturizer. Inexpensive moisturizers include plain mineral oil or petrolatum jelly applied over moist skin. Baumann (2010) has categorized several skin types and how to manage them.

Dietary measures include fish, rolled oats, and ground flaxseed, carrots, tomatoes, cantaloupe, green leafy vegetables, whole grains, and legumes. Nutritional supplements include flaxseed oil 1 or 2 tablespoons/day or evening primrose oil 3,000 mg/day, vitamin B complex, and vitamin C with bioflavonoids 1,000 to 3,000 mg/day. Herbal treatments include topical olive oil, almond oil, aloe vera cream, calendula ointment, or comfrey cream.

Folliculitis

Folliculitis is an inflammation of the individual hair follicles, usually due to a bacterial infection and less commonly due to a *Pityrosporum* yeast infection. It presents as folliculocentric red papules with or without pustules. Bacterial culture can identify problematic bacteria. If that is negative, a biopsy can demonstrate whether there is yeast present in larger than normal amounts. Conventional treatment for bacterial folliculitis includes topical antibiotics such as clindamycin. For *Pityrosporum* folliculitis topical ketoconazole may be effective or oral fluconazole may be necessary. Keeping the area dry and friction free may help. Scratching tends to spread the organisms and should be discouraged. Dietary measures include avoiding proinflammatory foods and eating anti-inflammatory foods as discussed earlier under acne. Nutritional supplements include β-carotene 25,000 IU, vitamin C 1,000 mg with bioflavonoids, vitamin E 400 IU, zinc 25 mg, and selenium 200 mcg per day, and flaxseed or evening primrose oil 2 teaspoons per day. Herbal treatments topically include calendula soap and tea tree oil.

Fungus, Ringworm, Jock Itch, Athlete's Foot, and Sunspots (Tinea Corporis, Capitis, Cruris, Pedis, and Versicolor)

Tinea fungal infections can involve skin, hair, and nails. Scraping the edge of the lesion and examining the scrapings under the microscope in a potassium hydroxide wet mount can often identify the presence of fungus, which typically is thread-like and branching except for tinea versicolor, where it is more like meatballs and spaghetti. Pulled hairs can also be examined under the microscope for fungus. Nail clippings sent in formalin can be stained for fungus by pathology labs. Fungal cultures may also be performed to confirm and identify the fungus. Conventional treatment is with topical antifungals, or with scalp fungus and in other severe cases with oral antifungals. The area should be kept dry. Dietary measures include a balanced diet with vegetables and avoidance of sugary foods and drinks. Nutritional supplements include a multivitamin, vitamin C with bioflavonoids 3,000 mg/day, and zinc 50 mg/day. Herbal treatments include calendula cream, garlic orally or topically, tea tree oil topically, licorice tea applied topically, myrrh paste topically, olive leaf extract orally, or tumeric extract topically and orally.

Hair Loss (Alopecia)

The most common patterns of hair loss are male-pattern alopecia with bitemporal and crown thinning, alopecia areata with patchy hair loss, and telogen effluvium with diffuse hair thinning. Black dot tinea capitis can also cause patchy hair loss. Some prescription drugs and many anticancer drugs can also cause hair loss. Most men experience some degree of male-pattern alopecia. Conventional treatments include topical minoxidil applied twice daily and oral finasteride. Hair transplants and wigs or hair weaves are also available. For alopecia areata, topical or intralesional corticosteroids may be effective. Black dot tinea capitis should be treated with oral antifungals.

Dietary measures for hair loss include a balanced diet with a good intake of protein. Nutritional supplements include a multivitamin, biotin 2 mg/day, vitamin C with bioflavonoids 3,000 mg/day, vitamin E 400 IU/day, iron 50 mg/day, and zinc 50 mg/day. Herbal treatments include oral saw palmetto, topical arnica cream or rinse, sage extract topically, or safflower oil scalp massage.

Hives (Urticaria)

Hives or urticaria is very itchy red swellings that typically last for less than a day at a particular location. Acute hives last less than 6 weeks, whereas chronic hives last for more than 6 weeks. Certain foods such as fresh tomatoes, nuts, seafood, fresh strawberries, and certain medicines such as aspirin can trigger hives on a nonallergic pharmacologic basis. The person can also be allergic to a food, food additive, drug, or herb. Stress, physical pressure, sunlight, heat, cold, and water can also sometimes trigger hives. Some chronic urticaria has an autoimmune mechanism (Grattan, 2004). If difficulty breathing or feeling faint develops, seek emergency medical help immediately. Conventional treatment consists of attempting to determine and eliminate the causal factors through physical examination and history and laboratory work; discontinuing all nonessential drugs; avoiding fresh tomatoes, nuts, seafood, and fresh strawberries; and taking oral antihistamines. In severe cases, oral prednisone may be necessary.

Dietary measures include avoiding suspected foods or doing an elimination diet. The elimination diet involves having only unflavored lamb, unflavored rice, and unflavored tea for 2 weeks. If the hives disappear with this diet, then add one new food back every 5 days and if the hives reappear, exclude that food from the diet. Nutritional supplements include a multivitamin, vitamin C with bioflavonoids 3,000 mg/day, vitamin E 400 IU/day, bromelain orally, and flaxseed or evening primrose oils 1 tablespoonful or equivalent per day. Herbal treatments include oral bilberry and oral stinging nettle. Acupressure sites include large intestine 4 and 11, spleen 7 and 10, and stomach 36 (Jacknin, 2001).

Itching (Pruritus)

Itching or pruritus is an unpleasant sensation conveyed by special nerves from the skin to the brain. The itch may occur as a result of skin inflammation, histamine release, peripheral neuropathy, metabolic problem, or central nervous system malfunction (Ständer et al., 2007). Conventional treatment consists of physical examination, history, laboratory work if indicated, and patch testing if indicated to determine the cause; elimination of contact with any identified irritants or allergens; application of cold packs; and use of topical corticosteroids where indicated. Also, oral antihistamines may reduce itching and promote sleep. Topical menthol and camphor in a moisturizing lotion may help to reduce itching. Ultraviolet light treatments may also reduce itching. Dietary measures include a balanced diet.

Nutritional supplements include a multivitamin, vitamin C with bioflavonoids 3,000 mg/day, and flaxseed or evening primrose oils 1 tablespoonful or equivalent per day. Herbal treatments include topical aloe vera gel, calendula cream, chamomile cream, and comfrey ointment. For persistent itching associated with peripheral neuropathy, careful use of topical capsaicin may be helpful. Acupressure sites include large intestine 4 and 11 and spleen 7 (Jacknin, 2001).

Lice

There are three kinds of lice, pubic, head, and body. Pubic lice affect the pubic region, armpits, eyebrows, and occasionally back of scalp. They are squat and slow with crab-like claws and are often called crab lice. Head lice are long and quick and affect the scalp, laying more nits usually on the occipital scalp. Both crab and head lice lay their nits attached with glue to hairs at the base of the hair. The egg or nit is usually brownish until the larva hatches, after which the egg or nit is whitish. Body lice look like head lice but live and lay their eggs in the seams of clothing. Conventional treatment for pubic or crab and head lice is permethrin shampoo or lindane shampoo. Recently Spinosad was approved for head lice. Nit removal can be performed with a fine-tooth nit comb. Applying petrolatum jelly twice a day for 3 days is messy but smothers the lice and their nits. For body lice very hot water laundering is usually sufficient. Dietary measures include a balanced diet. Herbal essential oils diluted in olive oil that help repel adult lice include rosemary, thyme, and lavender.

Moles (Nevi)

Moles or melanocytic nevi are common benign growths. In childhood and adolescence and early adulthood, sun exposure tends to induce more moles to form in susceptible individuals. Frequent strong intermittent sun exposure seems to trigger melanoma formation more than steady sun exposure. New, changing, irregular moles should be evaluated. The ABCDEs of potentially dysplastic moles or melanomas include asymmetry, border irregular, color irregular, diameter greater that a pencil eraser (6 mm), or enlarging. Conventional treatment for a mole or nevus that fits one or more of these danger signs is evaluation for the need to biopsy it. A mole or nevus that is otherwise okay but is in a bad location and gets injured or irritated can be flattened with a simple surgical procedure. Appropriate sun protection is key for prevention of melanomas and other skin cancers.

Nail Problems

Many different factors may affect nails. Repeated handwashing or use of solvents may contribute to brittle nails. Metabolic conditions may affect nail growth. Skin inflammatory conditions such as dermatitis, psoriasis, lichen planus, and alopecia areata may affect nails. Fungal or yeast infections may affect nails. Warts, squamous cell carcinoma, and melanoma can all affect nails. Conventional treatment includes determining and treating the specific causes. Physical examination, history, laboratory work, and biopsy may help to elucidate the cause.

Dietary measures include a balanced diet with adequate protein. Nutritional supplements include a multivitamin, biotin 2 mg/day, vitamin C with bioflavonoids 3,000 mg/day, iron 30 mg/day, and zinc 50 mg/day. Herbal treatments include topical myrrh, oral nettle, and horsetail.

Neurodermatitis (Skin Picking and Rubbing)

Neurodermatitis or psychogenic excoriations can produce scratch marks and scarring. Similarly, lichen simplex chronicus is a thickened itchy area of skin produced by chronic rubbing or scratching. Prurigo nodularis is discrete itchy nodules produced by picking.

Conventional treatments include topical and intralesional corticosteroids. Topical menthol and camphor in a moisturizing lotion may help to reduce itching. Dietary measures include a balanced diet.

Nutritional supplements include a multivitamin, vitamin C with bioflavonoids 3,000 mg/day, and flaxseed or evening primrose oils 1 tablespoonful or equivalent per day. Herbal treatments include aloe vera gel, calendula cream, chamomile cream, and comfrey ointment. For persistent itching careful use of topical capsaicin may be helpful. Acupressure sites include large intestine 4 and 11 (Jacknin, 2001). Cognitive-behavioral therapy may help to reduce the scratching and picking. Hypnosis and hypnoanalysis may benefit resistant cases (Shenefelt, 2010).

Psoriasis

Psoriasis is an inflammatory skin disease with an imbalance of lymphocytes producing IL-17 and related cytokines (Ortega et al., 2009). Red scaly plaques on elbows, knees, and scalp are typical, but psoriasis may only affect the nails, or inverse psoriasis may mainly affect the body fold areas. Some individuals may also have psoriatic arthritis. Conventional treatments include topical corticosteroids, topical vitamin D derivatives such as calcipotriene, topical vitamin A derivatives such as tazarotene, topical tar and anthralin, ultraviolet in the form of ultraviolet B (UVB), narrow-band UVB, or psoralens and ultraviolet A (PUVA). Oral medications include methotrexate, acitretin, and cyclosporine. There are several injectable biologics that inhibit psoriasis and psoriatic arthritis.

Dietary measures include avoiding proinflammatory foods such as sugar, processed foods, french fries, fast foods, white bread, pasta, whole milk, ice cream, cheddar cheese, snack foods, corn oil, soda, caffeine, and alcohol while including anti-inflammatory foods such as wild salmon, fresh whole fruits and bright multicolored vegetables, green tea, water, olive oil, lean poultry, nuts, legumes and seeds, dark green leafy vegetables, and old-fashioned oatmeal. Nutritional supplements include β-carotene 25,000 IU, vitamin C 1,000 mg with bioflavonoids, vitamin E 400 IU, zinc 25 mg, and selenium 200 mcg per day; flaxseed or evening primrose oil 2 tablespoons/day; or fish oil 1,000 mg 12 capsules/day. Herbal treatments topically include aloe vera cream, calendula ointment, chamomile cream, capsaicin cream, neem oil, and turmeric extract gel. Herbal treatments orally include burdock root 500 mg, garlic capsules, grapeseed or pine bark extract 250 mcg, or turmeric extract three times daily. Acupressure may be used to reduce stress, pressing for about 3 minutes each three times daily on large intestine 4, large intestine 11, liver 3, and stomach 36 on each side of the body. Acupressure on spleen 7 may help to relieve itching (Jacknin, 2001). Adequate sleep, adequate exercise, and daily use of relaxation or meditation techniques are also important.

Rosacea

Rosacea is an inflammatory condition of the central face with redness and/ or red papules with or without pustules. There are no blackheads with rosacea. Its cause is currently unknown (Crawford et al., 2004). Specific inflammatory cytokines are likely involved (Gerber et al., 2011). It is more common in fair-skinned people. Many people with rosacea experience easy blushing or flushing of the face, often triggered by sun exposure, heat, thermally hot food or beverages, spicy food, alcoholic beverages, or embarrassment. Uncommonly rhinophyma develops with a thickened enlarged nose. Conventional treatment includes metronidazole gel or cream, azelaic acid cream, topical clindamycin or erythromycin, oral tetracycline, doxycycline, minocycline, or erythromycin. For severe rosacea, isotretinoin may be considered. Laser treatments are available for the red blush and for dilated blood vessels. Rhinophyma can be improved with surgical or laser techniques. Dietary measures include avoiding proinflammatory foods and eating anti-inflammatory foods as discussed under acne. Also, avoid thermally hot foods and beverages, spicy foods, and alcoholic beverages. Nutritional supplements include β-carotene 25,000 IU, vitamin C 1,000 mg with bioflavonoids, zinc 25 mg, and selenium 200 mcg per day, and flaxseed or evening primrose oil 1 tablespoon per day. Herbal treatments orally include cats claw extract 500 mg and grapeseed or pine bark extract 250 mcg. Acupressure on small intestine 18, gallbladder 20, large intestine 4, and stomach 2 and 3 may be helpful (Jacknin, 2001). Adequate sleep, adequate exercise, and daily use of relaxation or meditation techniques are also important.

Scabies

Scabies is a mite infestation of the skin that produces intense itching. The red papules tend to occur around wrists and ankles, fingerwebs, waist, and genitals. A few of the latter sites may form persistent nodules. Burrows can sometimes be seen. The mite is about the size of a pinhead and the female lives in burrows in the skin. Skin scrapings placed in mineral oil wet mount and examined under the microscope can reveal mites, eggs, and scybala (feces). Itching begins about a month after the initial infestation. In adults the head is normally not involved. In normal people only a few mites are present due to the effectiveness of scratching at removing them. In immuno-compromised or mentally impaired individuals crusted scabies may develop with thousands of mites present. Conventional treatment for ordinary scabies is with permethrin cream followed by washing all recently exposed clothes and bed linens. Many scabies mites have become resistant to treatment with lindane lotion. It may take several weeks after treatment for the itching to abate. For crusted scabies oral treatment with ivermectin is often indicated. Alternative treatments include 6% precipitated sulfur in petrolatum jelly topi-cally daily for several days. The sulfur content in hot mineral spring baths was used in ancient times to help eliminate scabies. Herbal topical treatments for postmedical treatment relief include aloe vera gel, calendula cream, chamo-mile cream, and comfrey ointment. Acupressure site for itching is spleen 7 (Jacknin, 2001).

Scars and Keloids

A scar is formed in response to damage to the leathery dermis of the skin. In some individuals the scar may thicken into a hypertrophic scar or keloid. The earlobes, jawline, and upper chest and back tend to be more prone to form excess scar tissue. Most scars, hypertrophic scars, and keloids respond best if treated soon after formation. Conventional treatment for scars includes surgi-cal revision, dermabrasion, and deep peels. Conventional treatment for hyper-trophic scars and keloids includes topical and intralesional corticosteroids, surgical excision, and laser ablation (Vrijman et al., 2011). Nutritional supple-ments include vitamin E cream topically. Herbal treatments include topical onion extract (Mederma), calendula cream, and turmeric extract (curcumin) cream used several times a day for several months.

Shingles (Herpes Zoster)

Shingles or herpes zoster is a reactivation of the chickenpox virus that has lain dormant in a dorsal root ganglion. The reactivation occurs as natural immunity wanes or if immunosuppression occurs following organ transplant, cancer chemotherapy, or HIV infection. Both the nerve and the regional associated skin become inflamed from the infection, producing pain, itching, redness, and blistering. Untreated, it will resolve spontaneously in about 3 weeks. In older individuals postherpetic neuralgia may persist as a painful chronic condition. Conventional treatment includes oral episodic acyclovir, valacyclovir, or famciclovir (Lapolla et al., 2011) and topical lidocaine. In individuals 60 years and older, oral corticosteroids may be considered in addition to the antiviral treatment early in the course of the infection to reduce the chance of persistent pain. For postherpetic neuralgia oral gabapentin may be beneficial. Vaccination with Zostavax may help to prevent the development of herpes zoster and is recommended for those 60 years old and older.

Dietary measures include eating foods high in lysine such as dairy, seafood, chicken, turkey, eggs, beans, and potatoes and avoidance of foods high in arginine such as grains, seeds, nuts, peanuts, chocolate, coconut, beer, and raisins. Nutritional supplements include L-lysine 1,500 mg/day for 2 weeks, a multivitamin, vitamin B complex, vitamin C 3,000 mg/day, vitamin E 400 IU/day, zinc 50 mg/day, flaxseed oil 1 tablespoon daily, and selenium 100 mcg/day. Herbal treatments include echinacea, garlic, and lemon balm tea. For postherpetic neuralgia pain capsaicin cream used five times daily for several weeks may offer relief. Acupressure point for itching is spleen 7 (Jacknin, 2001).

Skin Cancer and Skin Cancer Prevention

The importance of skin cancer research, prevention, and therapy is underscored by the fact that the most common type of cancer in the United States is skin cancer (National Cancer Institute, n.d.). Although the mortality incidence due to cancer in the United States is declining, the incidence of skin cancer is steadily rising (Snowden, 2010). This is not surprising when taking into account the fact that many years ago the oncological potential of the sun was not well known nor was protection, such as sunscreen, widely promoted. Also, of all of the organs in the human body, skin is the largest, and due to its exterior protection it is more susceptible to environmental exposures (Marieb & Hoehn, 2009). Skin has many types of cells, including squamous, basal, and melanocytes. The three types of skin cancers, squamous cell carcinoma (SCC), basal cell carcinoma (BCC), and melanoma, are named after the cutaneous cell type that is affected, that is, squamous cells, basal cells, and melanocytes, respectively. In the United States, melanoma is a less common type of skin cancer but unfortunately is the most fatal type (National Cancer Institute, n.d.). Early detection is key to improving survival of melanoma. See the ABCDE warning signs listed under moles (nevi).

Basal cell carcinoma, the most common type of skin cancer, can be treated by surgical excision or in some cases by electrodessication and curettage (a scraping and cauterizing process). In areas such as the face, as special procedure called the Mohs microscopically controlled excision may be the best choice to preserve the most normal tissue while assuring that the skin cancer is fully removed. Squamous cell carcinoma is treated by excision. Malignant melanoma is treated by excision with a one or two centimeter margin depending on the depth of the lesion. Recently newer drugs have become available to help treat advanced basal cell carcinoma and to help treat metastatic melanoma.

According to the Skin Cancer Foundation, men have nearly double the rates of squamous and basal cell carcinomas that women have. With melanoma, the deadliest type of skin cancer, men have the highest chances of dying of the disease.

Why men? Men get more UV exposure because of their jobs, use sunscreen less, have higher rates of sunburn, and get later detection of skin cancer. Certain animal studies suggest that male skin may offer less innate protection from squamous cell carcinoma because of an apparent inability to retain adequate amounts of antioxidants. Though the researchers caution more research is needed to validate the findings, such research could lead to gender-specific sunscreen.

From a health care perspective, prevention is preferable to cure. Of course, an individual cannot prevent every disease, but steps can and should be taken to prevent diseases, especially when an individual is at high risk for a disease. The steps of prevention do not necessarily guarantee the individual will not get the disease but will only reduce the risk of getting the disease. Due to the various known and undiscovered risk factors for cancer, it should be stressed that prevention only reduces a person's chance of getting cancer and correspondingly lowers the incidence of cancer. Thus, cancer prevention will hopefully also reduce the mortality rate of cancer. When a skin tumor is caught early, the vast majority of cases—even cases of melanoma—are curable.

Skin cancer prevention can be approached from two directions: reducing the risk factors associated with skin cancer or increasing the protective factors associated with skin cancer. Certain skin cancer risk factors, such as hereditary traits, are unavoidable, whereas other risk factors, such as sun exposure, are avoidable. It should be noted that even avoidable risk factors are often impossible to avoid all the time. Plus, as the National Cancer Institute (n.d.) points out, there is insufficient evidence to prove that ultraviolet radiation (UVR) protection, such as avoiding sun exposure, decreases the risk of BCC and SCC, and preventive measures, such as using sunscreen, are not yet associated with a risk reduction for the development of cutaneous melanoma. For this reason, discovering and promoting protective factors for the development of skin cancer, which may also be beneficial for individuals with unavoidable risk factors, is a better research approach in the long run. Sunscreen with a sun protection factor (SPF) of at least 15 and protection against both UVA and UVB should be applied liberally every 2 hours during sun exposure and prior to sun exposure. Sunscreens that act as physical blockers, such as titanium or zinc, are effective immediately. Tightly woven clothing provides better sun protection than sunscreens. A hat with a 4 inch brim all of the way around also helps protect the scalp, face, ears, and neck.

Various studies have been conducted on the use of tea polyphenols in the treatment and prevention of many types of cancer, including cancer of the skin, esophagus, bladder, colorectum, lung, and breast (Arts, 2008; Bouzari et al 2009; Coyle et al., 2008; Sukhthankar et al., 2008; Velho et al., 2008; Wu et al., 2008). Polyphenols are a class of antioxidants that include tannins and flavonoids (Tangney & Rosenson, 2010) and are found in many plants. New medical research focuses on polyphenol extract from various types of tea. Tea is made from the tea plant, which is scientifically known as *Camellia sinensis*, and many tea varieties, including green tea and black tea, are derived from this plant (Sivasubramaniam et al., 2009). Teas and their beneficial properties differ by fermentation, processing, and added ingredients. Thus, herbal teas contain different properties because they are derived from herbs, fruits, and flowers but not from the tea plant; they may contain plant polyphenols depending on what herbs are used (Sivasubramaniam et al., 2009).

The multitudes of studies have been undertaken because the potential for cancer prevention using antioxidants has shown much promise. The current body of evidence to support the recommendation of the use of polyphenols in the field of oncology, specifically primary cutaneous melanoma, is insufficient, but the growing incidence of cancer and need for improved prevention and treatment modalities lends to the necessity of conducting more research in this field.

Although prevention and polyphenols are keys to working with an integrative approach to skin cancer, many other approaches exist. It is hard to test the role of nutrients in preventing various forms of skin cancer, but several studies have looked at antioxidants (including vitamin C, vitamin E, β-carotene, zinc, and vitamin A), folic acid, fats and proteins, and a variety of whole foods.

Antioxidants may offer some protection from skin cancer (Asgari et al., 2009a and 2009b; Baglia & Katiyar, 2006). Foods such as fish, beans, carrots, chard, pumpkin, cabbage, broccoli, and vegetables containing β-carotene and vitamin C may also help protect the skin (Birt et al., 1996). Studies on animals suggest that lignans, substances found in foods such as soy and flaxseed, may help fight cancer in general, including the spread of melanoma from one part of the body to another (Bain et al., 1993).

Substances found in plants that may help protect your skin from sun-related damage include apigenin, a flavonoid found in vegetables and fruits, including broccoli, celery, onions, tomatoes, apples, cherries, and grapes, and in tea and wine; curcumin, found in the spice turmeric; resveratrol, found in grape skins, red wine, and peanuts; and quercetin, a flavonoid found in apples and onions.

Skin Ulcers

Skin ulcers are more common in older adults and may be due to venous stasis, trauma, infection, skin cancer, neurologic disease, connective tissue disease, blood disorders, inflammatory processes such as pyoderma gangrenosum, arterial disease, or excessively prolonged pressure over bony areas (bedsores). Ulcers often are difficult to heal. Conventional treatment consists first of determining the cause of the ulcer through physical examination and history. Sometimes laboratory tests or biopsy is needed. Treatment is directed based on the cause of the ulceration. For stasis ulcers, support hose may be of benefit. Wound care centers are available for treating ulcers. Various soaks, dressings, topical agents, and systemic treatments may be indicated based on the type of ulcer. Dietary measures include a balanced diet with adequate protein. Nutritional supplements include a multivitamin, vitamin B complex, vitamin C with bioflavonoids 3,000 mg/day, vitamin D 400 to 1,000 IU/day, flaxseed oil 2 tablespoons/day, and zinc 50 mg/day. Herbal therapy includes honey applied three times daily to the ulcer, tea tree oil applied to the ulcer, calendula ointment or comfrey cream applied to dry areas, or oral horse chestnut for venous stasis ulcers. Acupressure to gallbladder 34, large intestine 4, liver 3, stomach 36, and the paraspinal bladder points helps to improve circulation (Jacknin, 2001).

Sunburn

Sunburn is an acute reaction to UVB spectrum excess irradiation from sunlight. UVC is the shortest portion of the UV spectrum (100 to 280 nm) that is blocked by the earth's atmosphere. UVB is next shortest portion of the UV spectrum (280 to 315 nm) and is blocked by ordinary window glass. It is the part that causes sunburn and is partially responsible for tanning. It also promotes skin cancers. UVA is the longest portion of the UV spectrum (315 to 400 nm) and passes through ordinary window glass. It is also partially responsible for tanning and over the long term promotes wrinkling and skin cancers. Certain oral drugs can be activated by UVA in the skin to produce phototoxic reactions. Skin exposure to certain plant juices such as lime juice can also be activated by UVA to produce phototoxic reactions. Sunburn can be first degree with redness or second degree with blistering. In severe cases systemic symptoms including fever, nausea, and malaise may occur. Prevention of sunburn is with sun avoidance, sun protective clothing, and sunscreen. Sunscreens are rated with SPF with respect to UVB. UVA protection may be rated by a one- to four-star rating. Sunscreen is imperfect, with high ratings required to protect pale skin. Skin types for sunburn are rated type 1: always burn, never tan; type 2: always burn, sometimes tan; type 3: sometimes burn, always tan; type 4: never burn, always tan; type 5: olive; and type 6: black. The darker the natural skin tone, the lower the SPF needed. Conventional and integrative treatments of sunburn are the same as for burns. In addition, topical corticosteroids may help suppress inflammation early in the course of the sunburn development.

Varicose Veins

Varicose veins occur in superficial leg veins when the one-way valves fail and the veins dilate. There often is a hereditary factor. Conventional therapies include support hose, sclerotherapy injections, and various surgical and laser procedures. Dietary measures include a high-fiber diet to avoid constipation and eating noninflammatory foods and avoiding inflammatory foods as listed under acne. If you are overweight, weight reduction will be helpful. Nutritional supplements include vitamin C and bioflavonoids 1,000 to 3,000 mg/day, vitamin E 200 to 400 IU/day, vitamin B complex, and β-carotene 25,000 IU/day. Herbal treatment with horse chestnut 500 mg two or three times a day may be as effective as support hose but takes up to 3 months to notice the benefit. Bilberry, gingko biloba, grapeseed extract, and hawthorn may also be beneficial. Acupressure on spleen 9 for 3 minutes three times a day may help to relieve water retention and varicose veins (Jacknin, 2001).

Vitiligo

Vitiligo is patchy complete pigment loss that occurs as an autoimmune attack by the body's immune system destroying pigment-producing cells.

Conventional treatments consist of cover-up dyes and cosmetics, topical corti-costeroids, topical tacrolimus, topical or oral PUVA therapy, minigrafting, or, in severely extensive cases, topical depigmentation of normal skin with mono-benzyl ether of hydroquinone. Nutritional supplements that may be of benefit include B-complex vitamins and vitamin C.

Warts (Verrucae)

Warts are a skin infection with human papilloma virus (HPV) resulting in a localized overgrowth of the skin. They are named by their appearance and location, with examples being common, flat, genital, plantar (on the sole), and filiform (thread-like). There are over 100 different HPV subtypes. Genital warts of certain HPV subtypes are associated with cervical, penile, and anal cancers. Vaccines have been developed against these carcinogenic subtypes and are rec-ommended for prepubescent girls and boys. Warts generally resolve sponta-neously after a number of months to a number of years. The body's immune system, especially the delayed cellular aspect, is what induces resolution of the warts. In immunocompromised individuals the warts often are multiple and resistant to resolution. Conventional treatments consist of topical salicylic and lactic acid solutions and plasters, freezing with liquid nitrogen, curettage or cutting (likely to leave scarring), or laser (HPV in smoke can be inhaled). Contact sensitization with squaric acid dibutyl ester, injection with candi-dal antigen, or topical imiquimod may help stimulate the immune system to respond against the HPV. Anticancer drugs can be injected into the wart and include bleomycin (painful) or 5-fluorouracil. Topical tretinoin can be used on flat warts, as can 5-fluorouracil cream. Podophyllin solution can be painted on genital warts. Trichloroacetic acid can also be painted on genital warts. Green tea extract sinecatechins can be applied to genital warts (Hara, 2011).

Dietary measures include foods high in vitamin A. Supplement options include vitamin A 25,000 IU daily for a month, B-complex vitamins, vitamin C with bioflavonoids 500 mg daily, vitamin E 400 IU daily, and zinc 50 mg daily. Herbal treatments include topical inner banana peel, fresh crushed basil, fresh crushed garlic, buttercup sap, dandelion sap, green tea concentrate, fresh pineapple slice, and inner bark of willow. Suggestion, guided imagery, hypno-sis, and hypnoanalysis may be beneficial (Ewin, 2011).

Wrinkles

Sun damage, heredity, and smoking account for most wrinkles. Smoking cessation is important. Prevention with high-SPF sunscreen use daily on sun-exposed areas, ultraviolet filtering sunglasses, sun-protective clothing and hats, sun avoidance, and eating antioxidant foods in the diet is important to reduce progression of wrinkling. Conventional treatments include glycolic and lactic acid creams and peels, trichloroacetic acid peels, topical tretinoin, injectable fillers, injectable dilute botulinum toxin, laser resurfacing, microdermabrasion, and surgical face lift.

Dietary antioxidant foods may be beneficial. Nutritional supplements include daily multivitamin, vitamin C with bioflavonoids 500 to 1,000 mg, vitamin E 400 to 800 IU, and selenium 100 to 200 mcg daily. Topical vitamin C and vitamin E may be of benefit, as may topical coenzyme Q10 cream. Topical preparations made from fruit juices or peels containing α-hydroxyl acids may be helpful. Moisturization with cocoa butter, coconut oil, olive oil, avocado oil, or almond oil may help to reduce the appearance of fine wrinkles.

Yeast *(Candida)*

Candidal yeast infections typically occur in moist areas such as the groin, axillae, uncircumcised foreskin, other body fold areas, or mouth (thrush). The infected skin is usually beefy red with satellite lesions near the edges. Oral lesions are usually whitish and can be scraped off. Potassium hydroxide (KOH) preparation examination under the microscope sometimes reveals the organism from cutaneous sites and usually reveals the organism from oral sites. Conventional treatments include topical antifungals such as ketoconazole and keeping the area dry. Dietary measures include a balanced diet with vegetables and avoidance of sugary foods and drinks. Nutritional supplements include a multivitamin, vitamin C with bioflavonoids 3,000 mg/day, and zinc 50 mg/day. Herbal treatments include calendula cream, garlic orally or topically, tea tree oil topically, licorice tea topically, myrrh paste topically, olive leaf extract orally, thyme oil topically, or tumeric extract topically and orally.

REFERENCES

Al-Niaimi F. Drug eruptions in dermatology. Expert Rev Dermatol. 2011;6(3): 273–286.

Arts IC. A review of the epidemiological evidence on tea, flavonoids, and lung cancer. J Nutr. 2008;138:1561S–1566S.

Asgari MM, Maruti SS, Kushi LH, White E. A cohort study of vitamin D intake and melanoma risk. J Invest Dermatol. 2009a;129(7):1675–1680.

Asgari MM, Maruti SS, Kushi LH, White E. Antioxidant supplementation and risk of incident melanomas: results of a large prospective cohort study. Arch Dermatol. 2009b;145(8):879–882.

Baglia MS, Katiyar SK. Chemoprevention of photocarcinogenesis by selected dietary botanicals. Photochem Photobiol Sci. 2006;5(2):243–253.

Bain C, Green A, Siskind V, Alexander J, Harvey P. Diet and melanoma: an exploratory case-control study. Ann Epidemiol. 1993;3:235–238.

Baumann L. *The Skin Type Solution*. New York, New York, Bantam, 2010.

Bedi MK, Shenefelt PD. Herbal therapy in dermatology. Arch Dermatol. 2002;138(2):232–242.

Birt DF, Pelling JC, Nair S, Lepley D. Diet intervention for modifying cancer risk. Prog Clin Bio Res. 1996;395:223–234.

Blumenthal M, Ed. *The Complete German Commission E Monographs: Therapeutic Guide to Herbal Medicines*. American Botanical Council, Austin, Texas, 1998.

Boguniewicz M, Leung DY. Atopic dermatitis: a disease of altered skin barrier and immune dysregulation. Immunol Rev. 2011;242(1):233–246.

Bouzari N, Romagosa Y, Kirsner RS. Green tea prevents skin cancer by two mechanisms. J Investigat Dermatol. 2009;129,1054. doi:10.1038/jid.2009.64

Cannon CP, Vierck E. *The Complete Idiot's Guide to the Anti-Inflammation Diet*. New York, New York, Alpha Books, 2006.

Choudhary S, McLeod M, Meshkov L, Nouri K. Lasers in the treatment of acne scars. Expert Rev Dermatol. 2011;6(1):45–60.

Coyle CH, Philips BJ, Morrisroe S, Chancellor MB, Yoshimura N. Antioxidant effects of green tea and its polyphenols on bladder cells. Life Sci. 2008;83:12–18. doi:10.1016/j.lfs.2008.04.010

Crawford GH, Pelle MT, James WD. Rosacea: I. Etiology, pathogenesis, and subtype classification. J Am Acad Dermatol. 2004;51(3):327–341.

Ewin DM. Treatment of HPV with hypnosis—psychodynamic considerations of psychoneuroimmunology: a brief communication. Internat J Clin Exper Hypn. 2011;59(4):392–398.

Gerber PA, Buhren BA, Steinhoff M, Homey B. Rosacea: the cytokine and che-mokine network. J Investig Dermatol Symp Proc. 2011;15(1):40–47.

Grattan CE. Autoimmune urticaria. Immunol Allergy Clin North Am. 2004;24(2):163–181.

Hara Y. Tea catechins and their applications as supplements and pharmaceu-tics. Pharmacol Res. 2011;64(2):100–104.

Ho SG, Yeung CK, Chan NP, Shek SY, Chan HH. A comparison of Q-switched and long-pulsed alexandrite laser for the treatment of freckles and lentigi-nes in oriental patients. Lasers Surg Med. 2011;43(2):108–113.

Jacknin J. *Smart Medicine for Your Skin*. New York, New York, Avery, 2001.

Khan AA, Khanum A, Eds, *Herbal Therapy for Skin Afflictions*. Hyderabad, India, Ukaaz Publications, 2009.

Lapolla W, Digiorgio C, Haitz K, Magel G, Mendoza N, Grady J, Lu W, Tyring S. Incidence of postherpetic neuralgia after combination treatment with gabapentin and valacyclovir in patients with acute herpes zoster: open-label study. Arch Dermatol. 2011;147:901–907.

Logan AC, Treloar V. *The Clear Skin Diet*. Naperville, Illinois, Cumberland House, 2007.

Marieb EN, Hoehn K. Human Anatomy & Physiology, 8th ed. San Francisco, California, Pearson Benjamin Cummings, 2009.

Muenke M, Draeger-Muenke R. Acupressure and hypnosis: healer, heal thyself (and thy patients). Contemp Hypn Integr Ther. 2011;23(3):224–134.

National Cancer Institute. (n.d.). Melanoma. Retrieved from http://www.cancer.gov

Nguyen N, Burkhart CN, Burkhart CG. Identifying potential pitfalls in conventional herpes simplex virus management. Int J Dermatol. 2010;49(9): 987–993.

Nobbe S, Dziunycz P, Mühleisen B, Bilsborough J, Dillon SR, French LE, Hofbauer GFL. IL-31 Expression by inflammatory cells is preferentially elevated in atopic dermatitis. Acta Derm Venereol. 2012;92:24–28.

Ortega C, Fernández AS, Carrillo JM, Romero P, Molina IJ, Moreno JC, Santamaría M. IL-17-producing CD8+ T lymphocytes from psoriasis skin plaques are cytotoxic effector cells that secrete Th17-related cytokines. J Leukoc Biol. 2009;86(2):435–443.

Preeti L, Magesh K, Rajkumar K, Karthik R. Recurrent aphthous stomatitis. J Oral Maxillofac Pathol. 2011;15(3):252–256.

Savage LJ, Layton AM. Treating acne vulgaris: systemic, local and combination therapy. Expert Rev Clin Pharmacol. 2010;13(4):563–580.

Shenefelt PD. Hypnosis in dermatology. Arch Dermatol. 2000;136(3):393–399.

Shenefelt PD. Hypnoanalysis for dermatologic disorders. J Altern Med Res. 2010;2(4):439–445.

Shenefelt PD. Psychodermatological disorders: recognition and treatment. Int J Dermatol. 2011;50(11):1309–122.

Sivasubramaniam S, Parrott-Sheffer C, Singh S, and the editors of Encyclopaedia Britannica. Tea. In Encyclopaedia Britannica, 2009. Retrieved from http://www.britannica.com/EBchecked/topic/585115/tea

Snowden RV. Annual report: US cancer death rates still declining, 2010. Retrieved from http://www.cancer.org/Cancer/news/annual-report-us-cancer-death-rates-still-declining

Ständer S, Weisshaar E, Mettang T, Szepietowski JC, Carstens E, Ikoma A, Bergasa NV, Gieler U, Misery L, Wallengren J, Darsow U, Streit M, Metze

D, Luger TA, Greaves MW, Schmelz M, Yosipovitch G, Bernhard JD, for the International Forum for the Study of Itch (IFSI). Clinical classification of itch: a position paper of the International Forum for the Study of Itch. Acta Derm Venereol. 2007;87:291–294.

Suárez AL, Feramisco JD, Koo J, Steinhoff M. Psychoneuroimmunology of psychological stress and atopic dermatitis: pathophysiologic and therapeutic updates. Acta Derm Venereol. 2012;92(1):7–15.

Sukhthankar M, Yamaguchi K, Lee S, McEntee MF, Eling TE, Hara Y, Baek SJ. A green tea component suppresses posttranslational expression of basic fibroblast growth factor in colorectal cancer. Gastroenterology. 2008;134:1972–1980. doi:10.1053/j.gastro.2008.02.095

Tangney CC, Rosenson RS. Lipid lowering with diet or dietary supplements, 2010. UpToDate. Retrieved from http://www.uptodate.com.ezproxylocal. library.nova.edu/online/content/topic.do?topicKey=lipiddis/6831&selected Title=1~150&source=search_result#H12

Tausk F, Elenkov I, Moynihan J. Psychoneuroimmunology. Dermatol Ther. 2008;21(1):22–31.

Velho AV, Hartmann AA, Kruel CD. Effect of black tea in diethylnitrosamine-induced esophageal carcinogenesis in mice. Acta Cirurgica Brasil. 2008;23(4):329–336.

Vrijman C, van Drooge AM, Limpens J, Bos JD, van der Veen JPW, Spuls PI, Wolkerstorfer A. Laser and intense pulsed light therapy for the treatment of hypertrophic scars: a systematic review. Brit J Dermatol. 2011;165(5):934–942.

Walling HW, Swick BL. Treatment options for hyperhidrosis. Am J Clin Dermatol. 2011;12(5):285–295.

Wu AH, Ursin G, Koh W, Wang R, Yuan J, Khoo K, Yu MC. Green tea, soy, and mammographic density in Singapore Chinese women. Cancer Epidemiol Biomarkers Prevent. 2008;17(12):3358–3365. doi:10.1158/1055-9965. EPI-08-0132

Yihou X. *Dermatology in Traditional Chinese Medicine*. St Albans, United Kingdom, Donica Publishing Ltd., 2004.

18

Healthy Aging

NEAL ROUZIER AND GEORGE E. MUÑOZ

The concept of healthy aging for men has been a historical non sequitur. Specifically, men tend to die sooner than women. Specific reasons have included war in medieval times and prior eras. World Wars I and II and modern-day conflicts would be the only other equivalents to medieval and ancient civilization conflicts. Having said this, what other factors contribute to shorter life spans in men versus women? Stress has to be considered one of the main contributors in modern eras; therefore, stress reduction interventions are key to reducing the health toll of this factor. Exercise, both cardiovascular and resistive weight training, and any enjoyable recreational physical activity are highly recommended as great coping strategies. A regular exercise plan with 30 minutes of cardiovascular and 20 to 30 minutes of weight training including a cool-down and flexibility activities is ideal for cardiovascular disease and cancer prevention. Additionally, endorphin generation from intensive exercise helps improve mood and is an essential aspect for preventing and treating depression. Coupling these lifestyle habits with mind–body interventions that enhance mindfulness, subconscious pathways, and autonomics can reduce the adrenalin-driven proinflammatory state of many men who are either in the alpha status professionally or the main bread winners. Breath work, mediation, guided imagery, progressive muscle relaxation, and the like are some but not all of the types of activities men should be encouraged to explore. The reflex prescriptive habit of writing nonstop anxiolytics and antidepressants for manageable stress scenarios should halt. Not only is this practice pervasive, but also it is essentially a band-aid approach and leads to at best more polypharmacy and at worst potential drug dependency or interactions that are unnecessary and avoidable. Using a diary for a multitude of health reasons including stress reduction, self-awareness, and personal growth is a proven tool in reducing depression. Stress reduction education is a powerful ally for the practitioner and his or her male patients.

Dietary patterns are equally important for healthy aging. As has been previously mentioned in this book, an anti-inflammatory Mediterranean diet with Paleolithic features is highly recommended. Diets that are high fiber, are micronutrient dense, have low to no processed carbohydrates, and are high in omega-3 and low omega-6 fats are recommended. The plate should have color! Vegetables, grains, limited nut portions, wild fatty fish, and poultry (preferably hormone free) are recommended. Cruciferous vegetables for men are protective against colon and prostate cancer as well as the rare event of breast cancer in men. Men who train and lift weights build muscle mass naturally, causing natural elevations of their own inherent testosterone and human growth hormone, which can occur when lactic acid builds up during intense workouts. For these men, cruciferous vegetables are very important to reduce pro-estrogenic tendencies and to help reduce body fat. Vitamins and supplements are another area where men may or may not be up-to-date in their knowledge base or habits. This will be covered in the appropriate section, but we recommend vitamin D 2000-10,0000 units daily depending on blood levels. Optimum serum level 60-80 ng ml. Vitamin E with mixed tocopherols 400 iudaily. Vitamin C buffered, esterified 1000-2000mg daily. Coenzyme Q10-100-2000 mg daily. Individualized and tailored recommendations can be made based on blood testing as well as transcutaneous spectrophotometric techniques that are quick and noninvasive and yield tissue results that are replicable. If men eat poorly, then I would recommend a good general multivitamin. Selenium for aging men is recommended for prostate health as well as for thyroid support. Conditions including metabolic syndrome, inflammation for any reason, and diabetes require broad ranges of B vitamins including folic acid, B_6, B_{12}, B_1, and B_2 in addition to the antioxidants mentioned previously. Similarly, very active men who train heavily form oxidant stress and radicals as well. They should also be supplemented.

Adequate hydration for men is underpublicized. Active men should be encouraged to "pee clear" when they are training. Urine color charts should reflect white clear urine, not yellow or darker shades, to signify maximal hydration status, especially if training outdoors in heat and/or humidity. Competitors should begin hydrating 24 to 48 hours before events as there are limits to comfortable fluid absorption in the setting of physical activities.

Sleep is another major area to emphasize as essential for healthy aging. Snoring or obstructive breathing patterns should be investigated, and men should be educated as to potential long-term sequelae including cardiovascular disease and central nervous system (CNS) effects. Specialists and testing are now more commonly utilized in conventional medical settings. In a culture where electronics abound, sleep hygiene should be taught to men, as this is not necessarily a concept men are routinely exposed to in their lives. Rituals, light dimming, and elimination of intrusive and pervasive electronics and their lighting should be done for restful sleep. Stimulants including caffeine should be eliminated or minimized after dinner for those who experience sleep disturbances.

Relationships are another key area for men to explore as part of their health. Forming intimate bonds with their spouse or significant other and close friends or family members is highly recommended. Disenfranchised individuals tend to have more health issues with aging and higher mortality statistically. The concept of "male bonding" has its merits in these regards as well for intimate sharing that may not occur in other settings. Spirituality has been discussed in Chapter 5 and will not be addressed here.

Having said all of this, healthy aging for men may necessitate support for low energy states or fatigue. The differential diagnosis of this complaint is quite broad yet common for men as they age. Assuming adequate diets and supplementation, adaptogens may be a useful approach for men. Ashwaganda, Rhodiola rosea, and Panax ginseng are example of botanicals that are effective and useful for improving low energy states. Once all these modalities and approaches have been exhausted, some men may want or need more intensive interventions if the problem remains such as hormone balancing.

Hormones

Although it is commonly accepted to replace hormones in women, it is just as important for health and well-being to also replace hormones in men when needed. There is an impressive amount of medical literature that demonstrates the health and longevity benefits of maintaining optimal hormone levels and the detrimental effects of hormone depletion. All of our hormone levels will fall with age, and there is no evidence at all that this is beneficial or necessary— all the data support significant harm from loss of hormones experienced by everyone as we age. The tremendous array of studies now support replacement of those lost hormones; however, more importantly is the concept of how they are replaced and to what level. Simply just replacing these hormones is not sufficient to maximize beneficial effects, yet the hormones must be replaced to the optimal, most effective levels, a concept not familiar to most physicians. We will explore the concept of optimization and the importance of understanding the difference or harm of maintaining low and midnormal levels of hormones in contrast to augmenting to higher or more optimal levels, defined as the upper range of normal for a young adult.

Conventional medicine has always held the belief that aging is inevitable and that the progressive deterioration that occurs in our adult years cannot be altered. This is simply not true. We have also been led to believe that the diseases of aging, such as heart disease, stroke, cancer, senility, and arthritis, are all a part of the normal aging process and nothing can be offered to slow down that process. Fortunately, there is now a scientific understanding and awareness that identifies hormone replacement as preventive medicine, or a therapy that forestalls the deterioration seen with aging. The downward spiral of physical and mental decline that we have come to accept as a natural part of growing older is becoming recognized as somewhat controllable and preventable. The most effective solution of any disease process is prevention of that illness. We are entering an era where patients now focus on slowing down aging and thereby achieve prevention of both illness and deterioration. More importantly, the demand is for wellness as well as improved quality of life. The medical community is becoming aware of the health benefits, but this push for optimal hormone supplementation comes mostly from patients who demand to feel and function better as well as maintain that quality of life. The tremendous health-protective benefits of hormones are growing in understanding, acceptance, and application. Research continues to show that maintaining our hormone levels in a youthful state can prevent the debility and illness that accompany the aging process. Obviously this will lead to increased longevity by preventing the illnesses that usually lead to our demise. However, most importantly from a patient perspective is the fact that our quality of life and wellness in our later years will be significantly enhanced (Winters, 1999).

Our hormone levels fall as we age (Carter et al., 1995). However, simply replacing hormone levels back to "normal" for the age of that person may not result in much of an effect in how one feels and functions. A decrease in the production of hormones begins in young adulthood and continues to diminish in a linear fashion until old age. However, that is not the only problem. In addition, as we age, the specific receptor sites in the cells tend to change and become not as receptive to the hormones as they once were in our younger years. This is commonly understood with type 2 diabetes, where there is an adequate amount of insulin yet the cell lacks sensitivity to insulin, which is commonly referred to as insulin resistance. This receptor site resistance is present when looking at other hormones also. Whatever the cause may be (low hormone level or otherwise), any decrease in stimulation of the receptor site will result in a decrease in stimulation of the cell, a decrease in signal transduction to inside the cell, a decrease in protein synthesis, and loss of effectiveness of the hormones. This is the very reason that we see and experience an improvement in symptoms in spite of the patient having "normal" levels in the first place. The treatment for the hormone resistance is to stimulate more receptor sites, which thereby requires increasing the hormone levels to a higher level, which stimulates more receptor sites, which increases hormone effectiveness. This is evidenced by studies showing that simply restoring levels to "normal" does not effect any change in how the patient feels or functions. However, optimizing or augmenting to higher or more optimal levels does effect a change. Therefore, simply restoring to normal levels is not adequate or effective. The medical literature overwhelmingly demonstrates this, and review articles in the Journal of Clinical Endocrinology and Metabolism (*JCEM*) and *New England Journal of Medicine* dictate that experienced practitioners replace levels to the upper range of normal of a young adult, a concept that most physicians are not taught or do not fully understand in spite of the overwhelming literature support for doing so.

With the advent of the Internet and patients becoming their own health advocates, we are now witnessing a growing change in how we practice medicine. Patients want to remain strong, healthy, and vigorous as well as preserve their physical and mental health. We can improve many of the symptoms that we have come to accept and associate with aging. We can also regain the youthful resilience that enables us to cope gracefully with the stressors that challenge us every day. For those of you already on hormone replacement therapy (HRT) and who have already experienced this boost of life, you will understand exactly to what I'm referring. For those of you who have not experienced this yet, this is your introduction to this life-changing phenomenon. This concept is so well embraced and promoted by patients yet so misunderstood or not embraced by physicians who are not aware of the concepts or scientific support for such a therapy.

HRT is not a panacea or fountain of youth, although it is promoted by some to be "antiaging." There is no scientific literature, support, or U.S. Food and Drug Administration (FDA) approval for use or promotion as an "antiaging" treatment, and it should not be promoted as such. We still continue to age and lose cells secondary to a process that is regulated genetically. Nothing reverses aging. However, with hormones we can slow down the precipitous decline that occurs after midlife and will remain resilient. Hormones help us maintain our good health, and loss of hormones adversely affects all tissues, organs, and systems. The purpose is to simply replenish the hormones that occur naturally in our body and boost them back up to the appropriate medically sound levels necessary to maintain youthful health and vigor. Which hormones to replenish, how much to replenish, and how to adjust the hormones so that they have a therapeutic effect are beyond the scope of this chapter and require that physicians attend training seminars to learn the nuts and bolts of this specialty. It is simply preventive medicine, all evidence based, but falls between the cracks in our training. Nevertheless, there are many medical conferences that offer training courses to any physician interested in preventive and quality-of-life medicine. We physicians can also slow down our own aging process, prevent deterioration, maintain a better quality of life, and feel and function better. This is true preventive medicine that we should all enjoy.

Testosterone

As we age, we experience changes in strength, endurance, muscle mass, bone density, energy, and sexual function. There is an increase in cardiovascular disease, cholesterol, body fat, and memory loss. Aging is associated with decreased sociability, decreased cognition, osteoporosis, and changes in body composition. Replacement of testosterone to optimal physiologic ranges (upper end of normal but not excessive) has been shown to slow down these age-related changes. Diseases of aging, such as heart disease, stroke (Fukui et al., 2003), hypertension, and diabetes, have all been associated with low levels of testosterone. Numerous medical journal articles, books, and lectures testify to the benefits of testosterone replacement and the harm of hormone deprivation (Winters, 1999). Patient testimonials praise the improvement in symptoms as well as energy, function, strength, motivation, libido, and sense of well-being. The increase in arthritis symptoms associated with andropause (loss of testosterone) and the improvement in symptoms with replacement may be due to the decrease in inflammatory cytokines demonstrated in the studies of testosterone. After 6 months of therapy, patients notice improved sense of well-being, improved outlook on life, reshaped bodies, fat disappearing, increased muscle tone, and return of lost energy, strength, and endurance. Physicians should be as ecstatic about the health benefits as patients are about the feel-good benefits.

Testosterone has been available for years but only in the form of an injection. It is now available commercially through three different pharmaceutical companies and advertised nightly on television. Oh how the pendulum swings. For years I heard that testosterone was bad for one's health, caused prostate cancer (Rhoden & Morgentaler, 2003), and made men berserk. Now the pharmaceutical industry advertises nightly the importance of replacing your "T." The pharmaceutical industry obviously understands the patient demand and importance of testosterone. Unfortunately, as evidenced by the subtherapeutic levels achieved by the commercial products, patients don't fare as well as they should. This is counterintuitive to what we are attempting to achieve with optimal replacement. To get FDA approval, the pharmaceutical manufacturers use low doses, which do not achieve levels into the upper range of normal for a young adult and therefore doesn't provide the optimal health benefits (Muller et al., 2005), nor symptomatic improvement, as demonstrated in the literature.

As a result many physicians, including myself, prescribe testosterone through compounding pharmacies at much more concentrated and user-friendly doses that achieve and maintain optimal levels much more effectively than the commercially available products. Symptomatic improvement is significant when a patient receives the correct doses that correlate with adequate optimal serum levels. For example, if the data support that total testosterone levels of 1,000 µg/ml are optimal for achieving therapeutic effectiveness and commercial testosterone preparations achieve levels of only 300 µg/ml, then it makes no sense from a scientific standpoint to utilize inferior products that do not optimize levels and effects. This is a prime example of the difference between optimal replacement and normal replacement and the importance of optimal replacement. If all the health benefits are achieved at levels of 1,000 and not at 300, then where would you like your levels to be? And from a patient perspective, patients will absolutely tell me vociferously the difference they feel. Once a man feels the effects of optimal levels, it is difficult for him to accept anything less.

There are a plethora of studies over the last 50 years demonstrating the health benefits of testosterone. The cardiovascular benefits are indisputable (English et al., 2000; Fukui et al., 2003; Muller et al., 2005). However, the rheumatology world is behind on their use and understanding of hormones for arthritis and degenerative joint changes and the accompanying loss of muscle mass and strength that accompany these disorders. The improved strength, energy, function, and quality of life and the decrease in pain are frequently not appreciated by my local rheumatologists. With the improved strength, energy, and endurance come an improved sense of well-being, less depressed mood, and renewed interest in life that are not possible with any other rheumatologic therapy. Many of my patients will voice that it wasn't until I put them on hormones that they began to feel better (Ginsberg & Cavalieri, 2008). The many rheumatologic agents help to relieve pain and inflammation, but none restore the well-being and quality of life that turns patients' lives around, which is what makes this a patient-driven therapy.

Testosterone is responsible for the sex drive of both men and women. As testosterone diminishes with age, so does sexual function. Restoring testosterone to youthful levels can reverse this situation. There is no need to accept this loss of sexuality. Patients, both men and women, do not hesitate to brag about their sex lives, and this is commonly seen in couples in their 80s. I hear it so often that I am no longer impressed. To hear an 87-year-old man request more testosterone because he is having trouble keeping up with his 87-year-old wife is truly impressive. For all that I do, the medicines and supplements and lifestyle changes I push, there is nothing more rewarding

Prinz PN, Scanlan JM, Vitaliano PP, Moe KE, Borson S, Toivola B, Merriam GR, Larsen LH, Reed HL. Thyroid hormones: positive relationships with cognition in healthy, euthyroid older men. J Gerontol A Biol Sci Med Sci. 1999;54(3):M111–M116. doi:10.1093/gerona/54.3.M111

Smallridge RC. Disclosing subclinical thyroid disease: an approach to mild laboratory abnormalities and vague or absent symptoms. Postgrad Med. 2000;107(1)143–146, 149.

19

Environmental Toxins and Men's Health

ALEXANDRA MUÑOZ

A t first glance the role of toxins in men's health may appear to be a highly specialized topic, applicable only to a few individuals with rare diseases—but in reality the information presented in this chapter is applicable to most men as environmental toxins can impact many aspects of men's health, from prostate cancer to reproductive health and aging. The toxins discussed in this chapter are only a selection from a panoply of toxins that now contaminate our natural and built environments. Environmental toxins impact human health through a wide range of physiological and molecular consequences, which involve long latency periods and mechanisms of action that are not yet elucidated, collectively making their impact difficult to detect and pinpoint. As the consequences of industrialization and worldwide pollution continue to be unveiled, understanding the impact of environmental toxins on men's health will prove to be increasingly relevant and necessary.

Toxins Specific to Men's Health

ENDOCRINE DISRUPTORS

Although there are many types of toxins that can impact health, endocrine disruptors (EDs) constitute a major concern for men because they can play an important role in prostate cancer, tumor progression, and sperm health. Endocrine disruptors are a category of toxins that interact with the hormone signaling systems and are defined by the Endocrine Society as "compound[s], either natural or synthetic, which through environmental or inappropriate developmental exposures alter the hormonal and homeostatic systems that enable the organism to communicate with and respond to its environment"

(Diamanti-Kandarakis, Bourguignon et al. 2009). During the last century industrialization and chemical manufacturing have altered the chemical landscape of our world, and many of the chemicals that have been released into the environment are highly persistent endocrine disruptors.

Endocrine disruptors influence molecular and systemic physiology through a variety of mechanisms. Originally, endocrine disruptors were thought to act exclusively through direct interactions with nuclear hormone receptors, and compounds were assessed based on their ability to structurally mimic steroid hormones. Now it is clear that endocrine disruption involves a broader range of receptors including nonsteroid receptors and orphan receptors, as well as interactions with enzymatic pathways involved in steroid biosynthesis/metabolism. In turn, EDs may interact with androgen, estrogen, and glucocorticoid receptors, and they can even alter metabolic pathways to promote the development of insulin resistance and obesity. Although a single ED may interact with multiple receptors and impact various avenues of physiology, the focus here will be on toxins that interact with androgen and estrogen pathways and their physiological consequences in relation to the prostate gland, tumor progression, and reproductive health.

The dose, duration, and timing of exposure influence the magnitude, duration, and type of effect an ED will have on the system. EDs exert the strongest influence during critical time periods of development and sexual maturation, which include exposures occurring in utero, in prepubescence, and at the beginning of puberty. During these critical windows of sensitivity, sexual organs are primed to developmentally respond to small alterations in the levels of circulating hormones, and an inappropriate input can alter the epigenetic pattern and the developmental course of the cells and the organ. This type of change can lead to lifelong consequences for health that may not be noticed until later in life when problems involving fertility or cancer manifest.

Two key features are important to note when considering the impact of endocrine disruptors. First, because many relevant exposures occur during childhood, there is a long latency period that often makes it difficult to connect exposures to health outcomes. Second, dose-response dynamics for EDs are distinct from those of traditional toxins where more toxin means more toxic. Low doses of EDs can promote strong responses and dangerous outcomes, because the endocrine system is primed to respond to small changes in hormone levels.

TOXINS AFFECTING THE PROSTATE GLAND
Prostate Cancer

Despite the high prevalence, the mechanisms of carcinogenesis surrounding prostate cancer have yet to be fully elucidated, and its development appears to be a multifactorial process. Although prostate cancers have a demonstrated sensitivity to androgens, and tumor growth often slows with androgen deprivation, circulating levels of androgen hormones lack consistent epidemiologic evidence supporting their role as a causative factor in prostate cancer. Similarly, there is also a lack of evidence supporting the role of circulating estrogen levels and the development of prostate cancers, despite the presence of higher estrogen levels in prostate cancers and the protective role of anti-estrogens. Debate over the role of hormones continues because as a proliferative disease these cancers tend to respond to hormones with increased growth. However, the role of hormones may be more difficult to fully understand than simple correlations between circulating levels and prostate cancer outcomes. Hormone levels present in utero, during early childhood, and in prepubescent growth may be most relevant to the development of prostate cancers. Within this area, questions of endocrine-disrupting toxins and their role in male prostate development and health come to bear on the discussion. Although the evidence is not definitive, there is substantial evidence to suggest, at minimum, the involvement of toxins in prostate cancer progression and severity. In turn, those looking to avoid prostate cancers should exercise caution and reduce their exposure to endocrine disruptors until their safety can be proven.

Farming

The strongest link between environmental exposures and prostate cancer can be found in the occupational exposure of farmers and their families, who are exposed to high levels of pesticides throughout the lifetime. Numerous human studies have demonstrated an increased risk for prostate cancer among farmers in North America. There are conflicting reports between studies, with some reporting a modestly increased association and others reporting no association. Difficulties in attaining consistent results may occur because farmers are exposed to a large group of chemicals that likely vary in dose, duration, and mixture across studies. If only a few chemicals are highly active with respect to the prostate, then conflicting results are expected.

Farming has been associated with an increased risk of mortality from prostate cancer (Morrison, Savitz et al. 1993), an increased risk of prostate cancer for those with a family history with exposures to chlorpyrifos, coumaphos, fonofos, phorate and permethrin, and butylate (Alavanja, Samanic et al. 2003, Barker, Alavanja et al. 2003, Mahajan, Bonner et al. 2006), and an increased risk of prostate cancer for Caucasians (Meyer, Coker et al. 2007).

Epidemiologic studies examining prostate cancer's relationship to single pesticides have yielded more concrete findings, including a direct link between the fungicide methyl bromide and prostate cancer risk (Alavanja, Samanic et al. 2003). Here the mechanisms of action are unknown, but it is suspected that such exposures interfere with hormone metabolism in the body, leading to abnormal steroid levels. The pesticides chlorpyrifos, fonofos, coumaphos, and phorate are suspected of interfering with the functioning of p450 enzymes, which metabolize hormones in the liver. The disruption of these enzymes would result in increased levels of circulating estrogens.

TOXINS AFFECTING TUMOR PROGRESSION

Some EDs may help prostate cancers to form and/or progress. Hormonally dependent tumors deprived of endogenous hormones may appear to have entered hormone-independent states of growth and be deemed androgen independent, when in reality they are utilizing toxins with endocrine activity to stimulate growth. The following section provides evidence suggesting that various toxins work by stimulating hormone-mediated growth in prostate tumors. Clinically, these findings may be relevant for individuals who have already been diagnosed with prostate cancer or for men who are looking to take preventive steps.

Bisphenol A

Bisphenol A (BPA) is an environmental estrogen capable of interacting with the estrogen receptors, ERα, ERβ, and GPR30, as well as with mutated forms of the androgen receptor (AR). In vitro studies have found that BPA is capable of interacting with mutated ARs found in prostate cancer cells and that such interactions may promote the therapeutic resistance of some forms of prostate cancer to androgen deprivation. It has been shown that tumor-derived mutant forms of AR are responsive to the noncanonical ligand binding with BPA (Wetherill, Fisher et al. 2005). In this study, environmentally relevant doses of BPA stimulated prostate cancer cells with mutated receptors to proliferate and bypass cell cycle checkpoints, facilitating androgen-independent growth and suggesting that tumor recurrence in patients receiving androgen deprivation therapy may be facilitated by exposure to BPA (Wetherill, Fisher et al. 2005, Wetherill, Hess-Wilson et al. 2006).

BPA exposure typically occurs via hard plastic water bottles and the epoxy resins found in tin can linings. See Tip #4 later in the chapter for exposure reduction information.

Cadmium

Cadmium may also play a role in the progression of tumor development. An in vitro study with prostate cancer cells demonstrated that cadmium treatment can lead to the development of androgen independence and an estrogen hypersensitivity, marked by increased levels of estrogen receptors and hyper-proliferation in response to E2 (Tallaa, Liu et al. 2007). In rats, oral exposure to cadmium induced prostatic tumors and preneoplastic lesions and also promoted the growth of pre-existing tumors (Waalkes 2000). Cadmium exposure can occur via cigarette smoke and contaminated food sources.

Arsenic

Arsenic can also interact via the estrogen receptors. Epidemiological evidence from both the United States and Taiwan (Chen, Kuo et al. 1988, Lewis, Southwick et al. 1999) demonstrates that exposure to arsenic may increase prostate cancer mortality. Increased rates of mortality may be due to the progression of prostate cancers toward androgen independence via arsenic exposure. In vitro studies involving arsenic-transformed prostate cells support this hypothesis and demonstrate that arsenic can promote androgen independence, which may be linked to activation of Ras signaling that enables activation of the AR in the absence of androgens (Tallaa, Liu et al. 2007).

Arsenic exposure occurs via drinking water. Certain regions of the United States, such as Vermont, are known for higher levels of arsenic in water. Patients may be advised to test their drinking water to determine levels of arsenic, utilize a reverse-osmosis filter, and increase consumption of methyl-donating supplements, folate, and B_{12} to aid in arsenic metabolism and excretion.

Polychlorinated Biphenyls

Polychlorinated biphenyls (PCBs) are a group of synthetic chemicals that were banned in the 1970s but whose high persistence maintains PCBs in active circulation in estuarine environments. Primary human exposure to PCBs occurs through the consumption of contaminated fish. Exposures increase generally with respect to fish size, as larger fish have the opportunity to bioaccumulate more PCBs over their lifetime. PCBs are highly lipophilic and the highest concentrations of PCBs are found in the fatty tissues of fish.

Many PCBs demonstrate estrogenic, antiestrogenic, and dioxin-like properties depending on the specific congener, where congeners vary based on molecular orientation and level of chlorination. Several human studies have found an increased risk of prostate cancer with exposure to PCBs. One study evaluated the levels of different persistent organic pollutants in adipose tissue of individuals with prostate cancer and found an association between levels of PCB153 and trans-chlordane and the occurrence of prostate cancer (Hardell, Andersson et al. 2006). Another study evaluating serum PCB levels found an association between PCB180 and prostate cancer (Ritchie, Vial et al. 2003).

Exposure to PCBs primarily occurs through the consumption of seafood. See Tip #5 later in the chapter for information about selecting seafood with lower levels of PCBs.

REPRODUCTIVE TOXINS FOR MEN

Over the last 50 years there has been a global decline in sperm counts occurring at a rate of about 1% per year and largely impacting developed regions such as North America and Europe (Swan, Elkin et al. 2000). Trend analysis of this process has led to controversial statements about the role environmental toxins play in the decline. The purpose of this section is to highlight the direct link between toxins and sperm health, which can be measured both by the number of sperm cells and by indices influencing pregnancy rates, including sperm motility and DNA damage to sperm. There is a substantial amount of epidemiologic evidence that links concentrations of particular toxins found in urine and seminal fluid to particular changes in sperm health— these studies will be reviewed here and collectively point to the growing, yet still underrecognized importance of men's preconception health. Living in an industrial world results in a multitude of environmental exposures that may influence sperm health and that can act through a variety of mechanisms to do so. Some toxins may be endocrine disruptors, whereas others may influence sperm health in situ as they alter the environment of the seminal fluid, creating adducts and DNA damage or leading to increased oxidative stress. These effects can influence the reproductive process at multiple stages, including increasing time to pregnancy, increasing spontaneous abortions, and even leading to birth defects and childhood cancers.

From a clinical perspective, the toxins outlined in this section are relevant to those couples who are having difficulty conceiving or who are seeking reproductive counseling.

TOXINS THAT IMPACT SPERM MOTILITY, SPERM COUNT, AND SPERM HEALTH
Sperm Health Criteria

The World Health Organization (WHO) reference values are typically used to evaluate sperm health, though there is some debate as to whether these values are appropriate (Nallella, Sharma et al. 2006, Cooper, Noonan et al. 2010). One complaint about the WHO reference values is that they cannot be used to clearly demarcate fertile men from infertile men, because sperm populations are considered heterogeneous and often, even normal sperm demonstrate some abnormal parameters. In a study designed to evaluate the WHO parameters (Nallella, Sharma et al. 2006), WHO reference values were compared to group means for individuals who were clearly identified as fertile with proven conception, as infertile due to male factor infertility (MFI), and as infertile with or without known female factor infertility. The study demonstrated that motility and concentration were better predictors of fertility than sperm morphology under both the WHO reference values and Tyberg's strict criteria. Motility and concentration had more distinct means with less overlap between the groups and the percent of MFI individuals with high motility was much smaller relative to sperm concentration and morphology. In general, sperm motility has proven to be a strong indicator of fertility in in vivo and in vitro fertilization scenarios and as a biomarker for normal development of both the seminal fluid and the spermatozoa occurring at multiple stages, including in the testis and epididymis. That said, there is also clear evidence that it is not the only predictor of fertility because some MFI cases demonstrate high levels of motility (Nallella, Sharma et al. 2006), whereas other studies have indicated that normal morphology is also a critical component (Coetzee, Kruge et al. 1998).

Another relevant criterion to assessing sperm health is assessing the level of DNA damage. Chromatin in sperm is highly compact due to the replacement of histones with protamines, which facilitates the formation of a unique chromatin structure consisting of toroidal forms. These forms are then protected with disulfide cross-links that stabilize, compact, and ultimately protect the DNA. A variety of factors can lead to DNA damage including endogenous damage, defects in DNA packaging, and high levels of oxidative stress. Infertile men often exhibit about two times as much DNA damage relative to fertile men (Zini, Bielecki et al. 2001), and such damage may influence reproductive outcomes via spontaneous miscarriages or idiopathic infertility (Zini 2011). At this time there is no definitive method for using levels of DNA damage to assess infertility, but many human studies support the association (Kodama, Yamaguchi et al. 1997, Spano, Bonde et al. 2000, Zini, Bielecki et al. 2001). At a mechanistic level, the association was further confirmed by an in vitro study in which sperm were exposed to various doses of radiation that consistently produced dose-dependent double-strand breaks in the DNA. DNA-damaged sperm were found capable of fertilizing the embryo, but the damage resulted in a low rate of embryonic development and high early pregnancy loss; researchers found that the oocyte has the capacity to repair the DNA damage so long as it is below the experimentally determined threshold value of 8% of DNA (Ahmadi and Ng 1999). Thus, DNA damage in spermatozoa is a potential source of prezygotic DNA damage.

Phthalates and Sperm Motility/Concentration

Phthalates are a group of chemicals used to make plastics more flexible and durable and are used as solvents in personal care products. Phthalates have a demonstrated effect on semen parameters, including sperm motility and semen concentration, and are suspected of impacting male testicular development in utero, an effect that has been documented extensively in animal models where the long-term impacts include reduced testosterone (T) levels, testicular malformations, and reduced sperm counts (Howdeshell, Furr et al. 2007, Howdeshell, Rider et al. 2008, Howdeshell, Wilson et al. 2008, Noriega, Howdeshell et al. 2009). Phthalates are antiandrogens that act through a variety of mechanisms and that are known to inhibit multiple enzymes in the testosterone synthesis pathway including CYP17A1, HSD3B, and HSD17B3 in rat models (Foster, Thomas et al. 1983, Ye, Zhao et al. 2011). Androgen signaling is highly conserved between rats and humans, suggesting that phthalates may impact human male development and testicular function.

Because phthalates can impact testosterone production in the testes, they may negatively impact spermatogenesis. Several epidemiologic studies have found evidence to support this conclusion. A fertility clinic in Massachusetts found an association between monobutyl phthalate (MBP) and sperm that was below WHO reference values for sperm motility and sperm concentration (Duty, Silva et al. 2003, Hauser, Meeker et al. 2006). Clinically, reducing body burden of phthalates may improve sperm counts and motility. See Tips #2 and #4 later in the chapter for ways to reduce exposure.

Polychlorinated Biphenyls and Sperm Motility

PCBs, as previously discussed, are synthetic halogenated aromatic compounds that are lipophilic and highly persistent in marine life. There are numerous studies that have demonstrated that the presence of PCBs is correlated with decreased sperm motility and sperm count (Dallinga, Moonen et al. 2002, Richthoff, Rylander et al. 2003). The consistency of this association varies depending on which congener is tracked: often an individual congener is chosen because it represents a reliable biomarker for total PCB exposure. Therefore, in some cases, studies present null or insignificant findings in the trend when tracking certain congeners (Rignell-Hydbom, Rylander et al. 2004, Hauser, Meeker et al. 2006), but the association is often upheld when PCBs are assessed as groups and with some individual PCBs, such as PCB-138 (Richthoff, Rylander et al. 2003). In Taiwan in 1979, large-scale exposure to PCBs occurred through contaminated rice oil that was used extensively in cooking. Twenty years later a human population study assessed the impact of the in utero exposure to PCBs and polychlorinated dibenzofurans (PCDFs) on the semen parameters of young men between the ages of 16 and 18 years old. Those exposed in utero demonstrated increased abnormal morphology and reduced motility (Guo, Hsu et al. 2000). In another study conducted in this population, men who were sexually mature at the time of exposure were evaluated to assess any long-term damage that may have resulted from the exposure. Exposed men aged 37 to 50 had sperm motility and counts similar to their age-matched controls but had significantly reduced capacity to bind and penetrate hamster oocytes, suggesting that long-term damage likely occurred (Hsu, Huang et al. 2003). This human case study demonstrates the concept that the timing of the exposure is critical in assessing its effect.

Exposure to PCBs can be reduced through changing fish consumption habits—see Tip #5 later in the chapter.

Dioxins Alter Sperm Count and Motility

Dioxins include a broad range of compounds, with the most toxic form being 2,3,7,8-tetrachlorodibenzo-*p*-dioxin (TCDD), whose toxicity is mediated through the aryl hydrocarbon receptor (AHR).

Epidemiologic evidence supporting dioxin's role in impacting male fertility comes from a chemical plant explosion that occurred in Seveso, Italy, in 1976, where high levels of TCDD massively contaminated the surrounding environment. In a study conducted 22 years after the explosion, sperm counts were assessed of young men who were different ages at the time of the explosion, and researchers found that the impact of TCDD on sperm count and motility depended on the age at the time of exposure (Mocarelli, Gerthoux et al. 2008). Those who were 1 to 9 years of age (infancy/prepuberty) had reduced sperm count and motility, whereas those who were 10 to 17 years of age (puberty) had an inverse effect of elevated sperm counts and motility relative to age-matched controls from nearby uncontaminated areas. Exposure in both age groups resulted in decreased levels of estradiol and follicle-stimulating hormone—an effect that occurred at 68 ppt, a dose that is within one order of magnitude of the dose found environmentally in the industrialized world. Numerous rat studies have also been performed to evaluate the impact of TCDD exposure that occurs in utero, and although the results are at times inconsistent, there is sufficient evidence to support the idea that exposure in utero in rats is associated with decreased sperm counts and that the interaction is likely occurring through epididymal function (Foster, Maharaj-Briceno et al. 2011).

Nonpersistent Pesticides and Semen Quality

Nonpersistent pesticides are considered "contemporary" pesticides and exist in contrast to persistent pesticides of the organochlorine variety, including DDT. The three main groups of nonpersistent pesticides include organophosphates, carbamates, and pyrethroids. Studies assessing occupational exposure to pesticides in farmers and their semen quality have had mixed results, with some studies finding a strong association (Abell, Ernst et al. 2000, Padungtod, Savitz et al. 2000) and others finding weak (Juhler, Larsen et al. 1999) or no association (Whorton, Milby et al. 1979, Larsen, Giwercman et al. 1998). In the general population, pesticide biomarkers have been associated with reduced sperm concentration and motility (Swan, Kruse et al. 2003, Meeker, Ryan et al. 2004). Variation in study results may be attributed to variations in exposure constituents, where the mixture of pesticides varies from study to study. This may be an example of the importance of the mixture of toxins present, where changes in the composition of the mixture alters toxicity.

Other Toxins That May Impact Sperm Counts

The toxins included in this section are only a selection of the ensemble of toxins that may impact spermatogenesis. There are a number of antiandrogens that may impact spermatogenesis and testes development by inhibiting testosterone. Testosterone inhibition in utero can potentially alter male reproductive abilities throughout the lifetime and interfere with the continued testosterone production that occurs in utero and in the Leydig cells. These toxins are classified as antiandrogens due to their ability to bind the AR in rat models or inhibit testosterone synthesis in rat models (Ye, Zhao et al. 2011). The high homology between the AR signaling systems in mammals suggests that these toxins may have similar effects on humans.

Methoxychlor (MXC), an organochlorine pesticide, interferes with testosterone production in rodent Leydig cells (Akingbemi, Ge et al. 2000). Organotins, chemicals used as agricultural fungicides and rodent repellents, inhibit multiple enzymes in T biosynthesis (Lo, Allera et al. 2003, McVey and Cooke 2003, Ohno and Nakajima 2005). 1,2-Dibromo-3-chloropropane (DBCP), a pesticide used to control plant worms, has resulted in male infertility in exposed workers (Potashnik, Yanaiinbar et al. 1979) and inhibits testosterone production in rats (Kelce, Raisbeck et al. 1990). Benzophenes are synthetic chemicals that block ultraviolet (UV) light and are used in food packaging printing and sunscreens (benzophonene-3/oxybenzone). Most benzophonenes demonstrate in vitro ability to inhibit enzymes involved in testosterone production, with BP-1 being the most potent and active in rodent models (Nashev, Schuster et al. 2010).

As previously mentioned, BPA is largely considered an estrogenic compound because it binds the estrogen receptors, but it is also an antiandrogen due to its ability to bind the androgen receptor with a potency level on par with that of flutamide, which is used as a negative control in experimental studies for androgen antagonists (Sohoni and Sumpter 1998). BPA has been shown to inhibit T production in vitro and in vivo and has been shown to inhibit human enzymes involved in T production including CYP17A1 and HSD3B (Niwa, Fujimoto et al. 2001, Ye, Zhao et al. 2011).

TOXINS IN THE SEMINAL FLUID

In addition to EDs, numerous other toxins can impact the reproductive process. Many types of toxins have been found in the seminal fluids including lead, cadmium, mercury, and nicotine (and cotinine, its metabolite), as well as chlorinated solvents such as trichloroethylene. These toxins work through a variety of mechanisms and can alter spermatogenesis, sperm morphology, and sperm motility, and can induce DNA damage that may be passed on to the developing embryo and result in abortion of the fetus or congenital birth defects.

Toxins in the seminal fluid may act via oxidative stress. Oxidative stress is implicated in many diseases, is a condition that occurs across all cell types, and is a major driver for aging and cancer. A cell's antioxidant defense systems are composed of scavenger molecules such as glutathione and catalase, which protect cells from reactive oxygen species (ROS). Oxidative stress occurs when these systems become overwhelmed by excess generation of ROS, which may be prompted by exposure to certain toxins, stress, or environmental factors such as heavy metals that engage in Fenton reactions. Once oxidative stress overwhelms these scavenging systems, ROS can lead to multiple types of cellular damage, including damaging DNA, proteins, and lipid peroxidation, a chain reaction that can severely damage membranes.

Investigations on the role of oxidative stress and sperm health have been occurring since 1943, when John Macleod demonstrated that spermatozoa incubated in an oxygen-rich environment demonstrated a significant and rapid loss in motility that was reversed by the addition of catalase to the system (MacLeod 1943). Since then, several forms of male infertility have also demonstrated high levels of ROS, and it is generally accepted that high levels of ROS result in DNA damage and lipid peroxidation in spermatozoa. DNA damage in spermatozoa has been linked to infertility, impaired embryonic development, pregnancy loss, birth defects, and in some cases childhood diseases such as cancer and autism (Gharagozloo and Aitken 2011). Although many studies point to the importance of oxidative stress and male sperm health, clinical attitudes toward this practice remain controversial (Zini 2011). The debate on this subject is centered around the lack of consistency in clinical trials to demonstrate that oxidative stress is a marker of male infertility and the challenges associated with clinical treatments using antioxidants.

Although appealing in theory, the use of antioxidant therapies presents several challenges in practice. First, it is difficult to attain the correct level of antioxidants needed to reduce the load of ROS to improve sperm function, but to not completely eliminate ROS. Sperm require ROS at some level for their signal transduction mechanisms, and ROS are critically involved in the rate of hyperactivation and the ability to undergo the acrosome reaction, which are important steps in penetrating the zona pellucida of the egg and achieving fertilization (Sharma and Agarwal 1996). Second, at higher concentrations and in certain combinations, some antioxidants such as vitamin C and E in high doses coadministered can go on to have pro-oxidant effects, which may further compromise sperm function (Donnelly, McClure et al. 1999).

Trichloroethylene

Trichloroethylene (TCE) is a chlorinated solvent used extensively in the 1950s as a dry cleaning agent and is currently used as a metal degreaser. TCE exposure can occur via contaminated drinking water; in a survey of eight states conducted by the Environmental Protection Agency (EPA), 46% of people were found drinking water with TCE.

Most evidence points to the fact that TCE is not a reproductive toxicant. However, there are limited studies on this topic, and there is some evidence indicating an association between exposure to TCE and time to pregnancy (Sallmen, Lindbohm et al. 1998). An occupational study conducted on workers from an electronics factory where TCE was used as a degreaser employed extensive medical examination along with a questionnaire. There were no differences found between the two groups with the exception of a dose-dependent increase in hyperzoospermia, which in some cases is related to infertility (Chia, Ong et al. 1996). Animal studies indicate that TCE does alter sperm viability in a dose-dependent manner and effectively reduces the ability to fertilize oocytes in unexposed females (DuTeaux, Berger et al. 2004).

Air Pollution

Air pollution is composed of a number of elements that vary based on location, time of year, and other environmental and industrial factors. Exposures occurring from air pollution may include exposure to metals such as lead, nickel, and cadmium; gases including nitrogen oxide, carbonium oxide, and sulphur oxide; and a variety of particulate matter including particles less than 2.5 microns in size (PM 2.5). Thus, the effect of air quality on changes in sperm health may vary depending on the abundances of different toxins and their relative concentrations over time.

Occupational studies have utilized toll workers as study populations because their exposure to vehicle-generated air pollution is concentrated and consistent. Motorway tollgate workers were found to have significantly lower sperm motility and kinetics relative to their age-matched controls (De Rosa, Zarrilli et al. 2003) as well as increased DNA fragmentation and chromatin damage (Calogero, La Vignera et al. 2011). Concentrations of lead and nitrogen oxide were inversely correlated with the sperm motility parameters, suggesting that increases in their concentration have a negative impact on semen quality (De Rosa, Zarrilli et al. 2003). The impact of air pollution may not be limited to those with occupational exposure, as PM 2.5 levels have been correlated with sperm motility in residents of Salt Lake City (Hammoud, Carrell et al. 2010). Interestingly, this correlation occurred with a temporal delay—where the relevant exposure occurred 3 months prior to the changes in sperm motility, suggesting that exposures that occur during spermatogenesis are most relevant to sperm health.

Smoking

Smoking exposes men to a large number of carcinogens, including cadmium, lead, and benzo-a-pyrene. One cigarette contains 0.6 to 2.0 µg Pb^{2+} and 1.0 to 4.5 µg Cd, of which about one tenth is inhaled. Smoking on the order of 20 cigarettes to 1 pack of cigarettes produces a measurable increase in the level of seminal Cd (Oldereid, Thomassen et al. 1994, Benoff, Cooper et al. 2000), as well as a significant decrease in the level of semen zinc. Cadmium can increase the level of oxidative stress, leading to DNA damage, a process that may be augmented by zinc deficiency, which plays a role in protecting DNA via chromatin compaction and stabilization.

The evidence linking smoking to male factor infertility is strong—smokers have been associated with sperm possessing lower rates of respiration (Chohan and Badawy 2010), increased benzo(a)pyrene diolepoxide (BPDE)-DNA adducts (Zenzes 2000), increased DNA fragmentation (Sepaniak, Forges et al. 2006), increased incidence of meiotic spindle dysfunction leading to aneuploidy (Rubes, Lowe et al. 1998, Robbins 2003), lower sperm concentration (Kunzle, Mueller et al. 2003, Chen and Kuo 2007, Ramlau-Hansen, Thulstrup et al. 2007), less motility (Kunzle, Mueller et al. 2003, Chen and Kuo 2007), and increased abnormal morphology (Chen and Kuo 2007). Smoking then leads to various forms of genetic damage that impair sperm function, reducing chances of fertilization but also decreasing genomic stability in sperm and thereby increasing chances of unsuccessful pregnancies. For example, BPDE-DNA adducts can be passed on to embryos even when only the father is a smoker (Zenzes, Puy et al. 1999). This genetic damage to embryos in the form of DNA adducts and aneuploidy may impact embryonic development and lead to failed implantation or loss of pregnancy. It may also explain the observation of some studies that link smoking with elevated rates of spontaneous abortion in smoking couples (Zenzes 2000). Most frightening is the association between paternal smoking and childhood diseases. In a human study conducted in China, paternal smoking occurring during the preconception period was associated with an increased risk of childhood cancers, including acute lymphocytic leukemia, lymphoma, and brain tumors (Ji, Shu et al. 1997). The rate of occurrence rose in accordance with pack-years of paternal smoking for acute lymphocytic leukemia, lymphoma, and all other cancers.

Lead

Lead exposure occurs via inhalation and ingestion. It is highly prevalent in the ambient air due to combustion of petroleum products and can be ingested through food products or water contaminated by lead-lined pipes. Because lead resembles calcium, it is often incorporated into bones where it remains bound until mobilization of calcium and phosphate occurs. It can also interfere with calcium transport in cells, which is integral in maintaining many normal cellular functions.

The role of lead exposure remains controversial and has been extensively reviewed (Benoff, Jacob et al. 2000), with the controversy ranging from conflicting results in human studies likely resulting from a host of confounding variables, as well as a lack of clarity regarding the appropriate way to assess levels of lead (in seminal fluid or in spermatozoa). A recent human study has found a significant correlation between the percentage of immotile sperm and seminal plasma levels of lead and calcium (Mendiola, Moreno et al. 2011). Further, seminal lead concentrations negatively affect outcomes of artificial insemination (Benoff, Hurley et al. 2003).

Clinical Tools

MINIMIZING EXPOSURES: IMPLEMENTING A PRECAUTIONARY APPROACH THROUGH LIFESTYLE CHOICES

The evidence presented here demonstrates that exposures to numerous toxins occur on a daily basis and are *not* benign in nature. In some cases, evidence may be lacking to support a clear mechanism or outcome, but historically many cases of weak evidence have later become definitive evidence. Therefore, a precautionary approach is advisable until potential toxins are definitively shown to be nontoxic.

We are exposed unwittingly and unknowingly to a vast array of toxins found in nearly every aspect of modern life. The task of minimizing these exposures is admittedly daunting. Although there are some cases where we have little control over our exposure, as with ambient air pollution, there are other cases where we can make choices that will significantly mitigate our exposures.

One major resource people can use while working to minimize exposures is the Environmental Working Group (EWG) website. This nonprofit group offers a number of easy-to-use Internet tools that link scientific research on toxins and useful consumer information. They have also conducted their own surveys on toxic loads in drinking water and beauty products that provide a reliable assessment from a third party.

Tip #1: Eat Certified Organic Foods

Basic idea. Conventional foods are often contaminated with a number of pesticide residues that cannot be removed with washing or peeling (Lu, Schenck et al. 2010). As discussed, even modern pesticides that are nonpersistent can have deleterious effects on men's health, including risk and outcome of prostate cancer as well as sperm health. Men experiencing difficulty conceiving may benefit from changing their diet.

Evidence. Changing from a nonorganic diet to an organic diet can reduce exposure to pesticides. In an intervention study with 23 elementary school children, organic foods were substituted for nonorganic foods for 5 days during a 15-day study in which urinary excretion of pesticides was measured in the morning and evening. Children enrolled in the study were consuming strictly organic diets that included regular consumption of fresh fruits and vegetables, fruit juices, and wheat-containing foods. Prior to the intervention, all the children had metabolites of organophosphorus pesticides, including metabolites of malathion and chlorpyrifos, in their urine. Immediately after switching to organic foods, detection of the pesticides decreased to undetectable levels and returned to the original levels when the nonorganic diet was resumed (Lu, Toepel et al. 2006).

Resource. The EWG provides a shopper's guide to food consumption utilizing data from the Pesticide Data Program to provide a comparison of the load of pesticides in commonly consumed foods. The data used to establish their shopping guides is derived from 51,000 tests for pesticides conducted between 2000 and 2009 in which nearly all of the foods had been rinsed or peeled prior to testing. Their "Dirty Dozen" contains the most contaminated foods and includes apples, celery, strawberries, peaches, spinach, nectarines (imported), grapes (imported), sweet bell peppers, potatoes, blueberries (domestic), lettuce, and kale/collard greens. Their "Clean 15" includes foods least likely to test positive for the presence of pesticides and includes onions, sweet corn, pineapples, avocado, asparagus, sweet peas, mangoes, eggplant, cantaloupe (domestic), kiwi, cabbage, watermelon, sweet potatoes, grapefruit, and mushrooms. These lists may be useful for individuals looking to reduce pesticide exposure but unable to afford all organic produce: http://www.ewg.org/foodnews/summary.

TIP #2: ASSESS THE SAFETY OF PERSONAL CARE PRODUCTS

Basic idea. Personal care products such as shampoos, conditioners, moisturizers, deodorants, shaving creams, aftershave gels, and fragrances often contain long lists of ingredients. These ingredients are largely unregulated—such that manufacturers can put nearly any chemical into personal care products and are not required to test its safety. Furthermore, labeling regulations for these products allows incomplete or misleading labeling of ingredients—so avoiding specific compounds listed on the label may not mean that you are not being exposed to them anyway under the guise of a vague ingredient such as "fragrance."

Evidence. Many personal care products test positive for the presence of endocrine-disrupting compounds. The evidence linking these compounds to reproductive dysfunction and prostate health has been presented in this chapter. According to the EWG, personal care products often contain phthalates such as diethyl phthalate and dibutyl phthalate, which are linked to adverse changes in sperm health. Many personal care products often contain parabens, which are estrogen mimics and are widely used as a preservative in personal care products.

Resource. The EWG has established a comprehensive database in which they have independently tested over 69,000 products for the presence of numerous chemicals and ranked them with hazard scores: http://www.ewg.org/skindeep. Individuals looking to reduce their exposure can query this database to find the safest products available.

TIP #3: DRINK CLEAN WATER

Basic idea. Drinking water represents a source of exposure to numerous toxins including metals, chlorinated compounds, industrial chemicals, and pharmaceuticals. Due to the vast array of contaminants found in drinking water and the resulting health effects, it is advisable to obtain a high-quality water filter with which to filter tap water. Use of bottled water is not an appropriate alternative due to the lack of testing on bottled water quality and the leaching that occurs from packaging materials (evidence and discussion in Tip #4).

Evidence. The EWG provides excellent information regarding the ubiquitous contamination of U.S. water sources. Although there is some regulation monitoring tap water contaminants, the EWG reports found 315 contaminants when they tested multiple water sources. Of these contaminants, only half were regulated by laws—meaning that municipal water sources test for their presence and take action if the levels are above certain thresholds. For those unregulated contaminants, these testing procedures are not performed, meaning that they can be present in drinking water at any level. Unfortunately, even the regulations already in place do not guarantee safe levels, as the EWG found that 49 regulated contaminants were present at concentrations above the acceptable limits in certain locations (EWG 2009)

Resources. The best option appears to be filtering tap water. Many water filters use carbon technologies, which vary in effectiveness based on the brand and type—meaning that the sort of contaminants removed will also vary. The most comprehensive filter is a reverse-osmosis system combined with a fine carbon filter. These systems can remove the inorganic contaminants in water, including metals such as arsenic and hexavalent chromium as well as chlorinated compounds. Also, look for product certifications such as the California certification and NSF certification, which require evaluation of the manufacturer's claims about toxin removal. See the EWG's water filter buying guide for more detailed information (http://www.ewg.org/tap-water/getawaterfilter).

Drinking bottled water isn't necessarily a safe alternative. The EWG found 38 contaminants when it tested 10 brands of bottled waters. Bottled water is held to the same contaminant standards as tap water, but unlike with municipal sources of water, water quality test results of bottled water do not have to be made public. The image of bottled water from pristine mountain springs is inaccurate at best and pure fabrication at worst—bottled water is often municipal water packaged and sold with less testing than that required for tap water, resulting in higher levels of contamination. The U.S. Food and Drug Administration (FDA) does not carefully regulate the contents of tap water, with the result that its pollutants may include radioactive pollutants, synthetic chemicals including hexane and acetaldehyde, pharmaceutical residues, and disinfectant byproducts (EWG 2008).

TIP #4: REDUCE OR ELIMINATE USE OF PLASTICS

Basic idea. Plastics are ubiquitous. Our bottled water, soft drinks, juices, nutritional supplements, and foods are packaged in plastics or stored in cans lined with epoxy resins. Most people view these containers as inert. Studies have demonstrated that even under normal storage conditions these containers can release toxins. Most chemicals leaching from plastics haven't been tested for their safety or extensively studied. Of those chemicals that have been studied, many are endocrine disruptors, which makes them important to men's health. Because we consume plastics every day, we are at risk for some known and likely many unknown health risks; therefore, it is important to make choices that reduce exposure. Some of the major toxins from plastics include bisphenol A, phthalates, antimony, and brominated compounds and ways to reduce exposure to them will be discussed here.

Basic Safety Tips for Plastic Use

Chemical leaching is increased from plastics that are heated or undergo a lot of use and demonstrate signs of wear. Avoid things like heating foods up in plastic containers, pouring hot beverages into plastic cups or travel mugs, and using water bottles that have scratches and other signs of abrasion.

Bisphenol A

BPA is a common component in polycarbonate (hard) plastics and epoxy resins. BPA leaches from plastics in contact with food and beverages. Exposure via this route likely explains the fact that 92.6% of the U.S. population has detectable levels of BPA in their urine (Calafat, Ye et al. 2008).

EVIDENCE
Water bottles. Patients may be able to reduce their exposure to BPA by eliminating the use of hard plastic drinking bottles and Tupperware. In an intervention study conducted by Harvard School of Public Health, participants

consumed all cold beverages out of BPA containers for 1 week and urine concentrations of BPA increased by two thirds (Carwile, Luu et al. 2009).

Food packaging. BPA is also found in the epoxy resin that lines tin cans and plastic food packaging. In another intervention study where families consuming canned and packaged foods on a daily basis were asked to consume fresh foods for 3 days, urinary levels of BPA were reduced by 76% (Rudel, Gray et al. 2011).

Since 2008, polycarbonate water bottles have been quickly replaced with BPA-free water bottles. However, the contents of these new BPA-free plastics often remain an industry secret. From a precautionary and historical standpoint, it would be naïve to assume that these new polycarbonate plastics are safe—there may be other unidentified toxins leaching from them.

Phthalates

Phthalates are found in highly flexible plastics and are not chemically bound to those plastics, thereby allowing them to leach into ambient air, dust, and food (Crinnion 2010). They are also found in many personal care products, children's toys, and enteric coatings of pharmaceutical pills and are used to soften polyvinyl chloride (PVC).

EVIDENCE
Families consuming canned and packaged foods on a daily basis were asked to consume fresh foods for 3 days, after which urinary levels of a phthalate metabolite from PVC was reduced by more than 50% (Rudel, Gray et al. 2011).

Water Bottles

Water bottles release EDs into water including BPA and other alkyl phenols such as 4-nonylphenol, adipates, phthalates, and antimony (Sb) (Amiridou and Voutsa 2011).

EVIDENCE
Studies have indicated that when water bottles are exposed to environmental stressors such as UV exposure and elevated temperatures, there is increased leaching of contaminants such as antimony into the water (Shotyk, Krachler et al. 2006, Keresztes, Tatar et al. 2009). Leaching of antimony and brominated compounds has also been observed to increase in response to the type of water—for carbonated waters and those enriched with other substances, there is an observed increase in leaching (Andra, Makris et al. 2012). The level of leaching also varies in response to the type of plastic being used—where polyethylene

terephthalate (PET) had the highest level of leaching for antimony and brominated compounds including BDE-209, a flame retardant used in the manufacturing of plastics, whereas polycarbonate (PC), high-density polyethylene (HDPE), and polystyrene (PS) had significantly lower levels (Andra, Makris et al. 2012). Recent studies assessing the estrogenic activity of bottled water samples found that water packaged in PET demonstrated three times higher estrogenic activity than the same water packaged in glass (Wagner and Oehlmann 2011).

TIP #5: MODIFY FISH CONSUMPTION

The fish we consume often contains a number of pollutants, including lipid-soluble persistent organic pollutants such as PCBs, PCDDs (polychlorinated dibenzo-p-dioxins), PCDFs, PBDEs (polybrominated diphenyl ethers), OCs (organochlorine pesticides), and PFAs (perfluorinated acids). Fish may also have high levels of mercury, which is concentrated in their muscle. As previously discussed, PCBs may impact reproductive and prostate health. They are highly lipophilic and therefore are concentrated in fat tissues. Modifying fish consumption is an important way of reducing PCB exposure.

One way to reduce exposure to PCBs is to trim the fat from fish before cooking or to cook the fish by broiling, baking, or grilling it in order to cook the fat off. These methods of cooking are preferable to frying or sautéing, where fats remain in the pan and are incorporated into any other foods you may be cooking with, such as vegetables (EWG 2003).

Another way to reduce PCB exposure is to alter your selection of the fish you eat, avoiding those fish and marine mammals that are highest in PCBs. General guidelines about selecting fish low in PCBs are difficult to outline, as it is always difficult to know exactly what you are getting and from where.

If you are catching your own fish or obtaining fish from local fisheries, it is best to consult state- or region-specific guidelines for fish consumption as these will vary depending on the local levels of water pollution. For example, the Hudson River, which has had a long history of PCB contamination initiated by a power plant in the upper Hudson region, is a region where officials still consider the fish uneatable. The New York State Department of Health provides guidelines for fish consumption from lower regions of the Hudson based on proximity to the source of pollution and known PCB concentrations of fish.

Though specific choices will vary based on the source of fish and also the life stage of the person consuming it, there are some general recommendations that can be made when sufficient information is not available. The first general rule is to choose fish that are smaller and from cold-water areas. The second general rule is to avoid farmed salmon unless it comes from Canada.

Most farmed salmon is extremely high in PCBs because the feed used for the fish is composed of other seafoods rich in lipids and concentrated with PCBs. Canadian fisheries have rectified this problem by testing feed for PCB levels and choosing options with low or no PCB. When possible, choose wild and canned Alaskan salmon rather than the farmed variety (EWG 2003).

The third way to lower PCB exposure is to evaluate the safety of your fish oil supplements. Depending on the source, PCB levels in fish oil can range from low to extremely high. A study evaluating the PCB levels of 17 n-3 polyunsaturated fatty acid (PUFA) supplements in Canada found that those derived from seal had the highest levels of PCBs and those from small, cold-water, fatty fish such as krill had the lowest (Bourdon, Bazinet et al. 2010). Selecting fish on the lower end of the food chain for both supplements and consumption reduces PCB exposure because PCBs bioaccumulate and dramatically increase as one moves up the food chain.

TIP #6: INVESTIGATE OTHER POSSIBLE SOURCES OF TOXINS

The important thing to remember about toxin identification is that many toxins may not be easy to identify. Here are some important questions to ask when considering toxins that may be specific to an individual's history:

1. Obtain a geographical history from the person by finding out where he or she was born and where he or she has lived. Then do the necessary detective work to obtain information about those areas. Are there any known cancer clusters in those areas? Are there any notable superfund sites or chemical accidents? Are there any major sources of pollution—power plants, air pollution, pesticide usage, refineries, contaminated drinking water?

2. Obtain an occupational history from the person. What exposures have occurred via work, hobbies, or other activities? Was there exposure to any known chemicals or fumes? Possible considerations include pesticides, construction materials, refining byproducts, and radioactive materials. Hobbies such as gardening, metal sculpture, woodworking, and other arts may implicate specific exposures.

Aging and Cancer

HOW TOXINS PROMOTE CARCINOGENESIS

Exposure to toxins can impact cellular health through many mechanisms. Current research is asking how aging and cancer—perennial concerns—may be related to toxin exposure.

There are many ways to answer this question and many lenses through which to view it—the focus here will be on *genomic instability* and *epigenetic regulation*. Genomic instability is the large-scale damage to DNA and chromosomes that results from repeated damage to DNA, inhibition of DNA repair pathways, and disruption of mitotic DNA replication (Aguilera and Gomez-Gonzalez 2008). Epigenetic regulation is the cell's way of adapting its software to meet a changing environment, and toxins can alter the software in a variety of ways. This discussion will provide an overview of these processes and some toxins that promote the progression of genomic instability and epigenetic deregulation.

During cellular proliferation, during reproduction, and during life, faithful replication of DNA is integral in maintaining not only health but also functionality. Every cellular activity requires faithful replication of DNA: the formation of proteins and enzymes, the regulation of signaling pathways, and the progression through the cell cycle all require the genetic information encoded in the DNA. Faithful replication of the genome is integral and there are a multitude of redundancies in place to ensure that damaged DNA is repaired, that cell cycle progression waits for DNA to be repaired, and that during the delicate process when replicated strands of DNA are separated from each other during anaphase, their segregation is exact, with no lagging strand, and no broken fragments. Despite this system of redundant checks, genomic instability can and does occur. Genomic instability happens through a variety of events that alter DNA and chromosomal structures and base patterns—these events lead to mutations in the DNA, inappropriate chromosome numbers (aneuploidy), and chromosomal structural aberrations such as inversions, deletions, duplications, and translocations (Rajagopalan and Lengauer 2004, Aguilera and Gomez-Gonzalez 2008, Holland and Cleveland 2009).

Environmental toxins can interact at every level of the various processes that maintain genomic stability, both by injuring the DNA and by interfering with its repair. Mutagens are toxins that directly damage DNA. Some mechanisms of damage include inducing oxidative damage (nickel and cobalt) (Kasprzak 2002), the formation of bulky DNA adducts (benzo-a-pyrene) (Hsu, Poirier et al. 1981), cross-links in the DNA (UV radiation) (Ravanat, Douki et al. 2001), and double-strand breaks (ionizing radiation) (Mahaney, Meek et al. 2009). The cell's natural defense systems are capable of dealing with each of these types of damage, and under normal conditions in the absence of environmental toxins these types of damage are often successfully repaired. But when the extent of damage exceeds the endogenous levels of the DNA damage response, DNA damage may go unrepaired, leading to mutations in the DNA, strand breaks, and inappropriate fusion events. Moreover, if other toxins are present, mechanisms of DNA damage sensing and repair may be inhibited, further exacerbating the level of damage. For example, arsenic can inhibit base excision repair and nucleotide excision repair; it can also block p53 (a safeguard against the proliferation of damaged cells) and thereby promote cell cycle progression even when DNA damage has occurred. Therefore, arsenic alone can increase the rate of spontaneous mutagenesis by inhibiting repair. In combination with a mutagen like UV radiation, it can lead to rapid progression of skin cancer (Burns, Uddin et al. 2004, Rossman, Uddin et al. 2004).

Other toxins may work through epigenetic routes to alter gene expression and promote carcinogenesis. The epigenetic impact of certain toxins extends beyond genomic instability to include heritable changes in gene expression, a process that is akin to changing the software of the cell. Researchers in this field place emphasis on the fact that the changes produced in the software must be heritable, but long-term exposures can consistently alter the software as well and are worth consideration. In the broadest sense, then, epigenetic toxins alter the likelihood of certain genes being transcribed into proteins. Control of gene transcription is not a one-to-one correlate as previously thought: all genes are not transcribed equally. Research in this area indicates that epigenetic programs that determine whether genes are transcribed are of equal or greater importance in maintaining health than individual genetic predispositions (Feinberg 2007). Therefore, the study of epigenetics has recently exploded and with the development of new technologies, we will likely spend at least the next decade exploring this system and its impact on our health.

Epigenetic regulation of DNA expression occurs at multiple levels and is a highly physical and structural event (Qiu 2006). Visualizing DNA structure is important in understanding epigenetic events, because DNA structure is not static in the cell: it moves between being fully unwound, to slightly wound, to highly compacted. Just as a rubber band continues to fold over on itself the more you twist it, so too does DNA. DNA is often found in its most twisted form, which is considered a chromosome. When the DNA in a single human cell is fully unwound and stretched out it is 2 meters long—so keeping DNA compact *and* making routinely important genes easily accessible are critical, and that's what epigenetic modifications do. These modifications are used on DNA at all the levels of compaction, influencing the degree to which it continues to compact or unwind, and in turn the extent to which DNA transcriptional machinery can access certain genes.

From a visual perspective epigenetic modifications occur at different levels of scale. At the smallest scale, strands of DNA that are fully open and available for transcription can undergo the addition of methyl groups. When methyl groups are added at the promoter of a gene, their presence physically blocks the DNA reading machinery from binding to the DNA and therefore prevents the gene from being expressed into RNA and protein. Zooming out a bit, the DNA is wrapped around histone proteins that serve an integral purpose in keeping the DNA organized as it is folded into higher order structures—much like the reels around film, DNA spools and unspools around histone proteins, where each protein manages about 146 base pairs of DNA; thus, there are millions of histone proteins in a single chromosome. When visualized at this scale DNA looks like beads on a string, where DNA is the string and histone proteins are the beads. Another avenue through which epigenetic regulation occurs is through posttranslational modification of these histone proteins that influence how tightly wound the DNA is, as well as how attracted the histone proteins are to each other. Toxins like nickel can interact with epigenetic enzymes and alter the abundance of histone marks, leading to systemic repression and overexpression of certain genes (Arita, Niu et al. 2012, Arita, Muñoz et al. 2013).

The epigenetic activity of many known toxins is now being evaluated and explored through gene expression analysis, where cells exposed to a toxin demonstrate markedly different gene expression profiles, indicating that changes in the software are occurring. Cancers are known to have altered gene expression profiles, and although these changes occur globally throughout the genome, there are certain genes that have garnered special attention. Some changes in gene expression confer special abilities to cells, allowing them to proliferate uncontrollably. Repression of tumor suppressor genes allows cells to evade normal pathways and checkpoints that would ordinarily halt their proliferation, whereas overexpression in oncogenes enhances their ability to grow, proliferate, and obtain nourishment.

DNA mutations are critical in the formation of cancers; so too is the ability to proliferate uncontrollably. Telomeres usually prevent this uncontrolled replication. Functionally, telomeres serve to protect the ends of chromosomes so that DNA repair machinery doesn't treat the end of a chromosome as a strand break and fuse it to another chromosome, which would increase genomic instability. As cells divide, telomeres naturally shorten due to their method of replication. Based on the length of the telomeres, one can determine approximately how many more divisions the cell will live for before it goes into senescence, where it stops dividing; although senescence may be associated with old age, here it is truly a sign of health. Short telomeres trigger cellular senescence, and cells that are senescent or die cannot be cancerous (Deng, Chan et al. 2008). Therefore, it is believed that all cancers must bypass this senescence barrier to gain the ability to proliferate uncontrollably and beyond the length of their telomeres. This bypass event occurs when a mutation in the DNA activates the telomerase gene, which is capable of maintaining telomere length during cellular division. When a cancer cell has telomerase activated, all of its mutations and its new genetic landscape are propelled forward in a course of aggressive proliferation (Stewart and Weinberg 2006).

Importance of Micronutrients

Integral to maintaining genomic stability and proper gene expression is the functionality of the enzymes and proteins involved in DNA repair, epigenetic regulation, and cell cycle progression. At various stages in these processes, biochemical reactions rely on nutritional inputs in the form of specific nutrients. In 2006, Bruce N. Ames presented the triage theory, in which he suggested that humans have adapted to live through periods of food scarcity by allocating scarce micronutrients to areas that need them for short-term survival (Ames 2006). The essential micronutrients that are critical for enzyme function, cellular maintenance, and DNA repair may be prioritized to support short-term function over long-term longevity. At a cellular level, this translates to favoring enzymes involved in adenosine triphosphate (ATP) production over those enzymes involved in DNA repair. Recently, research in this area has demonstrated that micronutrient deficiencies can produce DNA damage that is of the same magnitude as exposures to toxins (Branda and Blickensderfer 1993).

There are many vitamins that are integral to genome stability. Magnesium, niacin, folate, and vitamin B_6 and B_{12} are all necessary for effective DNA repair. Vitamin C, vitamin E, and antioxidants prevent damage to DNA and lipid peroxidation. Niacin is necessary to maintain telomere length, zinc for proper function of p53, zinc and manganese for superoxide dismutase, and calcium for the regulation of chromosome segregation during mitosis; selenium is involved in methionine metabolism, and deficiency in it can lead to telomere shortening (Fenech 2010).

Deficiency in any of these micronutrients results in observable changes in the levels of DNA damage; therefore, maintenance of the appropriate vitamin levels is a critical tool for maintaining lifelong health. However, caution must be used because at inappropriately high concentrations, many of these micronutrients can also have the reverse effect—they demonstrate U-shaped toxicity curves, where extremely low doses elevate the level of DNA damage, moderate doses decrease the level of damage, and high doses promote it. In some cases, as with metals such as iron and copper, elevated doses may increase the concentration of ions beyond the available protein binding sites, leaving them free to participate in oxidative chemistry, where they generate hydroxyl radicals that go on to produce damage to lipid membranes and DNA.

Conclusion

Maintaining cellular health and DNA integrity are integral components of cancer prevention, reproductive health, and overall well-being. Protecting DNA and repairing damaged DNA are necessary steps in any comprehensive health plan, requiring careful thought by both the practitioner and patient involved. In short, we must avoid those substances that are toxic to cellular health and DNA integrity and remember to include the necessary vitamins and micronutrients that repair damage when it does occur. Avoiding toxins may be a daunting task, but there are many easily implementable ways to reduce exposure to many toxins.

DNA integrity and cellular health are important for men's health concerns as they may impact the progression of prostate cancer and contribute to male infertility. Preconception health for men requires more attention as there are many toxins that may impact the quality of sperm and reduction of these exposures may improve fertility in many men.

REFERENCES

Abell A, Ernst E, Bonde JP. Semen quality and sexual hormones in greenhouse workers. Scandinavian Journal of Work Environment & Health. 2000;26(6):492-500.

Aguilera A, Gomez-Gonzalez B. Genome instability: a mechanistic view of its causes and consequences. Nature Reviews Genetics. 2008;9(3):204-217.

Ahmadi A, Ng SC. Fertilizing ability of DNA-damaged spermatozoa. Journal of Experimental Zoology. 1999;284(6):696-704.

Akingbemi BT, Ge RS, Klinefelter GR, Gunsalus GL, Hardy MP. A metabolite of methoxychlor, 2,2-bis(p-hydroxyphenyl)-1,1,1-trichloroethane, reduces testosterone biosynthesis in rat leydig cells through suppression of steady-state messenger ribonucleic acid levels of the cholesterol side-chain cleavage enzyme. Biology of Reproduction. 2000;62(3):571-578.

Alavanja MCR, Samanic C, Dosemeci M, et al. Use of agricultural pesticides and prostate cancer risk in the agricultural health study cohort. American Journal of Epidemiology. 2003;157(9):800-814.

Ames BN. Low micronutrient intake may accelerate the degenerative diseases of aging through allocation of scarce micronutrients by triage. Proceedings of the National Academy of Sciences. 2006;103:17589-17594.

Amiridou D, Voutsa D. Alkylphenols and phthalates in bottled waters. Journal of hazardous materials. 2011;185(1):281-286.

Andra SS, Makris KC, Shine JP, Lu C. Co-leaching of brominated compounds and antimony from bottled water. Environment International. 2012;38(1):45-53.

Arita A, Muñoz A, Chervona Y, Niu J, Qu Q, et al. Gene expression profiles in peripheral blood mononuclear cells of Chinese nickel refinery workers with high exposures to nickel and control subjects. Cancer Epidemiology Biomarkers & Prevention. 2013;22:261-269.

Arita A, Niu JP, Qu QS, et al. Global Levels of Histone Modifications in Peripheral Blood Mononuclear Cells of Subjects with Exposure to Nickel. Environmental Health Perspectives. 2012;120(2):198-203.

Barker J, Alavanja M, Coble J. Use of Agricultural Pesticides and Prostate Cancer Risk in the Agricultural Health Study Cohort. American Journal of Epidemiol. 2003;157(9):800–814.

Benoff S, Cooper GS, Centola GM, Jacob A, Hershlag A, Hurley IR. Metal ions and human sperm mannose receptors. Andrologia. 2000;32(4-5):317-329.

Benoff S, Hurley IR, Millan C, Napolitano B, Centola GM. Seminal lead concentrations negatively affect outcomes of artificial insemination. Fertility and Sterility. 2003;80(3):517-525.

Benoff S, Jacob A, Hurley IR. Male infertility and environmental exposure to lead and cadmium. Human Reproduction Update. 2000;6(2):107-121.

Bourdon JA, Bazinet TM, Arnason TT, Kimpe LE, Blais JM, White PA. Polychlorinated biphenyls (PCBs) contamination and aryl hydrocarbon receptor (AhR) agonist activity of Omega-3 polyunsaturated fatty acid supplements: Implications for daily intake of dioxins and PCBs. Food and Chemical Toxicology. 2010;48(11):3093-3097.

Branda RF, Blickensderfer DB. Folate-deficiency increases genetic-damage caused by alkylating-agents and gamma-irradiation in chinese-hamster ovary cells. Cancer Research. 1993;53(22):5401-5408.

Burns FJ, Uddin AN, Wu F, Nadas A, Rossman TG. Arsenic-induced enhancement of ultraviolet radiation carcinogenesis in mouse skin: A dose-response study. Environmental Health Perspectives. 2004;112(5):599-603.

Calafat AM, Ye X, Wong L-Y, Reidy JA, Needham LL. Exposure of the US population to bisphenol A and 4-tertiary-octylphenol: 2003-2004. Environmental Health Perspectives. 2008;116(1):39-44.

Calogero AE, La Vignera S, Condorelli RA, et al. Environmental car exhaust pollution damages human sperm chromatin and DNA. Journal of Endocrinological Investigation. 2011;34(6):E139-E143.

Carwile JL, Luu HT, Bassett LS, et al. Polycarbonate Bottle Use and Urinary Bisphenol A Concentrations. Environmental Health Perspectives. 2009;117(9):1368-1372.

Chen CJ, Kuo TL, Wu MM. Arsenic and cancers. Lancet. 1988;1(8582):414-415.

Chen HW, Kuo CT. Cotinine characterization and quality effect of sperm for smoking and nonsmoking students. Bulletin of Environmental Contamination and Toxicology. 2007;79(1):11-14.

Chia SE, Ong CN, Tsakok MFH, Ho A. Semen parameters in workers exposed to trichloroethylene. Reproductive Toxicology. 1996;10(4):295-299.

Chohan KR, Badawy SZA. Cigarette Smoking Impairs Sperm Bioenergetics. International Braz J Urol. 2010;36(1):60-64.

Coetzee K, Kruge TF, Lombard CJ. Predictive value of normal sperm morphology: a structured literature review. Human Reproduction Update. 1998;4(1):73-82.

Cooper TG, Noonan E, von Eckardstein S, et al. World Health Organization reference values for human semen characteristics. Human Reproduction Update. 2010;16(3):231-245.

Crinnion WJ. Toxic Effects of the Easily Avoidable Phthalates and Parabens. Alternative Medicine Review. 2010;15(3):190-196.

Dallinga JW, Moonen EJC, Dumoulin JCM, Evers JLH, Geraedts JPM, Kleinjans JCS. Decreased human semen quality and organochlorine compounds in blood. Human Reproduction. 2002;17(8):1973-1979.

De Rosa M, Zarrilli S, Paesano L, et al. Traffic pollutants affect fertility in men. Human Reproduction. 2003;18(5):1055-1061.

Deng Y, Chan SS, Chang S. Telomere dysfunction and tumour suppression: the senescence connection. Nat Rev Cancer. 2008;8:450-458.

Diamanti-Kandarakis E, Bourguignon J-P, Giudice LC, Hauser R, Prins GS, Soto AM, Zoeller RT, Gore AC. Endocrine-Disrupting Chemicals: An Endocrine Society Scientific Statement. Endocrine Reviews. 2009;30(4):293-342.

Donnelly ET, McClure N, Lewis SEM. The effect of ascorbate and alpha-tocopherol supplementation in vitro on DNA integrity and hydrogen peroxide-induced DNA damage in human spermatozoa. Mutagenesis. 1999;14(5):505-511.

DuTeaux SB, Berger T, Hess RA, Sartini BL, Miller MG. Male reproductive toxicity of trichloroethylene: Sperm protein oxidation and decreased fertilizing ability. Biology of Reproduction. 2004;70(5):1518-1526.

Duty SM, Silva MJ, Barr DB, Brock JW, Ryan L, Chen ZY, Herrick RF, Christiani DC, Hauser R. Phthalate exposure and human semen parameters. Epidemiology. 2003;14(3):269-277.

EWG. PCBs in Farmed Salmon: Recommendations. Retrieved January 18, 2012, 2012, from http://www.ewg.org/research/pcbs-farmed-salmon/recommendations. 2003.

EWG. Bottled water quality investigation:10 major brands, 38 pollutants. Retrieved January 25, 2012, 2012, from http://www.ewg.org/reports/BottledWater/Bottled-Water-Quality-Investigation. 2008.

EWG. Over 300 pollutants in U.S. tap water. Retrieved January 15, 2012, 2012, from http://www.ewg.org/tap-water/home. 2009.

Feinberg AP. Phenotypic plasticity and the epigenetics of human disease. Nature. 2007;447(7143):433-440.

Fenech MF. Dietary reference values of individual micronutrients and nutriomes for genome damage prevention: current status and a road map to the future. American Journal of Clinical Nutrition. 2010;91(5):1438S-1454S.

Foster PMD, Thomas LV, Cook MW, Walters DG. Effect of di-normal-pentyl phthalate treatment on testicular steroidogenic enzymes and cytochrome-p-450 in the rat. Toxicology Letters. 1983;15(2-3):265-271.

Foster WG, Maharaj-Briceno S, Cyr DG. Dioxin-induced changes in epididymal sperm count and spermatogenesis. Ciencia & Saude Coletiva. 2011;16(6):2893-2905.

Gharagozloo P, Aitken RJ. The role of sperm oxidative stress in male infertility and the significance of oral antioxidant therapy. Human Reproduction. 2011;26(7):1628-1640.

Guo YL, Hsu PC, Hsu CC, Lambert GH. Semen quality after prenatal exposure to polychlorinated biphenyls and dibenzofurans. Lancet. 2000;356(9237):1240-1241.

Hammoud A, Carrell DT, Gibson M, Sanderson M, Parker-Jones K, Peterson CM. Decreased sperm motility is associated with air pollution in Salt Lake City. Fertility and Sterility. 2010;93(6):1875-1879.

Hardell L, Andersson SO, Carlberg M, Bohr L, van Bavel B, Lindstrom G, Bjornfoth H, Ginman C. Adipose tissue concentrations of persistent organic pollutants and the risk of prostate cancer. Journal of Occupational and Environmental Medicine. 2006;48(7):700-707.

Hauser R, Meeker JD, Duty S, Silva MJ, Calafat AM. Altered semen quality in relation to urinary concentrations of phthalate monoester and oxidative metabolites. Epidemiology. 2006;17(6):682-691.

Holland AJ, Cleveland DW. Boveri revisited: chromosomal instability, aneuploidy and tumorigenesis. Nature Reviews Molecular Cell Biology. 2009;10(7):478-487.

Howdeshell KL, Furr J, Lambright CR, Rider CV, Wilson VS, Gray LE. Cumulative effects of dibutyl phthalate and diethylhexyl phthalate on male rat reproductive tract development: Altered fetal steroid hormones and genes. Toxicological Sciences. 2007;99(1):190-202.

Howdeshell KL, Rider CV, Wilson VS, Gray LE. Mechanisms of action of phthalate esters, individually and in combination, to induce abnormal reproductive development in male laboratory rats. Environmental Research. 2008;108(2):168-176.

Howdeshell KL, Wilson VS, Furr J, Lambright CR, Rider CV, Blystone CR, Hotchkiss AK, Gray LE. A mixture of five phthalate esters inhibits fetal testicular testosterone production in the sprague-dawley rat in a cumulative, dose-additive manner. Toxicological Sciences. 2008;105(1):153-165.

Hsu IC, Poirier MC, Yuspa SH, Grunberger D, Weinstein IB, Yolken RH, Harris CC. Measurement of benzo(a)pyrene-dna adducts by enzyme immunoassays and radioimmunoassay. Cancer Research. 1981;41(3):1091-1095.

Hsu PC, Huang WY, Yao WJ, Wu MH, Guo YL, Lambert GH. Sperm changes in men exposed to polychlorinated biphenyls and dibenzofurans. Jama-Journal of the American Medical Association. 2003;289(22):2943-2944.

Ji BT, Shu XO, Linet MS, Zheng W, Wacholder S, Gao YT, Ying DM, Jin F. Paternal cigarette smoking and the risk of childhood cancer among off-spring of nonsmoking mothers. Journal of the National Cancer Institute. 1997;89(3):238-244.

Juhler RK, Larsen SB, Meyer O, Jensen ND, Spano M, Giwercman A, Bonde JP. Human semen quality in relation to dietary pesticide exposure and organic diet. Archives of Environmental Contamination and Toxicology. 1999;37(3):415-423.

Kasprzak KS. Oxidative DNA and protein damage in metal-induced toxicity and carcinogenesis. Free Radical Biology and Medicine. 2002;32(10):958-967.

Kelce WR, Raisbeck MF, Ganjam VK. Gonadotoxic effects of 2-hexanone and 1,2-dibromo-3-chloropropane on the enzymatic-activity of rat testicular 17-alpha-hydroxylase c17,20-lyase. Toxicology Letters. 1990;52(3):331-338.

Keresztes S, Tatar E, Mihucz VG, Virag I, Majdik C, Zaray G. Leaching of antimony from polyethylene terephthalate (PET) bottles into mineral water. Science of the Total Environment. 2009;407(16):4731-4735.

Kodama H, Yamaguchi R, Fukuda J, Kasai H, Tanaka T. Increased oxidative deoxyribonucleic acid damage in the spermatozoa of infertile male patients. Fertility and Sterility. 1997;68(3):519-524.

Kunzle R, Mueller MD, Hanggi W, Birkhauser MH, Drescher H, Bersinger NA. Semen quality of male smokers and nonsmokers in infertile couples. Fertility and Sterility. 2003;79(2):287-291.

Larsen SB, Giwercman A, Spano M, Bonde JP, Grp AS. A longitudinal study of semen quality in pesticide spraying Danish farmers. Reproductive Toxicology. 1998;12(6):581-589.

Lewis DR, Southwick JW, Ouellet-Hellstrom R, Rench J, Calderon RL. Drinking water arsenic in Utah: A cohort mortality study. Environmental Health Perspectives. 1999;107(5):359-365.

Lo S, Allera A, Albers P, Heimbrecht J, Jantzen E, Klingmuller D, Steckelbroeck S. Dithioerythritol (DTE) prevents inhibitory effects of triphenyltin (TPT) on the key enzymes of the human sex steroid hormone metabolism. Journal of Steroid Biochemistry and Molecular Biology. 2003;84(5):569-576.

Lu C, Schenck FJ, Pearson MA, Wong JW. Assessing Children's Dietary Pesticide Exposure: Direct Measurement of Pesticide Residues in 24-Hr Duplicate Food Samples. Environmental Health Perspectives. 2010;118(11):1625-1630.

Lu CS, Toepel K, Irish R, Fenske RA, Barr DB, Bravo R. Organic diets significantly lower children's dietary exposure to organophosphorus pesticides. Environmental Health Perspectives. 2006;114(2):260-263.

MacLeod J. The role of oxygen in the metabolism and motility of human spermatozoa. American Journal of Physiology. 1943;138(3):0512-0518.

Mahajan R, Bonner MR, Hoppin JA, Alavanja MCR. Phorate exposure and incidence of cancer in the agricultural health study. Environmental Health Perspectives. 2006;114(8):1205-1209.

Mahaney BL, Meek K, Lees-Miller SP. Repair of ionizing radiation-induced DNA double-strand breaks by non-homologous end-joining. Biochemical Journal. 2009;417:639-650.

McVey MJ, Cooke GM. Inhibition of rat testis microsomal 3 beta-hydroxysteroid dehydrogenase activity by tributyltin. Journal of Steroid Biochemistry and Molecular Biology. 2003;86(1):99-105.

Meeker JD, Ryan L, Barr DB, Herrick RF, Bennett DH, Bravo R, Hauser R. The relationship of urinary metabolites of carbaryl/naphthalene and chlorpyrifos with human semen quality. Environmental Health Perspectives. 2004;112(17):1665-1670.

Mendiola J, Moreno JM, Roca M, et al. Relationships between heavy metal concentrations in three different body fluids and male reproductive parameters: a pilot study. Environmental Health. 2011;10(6).

Meyer TE, Coker AL, Sanderson M, Symanski E. A case-control study of farming and prostate cancer in African-American and Caucasian men. Occupational and Environmental Medicine. 2007;64(3):155-160.

Mocarelli P, Gerthoux PM, Patterson DG, et al. Dioxin exposure, from infancy through puberty, produces endocrine disruption and affects human semen quality. Environmental Health Perspectives. 2008;116(1):70-77.

Morrison H, Savitz D, Semenciw R, Hulka B, Mao Y, Morison D, Wigle D. Farming and prostate-cancer mortality. American Journal of Epidemiology. 1993;137(3):270-280.

Nallella KP, Sharma RK, Aziz N, Agarwal A. Significance of sperm characteristics in the evaluation of male infertility. Fertility and Sterility. 2006;85(3):629-634.

Nashev LG, Schuster D, Laggner C, Sodha S, Langer T, Wolber G, Odermatt A. The UV-filter benzophenone-1 inhibits 17 beta-hydroxysteroid dehydrogenase type 3: Virtual screening as a strategy to identify potential endocrine disrupting chemicals. Biochemical Pharmacology. 2010;79(8):1189-1199.

Niwa T, Fujimoto M, Kishimoto K, Yabusaki Y, Ishibashi F, Katagiri M. Metabolism and interaction of bisphenol A in human hepatic cytochrome p450 and steroidogenic CYP17. Biological & Pharmaceutical Bulletin. 2001;24(9):1064-1067.

Noriega NC, Howdeshell KL, Furr J, Lambright CR, Wilson VS, Gray LE. Pubertal Administration of DEHP Delays Puberty, Suppresses Testosterone Production, and Inhibits Reproductive Tract Development in Male Sprague-Dawley and Long-Evans Rats. Toxicological Sciences. 2009;111(1):163-178.

Ohno S, Nakajima Y. Triphenyltin and Tributyltin inhibit pig testicular 17 beta-hydroxysteroid dehydrogenase activity and suppress testicular testosterone biosynthesis. Steroids. 2005;70(9):645-651.

Oldereid NB, Thomassen Y, Purvis K. Seminal plasma lead, cadmium and sine in relation to tobacco consumption. International Journal of Andrology. 1994;17(1):24-28.

Padungtod C, Savitz DA, Overstreet JW, Christiani DC, Ryan LM, Xu XP. Occupational pesticide exposure and semen quality among Chinese workers. Journal of Occupational and Environmental Medicine. 2000;42(10):982-992.

Potashnik G, Yanaiinbar I, Sacks MI, Israeli R. Effect of dibromochloropropane on human testicular function. Israel Journal of Medical Sciences. 1979;15(5):438-442.

Qiu J. Epigenetics: Unfinished symphony. Nature, Nature Publishing Group. 2006;441:143-145.

Rajagopalan H, Lengauer C. Aneuploidy and cancer. Nature, Nature Publishing Group. 2004;432:338-341.

Ramlau-Hansen CH, Thulstrup AM, Aggerholm AS, Jensen MS, Toft G, Bonde JP. Is smoking a risk factor for decreased semen quality? A cross-sectional analysis. Human Reproduction. 2007;22(1):188-196.

Ravanat J-L, Douki T, Cadet J. Direct and indirect effects of UV radiation on DNA and its components. Journal of Photochemistry and Photobiology B: Biology. 2001;63:88-102.

Richthoff J, Rylander L, Jonsson BAG, Akesson H, Hagmar L, Nilsson-Ehle P, Stridsberg M, Giwercman A. Serum levels of 2,2',4,4',5,5'-hexachlor obiphenyl (CB-153) in relation to markers of reproductive function in young males from the general Swedish population. Environmental Health Perspectives. 2003;111(4):409-413.

Rignell-Hydbom A, Rylander L, Giwercman A, Jonsson BAG, Nilsson-Ehle P, Hagmar L. Exposure to CB-153 and p,p '-DDE and male reproductive function. Human Reproduction. 2004;19(9):2066-2075.

Ritchie JM, Vial SL, Fuortes LJ, Guo HJ, Reedy VE, Smith EM. Organochlorines and risk of prostate cancer. Journal of Occupational and Environmental Medicine. 2003;45(7):692-702.

Robbins WA. FISH (fluorescence in situ hybridization) to detect effects of smoking, caffeine, and alcohol on human sperm chromosomes. Advances in Male Mediated Developmental Toxicity. 2003;518:59-72.

Rossman TG, Uddin AN, Burns FJ. Evidence that arsenite acts as a cocarcinogen in skin cancer. Toxicology and Applied Pharmacology. 2004;198(3):394-404.

Rubes J, Lowe X, Moore D, et al. Smoking cigarettes is associated with increased sperm disomy in teenage men. Fertility and Sterility. 1998;70(4):715-723.

Rudel RA, Gray JM, Engel CL, et al. Food Packaging and Bisphenol A and Bis(2-Ethyhexyl) Phthalate Exposure: Findings from a Dietary Intervention. Environmental Health Perspectives. 2011;119(7):914-920.

Sallmen M, Lindbohm ML, Anttila A, Kyyronen P, Taskinen H, Nykyri E, Hemminki K. Time to pregnancy among the wives of men exposed to organic solvents. Occupational and Environmental Medicine. 1998;55(1):24-30.

Sepaniak S, Forges T, Gerard H, Foliguet B, Bene MC, Monnier-Barbarino P. The influence of cigarette smoking on human sperm quality and DNA fragmentation. Toxicology. 2006;223(1-2):54-60.

Sharma RK, Agarwal A. Role of reactive oxygen species in male infertility. Urology. 1996;48(6):835-850.

Shotyk W, Krachler M., Chen B. Contamination of Canadian and European bottled waters with antimony from PET containers. Journal of Environmental Monitoring. 2006;8(2):288-292.

Sohoni P, Sumpter JP. Several environmental oestrogens are also anti-androgens. Journal of Endocrinology. 1998;158(3):327-339.

Spano M, Bonde JP, Hjollund HI, Kolstad HA, Cordelli E, Leter G, Danish S. First Pregnancy Planner. Sperm chromatin damage impairs human fertility. Fertility and Sterility. 2000;73(1):43-50.

Stewart SA, Weinberg RA. Telomeres: Cancer to human aging. Annual Review of Cell and Developmental Biology. 2006;22:531-557.

Swan SH, Elkin EP, Fenster L. The question of declining sperm density revisited: An analysis of 101 studies published 1934-1996. Environmental Health Perspectives. 2000;108(10):961-966.

Swan SH, Kruse RL, Liu F, et al., and G. Study Future Families Res. Semen quality in relation to biomarkers of pesticide exposure. Environmental Health Perspectives. 2003;111(12):1478-1484.

Tallaa LB, Liu J, Webber MM. Estrogen signaling and disruption of androgen metabolism in acquired androgen independence during cadmium carcinogenesis in human prostate epithelial cells. Prostate. 2007;67(2):135–145.

Waalkes MP. Cadmium carcinogenesis in review. Journal of Inorganic Biochemistry. 2000;79(1-4):241-244.

Wagner M, Oehlmann J. Endocrine disruptors in bottled mineral water: Estrogenic activity in the E-Screen. Journal of Steroid Biochemistry and Molecular Biology. 2011;127(1-2):128-135.

Wetherill YB, Fisher NL, Staubach A, Danielsen M, White RWD, Knudsen KE. Xenoestrogen action in prostate cancer: Pleiotropic effects dependent on androgen receptor status. Cancer Research. 2005;65(1):54-65.

Wetherill YB, Hess-Wilson JK, Comstock CES, et al. Bisphenol A facilitates bypass of androgen ablation therapy in prostate cancer. Molecular Cancer Therapeutics. 2006;5(12):3181-3190.

Whorton MD, Milby TH, Stubbs HA, Avashia BH, Hull EQ. Testicular function among carbaryl-exposed employees. Journal of Toxicology and Environmental Health. 1979;5(5):929-941.

Ye LP, Zhao BH, Hu GX, Chu YH, Ge RS. Inhibition of human and rat testicular steroidogenic enzyme activities by bisphenol A. Toxicology Letters. 2011;207(2):137-142.

Zenzes MT. Smoking and reproduction: gene damage to human gametes and embryos. Human Reproduction Update. 2000;6(2):122-131.

Zenzes MT, Puy LA, Bielecki R, Reed TE. Detection of benzo a pyrene diol epoxide-DNA adducts in embryos from smoking couples: evidence for transmission by spermatozoa. Molecular Human Reproduction. 1999;5(2):125-131.

Zini A. Clinical Utility of Sperm DNA Integrity Tests. Sperm Chromatin, Springer New York: 2011;499-504.

Zini A, Bielecki R, Phang D, Zenzes MT. Correlations between two markers of sperm DNA integrity, DNA denaturation and DNA fragmentation, in fertile and infertile men. Fertility and Sterility. 2001;75(4):674-677.

20

The Future of Integrative Men's Health

MYLES D. SPAR AND GEORGE E. MUÑOZ

The field of men's health is nearing its adolescence. Clinicians, teachers, and researchers are starting to understand that there is a realm of medicine of special significance to men, and it is more specific than simply all medicine that is not women's health. The higher death rate of men from nine of the 10 leading causes of mortality (those that are not hormonally linked), the specific health concerns of the aging male, the lack of care-seeking behavior among men, and the higher rates of successful suicide and substance abuse among men are examples of male-specific health issues (Centers for Disease Control and Prevention, 2011).

Europe and the Pacific Rim have largely led the way in recognizing this field of men's health as a defined entity. The first three World Congresses on Men's Health have all been held in Europe. The European Commission of the European Union supported and published a summary of the state of men's health in Europe in 2011, and many European universities have departments of andrology, involving social science researchers, primary care, and a focus on men's health issues beyond the scope of practice typically found in American departments of urology.

The future for the United States depends on primary care providers, health service researchers, cardiologists, endocrinologists, and urologists working together to articulate what men's health clinical research and didactic programs would look like. The chapters in this book lay out some of the arenas that would be included in such programs. Men's health in general needs to mature to include such elements as more research into the causes of higher rates of death from heart disease among men, more effective outreach to men on when and why to see a health care provider, and better understanding of when and how to assess for and treat low testosterone (T). Integrative men's health, with its emphasis on a holistic approach to prevention and treatment, provides a model for successfully addressing the health needs of men.

The future of integrative clinical men's health can be modeled on the "executive physicals." These are comprehensive evaluations looking at all aspects of a patient's current state of health, including an attempt, as objectively as possible, to estimate the patient's risk for specific causes of morbidity or mortality down the road. Such a comprehensive evaluation can take into account all factors that impact a man's current state of health and future risk for disease and would include recommendations related to optimal nutrition, supplement use, physical activity/exercise, stress management, and sleep habits. Although women certainly undergo extensive evaluations and executive physicals, the concept of such an executive physical has been marketed successfully to men and often has elements that are especially germane to men's health concerns. An evaluation typically includes:

- Extensive cardiovascular disease risk assessment including stress testing
- Genomic testing for individualized risk reporting based on presence or absence or polymorphisms of certain genes (see Table 20.1 for specific genetic tests currently available)
- Nutritional assessment, which may include testing of micronutrient levels
- Stress management assessment and training
- Exercise tolerance testing including VO_2 max
- Hormonal analysis to include sex hormones, thyroid hormones and antibodies, adrenal hormones, and insulin

Table 20.1: Genetic Testing Currently Available

Genetic Test	Involved In	Condition Affected by Polymorphisms
MTHFR	Folate metabolism	Elevated homocysteine
ApoE	Fat metabolism	Risk for CAD and Alzheimer's
KIF6	Intracellular transport proteins	Risk of CHD and response to atorvastatin and pravastatin
SLCO1B1	Transportation for hepatic uptake of statins	Risk for myopathy from statin use
CYP2C19	Clopidogrel metabolism	Effectiveness of Plavix
LPA-aspirin response	Aspirin metabolism	Responsiveness to aspirin for reducing heart attack risk
4q25-AF	Heart development	Risk for atrial fibrillation
LPA-intron 25	Uncertain	Risk for heart disease
9p21-MI	Uncertain	Risk for CAD and AAA

AAA = abdominal aortic aneurysm; CAD = coronary artery disease; CHD = coronary heart disease.

Such personalized medicine may be one key way to compel men to schedule a health care visit. For example, genomic testing is now available to assess an individual's risk for many of the conditions that afflict men.

Hormonal analysis is key to making accurate recommendations aimed at improving a man's health. The increased recognition of the impact of low testosterone on overall health, beyond sexual health, is leading the way for primary care providers to be more likely to test for T levels and to appropriately treat low levels. Studies have shown that low T can increase rates of heart disease and diabetes as well as contribute to depression (Abate et al.; Hak et al., 2002; Traish et al., 2009). This recognition of the prevalence and impact of low T is leading to a greater understanding of issues related to the aging male, including andropause, brain aging, and mental illness.

Women's health has made great strides in advocacy and treatment, building research and treatment programs specifically designed around women's health needs. Men's health advocates can use this as a model in creating programs targeting the health needs of men. Successful men's health programs have some of the following characteristics:

- Partnership with a women's health center (as often the female partners are the best source of new patients for men's health centers)
- Inclusion of a sexual health program for issues such as low T and erectile dysfunction. Such programs assess testosterone and other male hormones, offering treatment for low T with appropriate follow-up. Many use sexual concerns (such as erectile dysfunction) as a point of entry to evaluate other issues such as undiagnosed hypertension or unhealthy body weight.
- Comprehensive health evaluation, as discussed previously, with concrete treatment/wellness plan based on the results
- Assistance with weight and primarily fat loss
- Partnership with sleep study center given the prevalence of sleep apnea among men

Besides the success of the field of women's health in growing into its own mature discipline for clinical medicine, research, and didactics, there are other ways men can learn from women when it comes to optimizing health. Attending shamanic and energy trainings, whether in the United States or abroad, one cannot help but notice that the vast majority of the attendees are female. These sessions are primarily geared for self-exploration, a sort of healing journey before one undertakes the trainings to help and attempt healing of others. This type of training is similar to what is practiced in psychoanalysis training. Male participants at these sessions ask themselves: "Why are there so few men at these training sessions? What is wrong with me? Am I missing something?" Our Western culture does not encourage men of any age past early childhood to display characteristics such as sensitivity or expressing a "softer" side that could be considered feminine. This may be for a variety of reasons including imposition of gender behavior differences that fathers and mothers feel should exist as a child grows from infant, to toddler, to young child, to school-age child and on through puberty, and so on. For some reason, displaying a softer side seems much more acceptable as a very young child than as an adolescent, especially in the world of competitive athletics. Competitive athletes, for example, don't often display this more sensitive side on or off the field. These are generalizations, and profoundly sensitive individuals do exist of both genders, but generally speaking, these behavioral norms are societal and affect attitudes that men are taught in either unspoken form, by inference, or overtly. The net effect then becomes for men almost a taboo area of the psyche where exploration of sensitivities and vulnerabilities and the ability to cry and become vulnerable are considered signs of "weakness' in a male-dominated society. Consequently, the concept of self-exploration and even personal growth seems not to be in line within the remotest thought of the average male through early adulthood on until, possibly, a life crisis occurs to jar this necessity.

Perhaps, then, a paradigm shift can be considered. Males could be taught to embrace the mind/body/spirit interaction along with the feminine and masculine aspects within their psyche regardless of age. There is a universal concept that is widely seen globally in indigenous cultures who routinely maintain both the feminine and masculine energies conceptually in their mysticism, planetary views, personal interactions, and universal cosmology. Along with this transcendence comes a deep care of "mother earth," which mirrors how we care for ourselves and families. Such respect for the need to nurture both masculine and feminine energies has led to more and more workshops and men's groups where vulnerability, sensitivity, and self-fears are explored.

These concepts of an unveiling and letting go of tenets that no longer serve our evolving cultures can then be expanded to men's health care views and access of care. The ideas of help seeking being a strength and knowing when to let go for the greater good are seen as feminine wisdom, yet hold great lessons for men. Traditionally, men don't seek medical care unless something is drastically wrong. This may be a habitual process in not wanting to appear vulnerable or needy and a resistance to asking for help. Certainly fear is a factor in limiting men from seeking medical care. The idea that men should "surrender" in order to win parallels the general concepts mentioned earlier regarding men being taught to accept vulnerabilities. Culturally doing so makes it more okay to seek help. Men should be encouraged to do so early in their transitions from pediatrics to adulthood in routine medical encounters.

The creation of men's life wellness plans could be a guide to keep men healthy as they progress from teens to early adulthood and through their future stages of life. Both pediatrics and adult medicine disciplines need to not only improve the transition-of-care process but also specifically address the issue that men traditionally aren't coming in for "check-ups." Establishing a life plan for men with recommendations for prevention of the major future health hazards including realms such as nutrition, supplement use, physical activity, and stress management could create a more inviting environment for men and change their views toward access. Such wellness plans would include hormone optimization using supplementation when needed and a plan to attenuate the impact of potential causes of inflammation or hormonal dysregulation such as heavy metals or toxins. The chapters on testosterone, nutrition, supplements, and environmental toxins all include recommendations for assessment, prevention, and treatment of conditions that highly impact men and that could be included in men's health wellness plans.

Finally, we have to ask men what they want and why they don't go to see their health providers. The lack of early detection and awareness of problems leads to many of the conditions that disproportionately impact men's life spans, from higher rates of death from heart disease to higher rates of death from cancer. Community- and practice-based populations should be surveyed especially at the health care juncture change in early adulthood. University health programs should be part of this process. For many males, this is their first significant independent time from parents. How they access and are accepted by the health care system at this time of life can be extremely impactful, especially with regard to sexually transmitted diseases, family planning, high-risk behaviors, and routine health issues that arise.

Shaping our health care system to continue to reach out to males from an early age is one possible solution. Advocacy and special awareness days such as "Men's' Health Month" in June of every year are great steps toward this goal. Education for men about regular prostate health issues at every age would help men be less shy, secretive, or embarrassed about having a dialog with their providers even during routine exams. Mothers should learn to encourage their sons to seek medical advice early in life and to engage the fathers in this process if appropriate to the son's wishes. Practitioners should seek to also involve the fathers in communication of their child's health, especially for a male reaching or in adolescence. Athletic training rooms and college health services for many young males may be the first major time young men have private health access. These encounters should be inviting to young men, encouraging open dialog and future education or prevention programs or behaviors.

The transition out of athletics and out of college settings for many men is the big "black hole" medically. Men don't have the pressing need for yearly exams such as women have with Pap smears, so the health care system must be welcoming to men in a way that addresses some emotional needs that are inherent in the male psyche. When all else failed, my grandmother just held me, comforted me, and made me tea or chicken soup. We as a society need to be able to create warm, hospitable environments with soothing messages for men as well as for women.

The future of integrative men's health can be modeled on the successful women's health movement in terms of recognizing the unique needs of men, utilizing a holistic biopsychosocial model of health care, and understanding the importance of hormone optimization as well as optimal lifestyle. Men will likely engage with the health care system with this approach coupled with a focus on performance optimization and prevention-oriented assessments including hormone and genomic testing. Recommendations on medications, supplements, optimal diet, physical activity, and the use of complementary modalities would make up a truly holistic and integrative wellness plan that could do much to improve the health of men.

REFERENCES

Abate N, Haffner SM, Garg A, et al. Sex steroid hormones, upper body obesity, and insulin resistance. J Clin Endocrinol Metab. 2002;87(10):4522–4527.

Centers for Disease Control and Prevention. CDC Summary Health Statistics for U.S. Adults: National Health Interview Study, 2011, series 10, number 256, December 2012.

Hak AE, Witteman JC, de Jong FH, et al. Low levels of endogenous androgens increase the risk of atherosclerosis in elderly men: the Rotterdam study. J Clin Endocrinol Metab. 2002;87(8):3632–3639.

Traish AM, Saad F, Guay A. The dark side of testosterone deficiency: II. Type 2 diabetes and insulin resistance. J Androl. 2009;30(1):23–32.

INDEX

In this index, "*b*" after the page number indicates a highlighted box; "*f*" after the page number indicates a figure; "*t*" indicates a table.